Encyclopedia of Public Health

Encyclopedia of Public Health

Principles, People, and Programs

VOLUME 1: A–L

SALLY KUYKENDALL, EDITOR

GREENWOOD™

An Imprint of ABC-CLIO, LLC
Santa Barbara, California • Denver, Colorado

Library of Congress Cataloging in Publication Control Number: 2017045280

ISBN: 978-1-61069-982-2 (set)
978-1-4408-4809-4 (vol. 1)
978-1-4408-4810-0 (vol. 2)
978-1-61069-983-9 (ebook)

22 21 20 19 18 1 2 3 4 5

This book is also available as an eBook.

Greenwood
An Imprint of ABC-CLIO, LLC

ABC-CLIO, LLC
130 Cremona Drive, P.O. Box 1911
Santa Barbara, California 93116-1911
www.abc-clio.com

This book is printed on acid-free paper ∞

Manufactured in the United States of America

Contents

Guide to Related Topics xv

Introduction xxi

Chronology xxvii

Volume 1

Acute Illnesses 1

Addictions 3

Administration, Health 7

Adverse Childhood Experiences (ACEs) 11

Affordable Care Act (ACA) 15

Aging 18

Agricultural Safety 22

Air Pollution 25

Alcohol 30

Alzheimer's Disease (AD) 33

American Journal of Public Health (AJPH) 37

American Medical Association (AMA) 38

American Public Health Association (APHA) 40

Americans with Disabilities Act (ADA) 41

Ancient World, Public Health in the 44

Anderson, Elizabeth Milbank (1850–1921) 47

Antibiotic Resistance 50

Association of Public Health Laboratories (APHL) 53

Association of State and Territorial Health Officials (ASTHO) 54

Attention-Deficit/Hyperactivity Disorder (ADHD) 57
Baker, Sara Josephine (1873–1945) 61
Beers, Clifford Whittingham (1876–1943) 64
Behavioral Health 69
Belmont Report, The 71
Biostatistics 73
Bioterrorism 75
Birth Defects 79
Blackwell, Elizabeth (1821–1910) 81
Body Mass Index (BMI) 86
Bousfield, Midian Othello (1885–1948) 88
Bowditch, Henry Ingersoll (1808–1892) 91
Cancer 97
Care, Access to 99
Causality 102
Centers for Disease Control and Prevention (CDC) 104
Centers for Medicare and Medicaid Services (CMS) 108
Certified in Public Health (CPH) 108
Chadwick, Edwin (1800–1890) 109
Child Maltreatment 113
Children's Health 116
Cholera 119
Chronic Illness 123
Code of Ethics 126
Collaborations 130
Community Health 133
Community Health Centers (CHCs) 136
Community Organizing 139
Core Competencies in Public Health 141

Cornely, Paul Bertau (1906–2002) 146
Council on Education for Public Health (CEPH) 150
Cultural Competence 152
Cutter Incident, The 154
Dean, Henry Trendley (1893–1962) 159
Degrees in Public Health 162
Diabetes Mellitus 164
Diffusion of Innovations Theory 167
Disability 170
Disability Movement 173
Disease 175
Dix, Dorothea Lynde (1804–1887) 178
Drew, Charles Richard (1904–1950) 183
Dritz, Selma Kaderman (1917–2008) 187
Dunham, Ethel Collins (1883–1969) 190
Eating Disorders 193
Elder Maltreatment 195
Elders, Joycelyn (1933–) 198
Eliot, Martha May (1891–1978) 199
Ellertson, Charlotte Ehrengard (1966–2004) 203
Emergency Medical Treatment and Labor Act (EMTALA) 205
Emergency Preparedness and Response 207
Environmental Health 210
Environmental Protection Agency (EPA) 213
Epidemic 216
Epidemiology 220
Ethics in Public Health and Population Health 223
Evaluation 226
Evidence-Based Programs and Practices 230

False Claims Act (FCA) 233
Family Planning 234
Fluoridation 237
Food and Drug Administration (FDA) 240
Food Insecurity 243
Food Safety 245
Genetics 249
Global Health 251
Goals and Objectives 255
Grants 258
Greco-Roman Era, Public Health in the 260
Hamilton, Alice (1869–1970) 263
Handwashing 267
Health 269
Health and Medicine Division of the National Academies of Sciences, Engineering, and Medicine 272
Health Belief Model 274
Health Care Disparities 276
Health Communication 281
Health Disparities 285
Health Education 291
Health Information Management (HIM) 295
Health Insurance Portability and Accountability Act (HIPAA) 295
Health Literacy 298
Health Policy 300
Health Resources and Services Administration (HRSA) 304
Healthy People 2020 306
Healthy Places 308
Heart Disease 311

Heart Truth® (Red Dress) Campaign, The 314
Hepatitis 317
Hinton, William Augustus (1883–1959) 321
Hippocrates (460–375 BCE) 323
Home Safety 326
Human Immunodeficiency Virus (HIV) and Acquired Immune Deficiency Syndrome (AIDS) 331
Human Trafficking 336
Hypertension (HTN) 339
Immigrant Health 343
Indian Health Service (IHS) 345
Infant Mortality 349
Infectious Diseases 352
Influenza 355
Injuries 359
Intervention 362
Intimate Partner Violence (IPV) 366
Jenner, Edward (1749–1823) 371
Kelley, Florence (1859–1932) 373
Koch, Heinrich Hermann Robert (1843–1910) 377
Leading Health Indicators 383
Lesbian, Gay, Bisexual, and Transgender (LGBT) Health 385
Locus of Control 389
Logic Model 390

Volume 2

Mallon, Mary (1869–1938) 393
Master Settlement Agreement (MSA) 396
Maternal Health 397
Measles 404

Medicaid 406
Medicare 408
Medicine 410
Meningitis 412
Men's Health 416
Mental Health 418
Mental Illness 420
Middle Ages, Public Health in the (500–1500 CE) 425
Modern Era, Public Health in the 428
Motor Vehicle Safety 430
Nader, Ralph (1934–) 435
National Association of County and City Health Officials (NACCHO) 438
National Cancer Institute (NCI) 439
National Center for Injury Prevention and Control (NCIPC) 441
National Health and Nutrition Examination Survey (NHANES) 443
National Heart, Lung, and Blood Institute (NHLBI) 444
National Institute on Drug Abuse (NIDA) 446
National Institutes of Health (NIH) 449
Nation's Health, The 451
Needs Assessment 452
Nightingale, Florence (1820–1910) 455
Nutrition 460
Obesity 465
Oral Health 468
Pandemic 473
Pasteur, Louis (1822–1895) 475
Patient Safety 478
Penicillin 481
Physical Activity 484

Planned Parenthood	488
Polio	491
Population Health	494
Precaution Adoption Process Model (PAPM)	498
PRECEDE-PROCEED Planning Model	500
Prescription Drugs	502
Prevention	505
Public Health Department Accreditation	508
Public Health in the United States, History of	511
Public Health Law	515
Quarantine	519
RE-AIM (Reach, Effectiveness, Adoption, Implementation, and Maintenance)	523
Reciprocal Determinism	525
Renaissance, Public Health in the	525
Research	529
Risk-Benefit Analysis	532
Roosevelt, Eleanor (1884–1962)	534
Roosevelt, Franklin Delano (1882–1945)	536
Rosen, George (1910–1977)	541
Rural Health	545
Sabin, Florence Rena (1871–1953)	549
Salk, Jonas (1914–1995)	552
Sanger, Margaret Louise Higgins (1879–1966)	554
School Health	559
Self-Efficacy	562
Shattuck, Lemuel (1793–1859)	564
Skin Cancer	567
Smallpox	570
Smith, James McCune (1813–1865)	573

Snow, John (1813–1858) 577

Social Cognitive Theory (SCT) 579

Social Determinants of Health (SDOH) 582

Social Ecological Model 586

Social Security Act (SSA) 589

Society of Public Health Education (SOPHE) 592

Spiritual Health 594

Sports-Related Concussions (SRCs) 597

Stark Law 600

State, Local, and Territorial Health Departments 602

Substance Abuse and Mental Health Services Administration (SAMHSA) 604

Surgeon General 607

Syringe Service Programs 609

Transtheoretical Model (TTM) 613

Truth Campaign, The 615

Tubman, Harriet (1822–1913) 618

Tuskegee Syphilis Study 620

Upstream Public Health Practices 625

U.S. Department of Agriculture (USDA) 626

U.S. Department of Health and Human Services (HHS) 628

U.S. Public Health Service (PHS) 630

Vaccines 633

Veterans' Health 636

Violence 639

Wald, Lillian (1867–1940) 643

Waterborne Diseases 645

Wegman, Myron Ezra (1908–2004) 648

Winslow, Charles-Edward Amory (1877–1957) 650

Women's Health 653
World Health Organization (WHO) 657
Wynder, Ernst Ludwig (1922–1999) 660
Zombie Preparedness 665
Controversies in Public Health 669
Directory of Organizations 711
Glossary 717
About the Editor and Contributors 723
Index 729

Guide to Related Topics

Diseases, Health Problems, and Wellness

Acute Illnesses
Addictions
Adverse Childhood Experiences (ACEs)
Air Pollution
Alcohol
Alzheimer's Disease
Antibiotic Resistance
Attention-Deficit/Hyperactivity Disorder (ADHD)
Bioterrorism
Birth Defects
Body Mass Index (BMI)
Cancer
Care, Access to
Child Maltreatment
Cholera
Chronic Illness
Diabetes
Disability
Disease
Eating Disorders
Elder Maltreatment
Environmental Health
Epidemic
Food Insecurity
Food Safety
Genetics
Global Health
Handwashing
Health Care Disparities
Health Disparities
Heart Disease
Hepatitis
Home Safety
Human Immunodeficiency Virus (HIV) and Acquired Immune Deficiency Syndrome (AIDS)
Human Trafficking
Hypertension (HTN)
Immigrant Health
Infant Mortality
Infectious Diseases
Influenza
Injuries
Intimate Partner Violence (IPV)
Maternal Health
Measles
Meningitis
Mental Illness
Obesity
Pandemic
Polio
Prescription Drugs
Rural Health
School Health
Skin Cancer
Smallpox
Social Determinants of Health (SDOH)
Sports-Related Concussions
Veterans' Health
Violence
Waterborne Diseases
Women's Health

Government Organizations

Centers for Disease Control and Prevention (CDC)

Centers for Medicare and Medicaid Services (CMS)
Community Health Centers (CHCs)
Environmental Protection Agency (EPA)
Food and Drug Administration (FDA)
Health Resources and Services Administration (HRSA)
Indian Health Service (HIS)
National Cancer Institute (NCI)
National Center for Injury Prevention and Control (NCIPC)
National Heart, Lung, and Blood Institute (NHLBI)
National Institute on Drug Abuse (NIDA)
National Institutes of Health (NIH)
State, Local, and Territorial Health Departments
Substance Abuse and Mental Health Services Administration (SAMHSA)
Surgeon General
U.S. Department of Agriculture (USDA)
U.S. Department of Health and Human Services (DHHS)
U.S. Public Health Service (PHS)
World Health Organization (WHO)

Laws and Guidelines

Affordable Care Act (ACA)
Americans with Disabilities Act (ADA)
Belmont Report, The
Emergency Medical Treatment and Labor Act (EMTALA)
Evidence-Based Programs and Practices
False Claims Act (FCA)
Health Insurance Portability and Accountability Act (HIPAA)
Master Settlement Agreement (MSA)
Public Health Law
Social Security Act (SSA)
Stark Law

Major Events in the History of Public Health

Agricultural Safety
Ancient World, Public Health in the
Americans with Disabilities Act (ADA)
Cutter Incident, The
Family Planning
Fluoridation
Food Safety
Greco-Roman Era, Public Health in the
Heart Disease
Infectious Diseases
Master Settlement Agreement (MSA)
Maternal Health
Medicaid
Medicare
Middle Ages, Public Health in the
Modern Era, Public Health in the
Motor Vehicle Safety
Oral Health
Pandemic
Penicillin
Polio
Public Health in the United States, History of
Quarantine
Renaissance, Public Health in the
Social Security Act (SSA)
Tuskegee Syphilis Study
Vaccines

People

Anderson, Elizabeth Milbank (1850–1921)
Baker, Sara Josephine (1873–1945)

Beers, Clifford Whittingham (1876–1943)
Blackwell, Elizabeth (1821–1910)
Bousfield, Midian Othello (1885–1948)
Bowditch, Henry Ingersoll (1808–1892)
Chadwick, Edwin (1800–1890)
Cornely, Paul Bertau (1906–2002)
Dean, Henry Trendley (1893–1962)
Dix, Dorothea Lynde (1804–1887)
Drew, Charles Richard (1904–1950)
Dritz, Selma Kaderman (1917–2008)
Dunham, Ethel Collins (1883–1969)
Elders, Joycelyn (1933–)
Eliot, Martha May (1891–1978)
Ellertson, Charlotte Ehrengard (1966–2004)
Hamilton, Alice (1869–1970)
Hinton, William Augustus (1883–1959)
Hippocrates (460–375 BCE)
Jenner, Edward (1749–1823)
Kelley, Florence (1859–1932)
Koch, Heinrich Hermann Robert (1843–1910)
Mallon, Mary (1869–1938)
Nader, Ralph (1934–)
Nightingale, Florence (1820–1910)
Pasteur, Louis (1822–1895)
Roosevelt, Eleanor (1884–1962)
Roosevelt, Franklin Delano (1882–1945)
Rosen, George (1910–1977)
Sabin, Florence Rena (1871–1953)
Salk, Jonas (1914–1995)
Sanger, Margaret Louise Higgins (1879–1966)
Shattuck, Lemuel (1793–1859)
Smith, James McCune (1813–1865)
Snow, John (1813–1858)
Tubman, Harriet (1822–1913)
Wald, Lillian (1867–1940)
Wegman, Myron Ezra (1908–2004)
Winslow, Charles-Edward Amory (1877–1957)
Wynder, Ernst Ludwig (1922–1999)

Principles

Behavioral Health
Belmont Report, The
Body Mass Index (BMI)
Causality
Code of Ethics
Collaborations
Community Health
Community Health Centers (CHCs)
Community Organizing
Core Competencies in Public Health
Cultural Competence
Diffusion of Innovations Theory
Disability Movement
Emergency Preparedness and Response
Ethics in Public Health and Population Health
Evaluation
Food Safety
Grants
Health
Health Belief Model
Health Communication
Health Education
Health Literacy
Health Policy
Healthy People 2020
Healthy Places
Intervention
Leading Health Indicators
Lesbian, Gay, Bisexual, and Transgender (LGBT) Health
Locus of Control
Logic Model

Maternal Health
Medicine
Men's Health
Mental Health
Needs Assessment
Nutrition
Patient Safety
Physical Activity
Population Health
Precaution Adoption Process Model (PAPM)
PRECEDE-PROCEED Planning Model
Prescription Drugs
Prevention
Quarantine
RE-AIM (Reach, Effectiveness, Adoption, Implementation, and Maintenance)
Reciprocal Determinism
Research
Risk-Benefit Analysis
Self-Efficacy
Social Cognitive Theory (SCT)
Social Determinants of Health (SDOH)
Social Ecological Model
Spiritual Health
Transtheoretical Model (TTM)
Veterans' Health
Women's Health

Professional Organizations and Resources

American Journal of Public Health (AJPH)
American Public Health Association (APHA)
Association of Public Health Laboratories (APHL)
Association of State and Territorial Health Officials (ASTHO)
Certified in Public Health (CPH)
Council on Education for Public Health (CEPH)
Degrees in Public Health
Grants
Health and Medicine Division of the National Academies of Sciences, Engineering, and Medicine
National Association of County and City Health Officials (NACCHO)
National Health and Nutrition Examination Survey (NHANES)
Nation's Health, The
Public Health Department Accreditation
Society of Public Health Education (SOPHE)

Programs

Affordable Care Act (ACA)
Centers for Disease Control and Prevention (CDC)
Centers for Medicare and Medicaid Services (CMS)
Community Health Centers (CHCs)
Environmental Protection Agency (EPA)
Evidence-Based Programs and Practices
Family Planning
Fluoridation
Food and Drug Administration (FDA)
Genetics
Global Health
Health and Medicine Division of the National Academies of Sciences, Engineering, and Medicine
Health Resources and Services Administration (HRSA)
Healthy People 2020
Healthy Places
Heart Truth® (Red Dress) Campaign, The
Home Safety

Indian Health Service (IHS)
Logic Model
Master Settlement Agreement (MSA)
Medicaid
Medicare
National Cancer Institute (NCI)
National Center for Injury Prevention and Control (NCIPC)
National Heart, Lung, and Blood Institute (NHLBI)
National Institutes of Health (NIH)
Needs Assessment
Planned Parenthood
Social Security Act (SSA)
State, Local, and Territorial Health Departments
Substance Abuse and Mental Health Services Administration (SAMHSA)
Surgeon General
Syringe Service Programs
Truth Campaign, The
Upstream Public Health Practices
U.S. Department of Agriculture (USDA)
U.S. Department of Health and Human Services (DHHS)
U.S. Public Health Service (PHS)
Vaccines
Zombie Preparedness

Specialty Areas of Practice

Administration, Health
Aging
Agricultural Safety
Behavioral Health
Biostatistics
Bioterrorism
Care, Access to
Children's Health
Community Health Centers (CHCs)
Community Organizing
Emergency Preparedness and Response
Environmental Health
Epidemiology
Ethics in Public Health and Population Health
Family Planning
Food Insecurity
Food Safety
Genetics
Grants
Health Communication
Health Education
Health Information Management (HIM)
Health Policy
Human Immunodeficiency Virus (HIV) and Acquired Immune Deficiency Syndrome (AIDS)
Immigrant Health
Infectious Diseases
Injuries
Maternal Health
Men's Health
Mental Health
Nutrition
Oral Health
Population Health
Public Health Law
Research
Risk-Benefit Analysis
Rural Health
School Health
Social Determinants of Health (SDOH)
Vaccines

Introduction

Public health encompasses a broad array of programs, principles, and professional disciplines. The field is a multidisciplinary science, drawing from medicine, biology, sociology, management, psychology, political science, communications, marketing, and engineering. Public health works with traditional medical practice to promote health and well-being and to prevent disease and injury. Although the two systems have similar goals, each uses different strategies to achieve the goals. Traditional Western medicine focuses on individuals. Public health focuses on groups of people. Western medicine is reactionary, responding to individual cases of injury or disease. Public health is proactive, identifying at-risk groups and working to stop a problem early, sometimes before the problem starts. Western medicine is treatment oriented. Public health strives for prevention. Although the traditional medical system treats individuals suffering from a health problem, public health intervenes to prevent potential problems. The two systems work together to alleviate human suffering and to promote quality of life.

The public health workforce is composed of diverse professionals who work together through many different agencies and organizations. Common functions are to monitor community health, investigate outbreaks of disease, empower communities, mobilize partnerships, and care for vulnerable populations. Over the past 100 years, public health has realized significant achievements, increasing life span and quality of life. Activities work at the macro-level with policies, regulations, and programs and at the micro-level of influencing individual health behaviors. Public health extends beyond the day-to-day tasks of disease prevention and health promotion. Public health is a frame of mind, a political advocacy, a social movement of advocating for others, especially those who lack the power and resources to secure their own health. Public health professionals work toward a common vision for equitable health and health care in the United States.

The origins of public health trace back to early humans who devised ways to dispose of human waste without contaminating drinking water. As bacteriology and immunology emerged as scientific disciplines, so did the multidisciplinary field of public health. The most commonly recognized definition of public health was penned by Charles-Edward Amory Winslow, founder of the Yale School of Public Health. In 1920, Winslow described the newly emerging public health profession as:

> The science and art of preventing disease, prolonging life, and promoting health and efficiency through organized community efforts for the sanitation of the environment,

> the control of communicable infections, the education of the individual in personal hygiene, the organization of medical and nursing services for the early diagnosis and preventive treatment of disease, and for the development of the social machinery to insure everyone a standard of living adequate for the maintenance of health, so organizing these benefits as to enable every citizen to realize his birthright of health and longevity. (Winslow, 1920, p. 183)

Winslow's definition is timeless. Key points are (1) public health uses systematic investigations and organized knowledge to understand, predict, and intervene in adverse health conditions; (2) public health uses creativity and collaboration to design effective prevention activities; (3) public health encompasses a wide array of topics including sanitation, hygiene, health education, administration of health services, and health policies; and (4) public health is founded in the basic principle of human rights. More recently, the Essential Services Working Group defined the purpose of public health as preventing the spread of disease; promoting safe environments for living, working, and recreating; preventing intentional and unintentional injuries; promoting and encouraging healthy behaviors and mental health; responding to natural and man-made disasters and assisting communities in recovery; and assuring readily accessible, quality health services. In summary, public health practice is a cross-disciplinary field, using science, creativity, and collaboration to promote human health.

Public health professionals firmly believe that physical and mental health is a basic human right, not a choice, not a reward, not a privilege. Toward this vision, public health is a social movement with health equity as the main objective. Just as early man recognized that it was the responsibility of each and every member of the society to safeguard the community well or sources of drinking water, modern man is responsible for the health of others in society. In the landmark document, *The Future of Public Health*, the Institute of Medicine (1988) defined the mission of public health as "the fulfillment of society's interest in assuring the conditions in which people can be healthy" (p. 40). The IOM points to the responsibility of government and society in supporting and promoting health. This concept may seem a little alien to American culture, which embraces the ideals of independence, individualism, and self-determination. The idea that members of a group have responsibility of caring for others in society requires individuals to consider the needs of others before their own. This means that companies cannot dump waste into the ground where toxic chemicals could potentially poison the water of local residents; tobacco companies cannot market addictive and harmful products to children; and bystanders cannot turn away when they hear domestic violence. Public health requires everyone, corporate leaders, businesses, politicians, communities, schools, police, parents, neighbors, and individuals to consider the short- and long-term impact of their own behaviors on others. Social justice requires society to balance benefits and burdens. Members of society who experience burdens due to a particular action deserve benefits, and those who enjoy benefits from a particular action should carry a fair share of the burden.

The precautionary principle is used to set the bar on social responsibility. The precautionary principle states that *if* an action is *believed* to cause harm, even when there is insufficient science to support a biological connection, the burden of proof is on the actor not on the potential victim. In the case of toxic waste, the business is responsible for proving that runoff is not hazardous. The company cannot dump waste until the runoff is deemed safe through rigorous, impartial scientific study. It is not the citizens' responsibility to prove that waste products are causing disease.

The duty of providing public health services rests primarily on state, tribal, local, and territorial health departments. These entities are managed and financed by different sources. The issue of financing is important because microorganisms do not recognize state, county, or city boundaries. Sufficient funding ensures problems are addressed before they escalate out of control. State health departments are funded by the federal government, Medicare, Medicaid, state funds, and monies collected from fines for public health violations. State departments perform epidemiological surveillance, disease screening, laboratory services, treatment, and technical assistance. If there is a major outbreak of tuberculosis, the state health department would investigate, test, and treat. The majority of local public health departments are governed by local government. For example, the San Francisco Department of Public Health is governed by the city of San Francisco through the San Francisco Health Commission. The mayor of San Francisco appoints health commissioners who oversee public health programs, hospitals, home health care, outpatient treatment, disease surveillance, vital records, primary care, dental services, and maternal health services. A few states—Kentucky, Georgia, and Florida—share governance with local authorities. Local health departments are financed through local, state, and federal sources. Public health in U.S. territories of Puerto Rico, Guam, Virgin Islands, American Samoa, and the Commonwealth of Northern Mariana Islands and Freely Associated States of the Republic of Marshall Islands, Federated States of Micronesia, and Republic of Palau is funded through federal grants and cooperative agreements. Tribal health departments operate within the jurisdiction of the tribal nations to serve the health needs of Native Americans.

In general, state, tribal, local, and territorial health departments provide many of the day-to-day functions of public health, such as managing immunization programs; communicable disease screening, surveillance, and treatment; food safety and nutrition education; and inspections of restaurants, schools, and day care centers. Different populations may also present unique geographic, cultural, or economic challenges. For example, the World Health Organization reports that replacing traditional diets of nutrient-dense foods with imported energy-dense foods is causing obesity and other major health problems among Pacific Islanders (WHO, 2010). Thus, public health departments serving Pacific Islanders must focus on the negative effects of acculturation. Federal agencies are responsible for ensuring that state, tribal, local, and territorial governments have the capability to provide needed services. The federal government will only intervene if health threats extend beyond the region, require solutions outside of state or local jurisdiction, or in which states do not have the capacity to act. A man-made or natural disaster, such as major flooding, will prompt action by federal public health agencies.

Beyond assisting in natural or man-made health emergencies, the federal government manages the health of the nation by setting goals, policies, and standards, managing resources and supporting scientific research toward health solutions. Federal agencies responsible for ensuring public health include the Centers for Disease Control and Prevention (CDC), Agency for Healthcare Research and Quality, Environmental Protection Agency, Food and Drug Administration (FDA), Substance Abuse and Mental Health Services Administration (SAMHSA), National Cancer Institute (NCI), National Institute on Alcohol Abuse and Alcoholism (NIAAA), National Institute on Drug Abuse (NIDA), Department of Agriculture (USDA), Office of Minority Health (OMH), and the U.S. Public Health Service Commissioned Corps (USPHSCC). Within the CDC is the Office for State, Tribal, Local, and Territorial Support; Office of Public Health Preparedness and Response; National Institute for Occupational Safety and Health; Center for Global Health; Office of Public Health Scientific Services; Center for Surveillance, Epidemiology, and Laboratory Services; National Center for Health Statistics; Office of Noncommunicable Diseases, Injury, and Environmental Health; National Center for Birth Defects and Developmental Disabilities; National Center for Chronic Disease Prevention and Health Promotion; National Center for Environmental Health; Agency for Toxic Substances and Disease Registry; National Center for Injury Prevention and Control; Office of Infectious Diseases; National Center for Immunization and Respiratory Diseases; National Center for Emerging and Zoonotic Infectious Diseases; and the National Center for HIV, Viral Hepatitis, STD, and TB Prevention. The multiple centers, institutes, and offices within the CDC enable effective and efficient responses to public health threats. Each group provides specialized expertise while still accessing valuable resources from across the network.

Public health services are delivered by individuals of many different backgrounds and skill sets working in for-profit and nonprofit agencies, communities, and all levels of government. The public health workforce is one of the most professionally diverse groups one could envision. Workers include physicians, nurses, nutritionists, health inspectors, occupational health and safety workers, social workers, dentists and dental assistants, emergency responders, health educators, journalists, laboratory workers, X-ray technicians, animal control, veterinarians, researchers, scientists, statisticians, administrators, and policy experts. Each group offers their own distinct professional skills and together, practitioners create a larger system of care. Partnerships with the private sector, civic groups, nongovernmental organizations (NGOs), faith communities, schools, hospitals, community centers, tribal health, law enforcement, transit organizations, and employers develop a network, reaching as many people as possible in as many ways as possible. Each entity contributes in a unique way. In the case of head injuries, the National Operating Committee on Standards for Athletic Equipment (NOCSAE) develops and publishes standards for helmet safety; helmet manufacturers make helmets that meet the standards; parents purchase safety helmets; athletic organizations require players to wear helmets consistently and correctly; and coaches develop maneuvers to avoid high-impact plays (National Center for Injury Prevention and Control, 2015). Creating systems of care, developing policies, providing direct care and education, and advocating for health and safety require many different skills and partnerships.

Over the past century, public health in the United States has emerged as a unique discipline. Major achievements in the control of communicable diseases, oral hygiene, family planning, motor vehicle safety, workplace safety, heart disease prevention, and smoking cessation have extended human life span by approximately 25 years. These achievements were accomplished by many people and groups working together toward the common goal of disease prevention and health promotion.

The *Encyclopedia of Public Health: Principles, People, and Programs* describes selected public health strategies, achievements, and challenges throughout U.S. history. The entries featuring *principles* describe basic and complex concepts, and models and theories that help to guide effective public health practice. These entries provide a deeper understanding and appreciation of the field, the logic behind why public health professionals do what they do. The entries on *programs* present a sample of important, evidence-based interventions, policies, and organizations. There are many, many health education and health promotion programs. Not every program works, and some programs can cause more harm than good. The encyclopedia entries highlight programs that serve as a positive model for other programs. The context of why and how these programs were developed and implemented provides an understanding of the history of public health and best practices for the future. The entries on *people* detail the lives and achievements of social reformers, biologists, microbiologists, medical doctors, nurses, dentists, and other health professionals. The unique contributions of these men and women foster respect for all public health professionals. The stories of these pioneers reveal insightful discoveries, dogged perseverance, and dignity despite racism, gender biases, and professional or scientific challenges. Their stories tell us where public health has been and where public health must go. Their stories encourage emerging professionals to pursue a career in public health, medicine, epidemiology, biostatistics, or research. The field offers so many opportunities and needs people from diverse backgrounds with different skills. Public health belongs to everyone, and everyone belongs in public health.

Sally Kuykendall

Further Reading

American Public Health Association. (n.d.). *What is public health?* Retrieved from http://www.apha.org/~/media/files/pdf/factsheets/whatisph.ashx.

Essential Services Work Group. (n.d.). *Ten essential services: Purpose and practices of public health.* Atlanta: Centers for Disease Control and Prevention. Retrieved from http://www.cdc.gov/stltpublichealth/hop/pdfs/Ten_Essential_Public_Health_Services_2011-09_508.pdf.

Healthy people: The Surgeon General's report on health promotion and disease prevention. (1979). Rockville, MD: Department of Health, Education, and Welfare, Public Health Service, Office of the Assistant Secretary for Health and Surgeon General.

Institute of Medicine. (1988). *The future of public health.* Washington, DC: The National Academies Press.doi:10.17226/1091. Retrieved from http://www.nap.edu/catalog/1091/the-future-of-public-health.

National Center for Injury Prevention and Control. (2015). *HEADS UP to youth sports.* Atlanta: Centers for Disease Control and Prevention. Retrieved from http://www.cdc.gov/headsup/youthsports/index.html.

Office of State, Tribal, Local and Territorial Support, Centers for Disease Control and Prevention. (2013). *United States public health 101.* Retrieved from http://www.cdc.gov/stltpublichealth/docs/usph101.pdf.

Winslow, C. E. A. (1920). The untilled field of public health. *Modern Medicine, 2,* 183–191.

World Health Organization. (2010). Pacific Islanders pay heavy price for abandoning traditional diet. *Bulletin of the World Health Organization, 88*(7), 481–560. Retrieved from http://www.who.int/bulletin/volumes/88/7/10-010710/en.

Chronology

c. 1754 BCE	Code of Hammurabi states laws of Mesopotamia including medical fees
c. 1000 BCE	*Sushruta Samhita* records Indian medical and surgical practices
c. 600 BCE	Early bioterrorism: Assyrians poison enemy wells with rye ergot fungus
c. 460 BCE	Hippocrates proposes that diseases are related to diet, activity, lifestyle, and environment rather than punishment from the gods
c. 300 BCE	*Yellow Emperor's Inner Canon* documents Chinese medical practices
583	Roman Catholic Church isolates people with leprosy
c. 860	*Al-Risalah al-Dhahabiah* (*The Golden Treatise*) records medicine and wellness in Persia (Iran)
1346	Plague extends to Europe initiating the Black Death
1403	Venice establishes the first quarantine station
1431	Joan of Arc is declared a witch and burned at the stake
1492	Christopher Columbus sails to the Caribbean Islands
1520	Cortez exploration unintentionally introduces smallpox to the Aztec
1620	Pilgrims establish Plymouth colony
1628	William Harvey describes the circulatory system
1632	King Charles I licenses The Guinea Company to export African slaves to America
1683	Anton Van Leeuwenhoek visualizes microscopic animals
1754	Indigenous Americans are intentionally infected by blankets from smallpox victims
1775	American Revolutionary War begins
1776	Declaration of Independence

1783	American Revolutionary War ends with an estimated 4,435 U.S. service member deaths; Yellow fever epidemic
1794	Philadelphia establishes the first local board of health
1796	Edward Jenner inoculates James Phipps with cowpox
1798	Marine Hospital Service is founded
1831	Forced removal of Native Americans begins with the Choctaw Nation
1837	Great Plains smallpox epidemic decimates Native American people
1838	Forced removal of the Cherokee Nation results in the Trail of Tears
1842	Edwin Chadwick publishes *The Report on the Sanitary Conditions of the Labouring Population of Great Britain*
1843	Dorothea Dix publishes *Memorial to the Legislature of Massachusetts* documenting the living conditions of mentally ill in Massachusetts
1847	American Medical Association is founded; Ignaz Semmelweis recommends that doctors wash their hands to reduce infections
1848	Women's rights convention held at Seneca Falls, New York
1849	Elizabeth Blackwell is the first female to earn a medical degree from a U.S. college
1850	Lemuel Shattuck releases *Report of the Sanitary Commission of Massachusetts*; Congress passes the Fugitive Slave Act mandating all states to cooperate in the capture and return of suspected slaves
1854	John Snow traces London cholera outbreak to the Broad Street pump; Florence Nightingale establishes the first school of nursing at Saint Thomas's Hospital
1869	Massachusetts establishes the first state board of health
1861	American Civil War begins
1863	President Lincoln signs the Emancipation Proclamation
1865	American Civil War ends with an estimated 498,332 deaths
1871	John Maynard Woodworth is appointed the first supervising surgeon (surgeon general) of the Marine Hospital Service
1876	Alexander Graham Bell invents the telephone; Robert Koch discovers *Bacillus anthracis*

1877	Louis Pasteur proves germ theory
1878	National Quarantine Act
1884	Robert Koch and Friedrich Loeffler propose Koch's postulates, scientific criteria used to determine causal organism of an infectious disease
1885	Karl Benz builds the first gasoline-powered automobile
1886	Labor protests at Haymarket Square escalate to violence and death
1889	Andrew Carnegie publishes *The Gospel of Wealth* encouraging philanthropy; Jane Addams establishes Hull House
1891	Florence Kelley investigates working conditions in the garment industry
1896	London pedestrian Bridget Driscoll is struck and killed by a gasoline-powered automobile, becoming the first recorded motor vehicle fatality; Wilhelm Conrad Roentgen discovers X-ray
1898	Spanish American War begins
1901	Oldsmobile introduces the speedometer
1902	Spanish American War ends with an estimated 2,446 U.S. service member deaths
1904	National Child Labor Committee organized
1906	Upton Sinclair describes the meatpacking industry in *The Jungle*; Meat Inspection Act and the Pure Food and Drugs Act are passed
1907	George Soper traces Oyster Bay typhoid outbreak to cook Mary Mallon
1908	Ford Motor Company produces the Model T; Clifford Beers writes *A Mind That Found Itself* describing his experiences as a mentally ill patient
1909	National Association for the Advancement of Colored People forms
1910	Flexner Report; Alice Hamilton investigates occupation-related diseases
1912	*Titanic* sinks
1913	American Society for the Control of Cancer (American Cancer Society) is founded

1914	World War I begins; Margaret Sanger publishes the birth control pamphlet *Family Limitation*
1917	United States joins allied troops in World War I
1918	Flu pandemic
1919	World War I ends with 116,516 U.S. service member deaths
1923	George Papanicolau creates the Pap smear to detect cervical cancer
1924	Martha May Elliot directs the National Children's Bureau Division of Maternal and Child Health
1928	Alexander Fleming discovers penicillin
1929	Great Depression starts with the stock market crash of October 29, Black Tuesday
1930	Veterans Health Administration (VHA) established
1931	FDR elected president
1932	Tuskegee Syphilis Study started
1933	Widespread amoebic dysentery cases traced to Chicago World's Fair hotel
1934	Midian Othello Bousfield advocates for health needs of African American people
1935	Social Security Act signed into law
1937	The National Safety Council creates a national plan for farm safety
1939	World War II begins
1941	Charles Drew creates blood storage and transfusion techniques; Japan attacks Pearl Harbor
1942	Explosion at the Benxihu Colliery in China kills 1,549 coal mine workers
1945	World War II ends with 405,399 U.S. service member deaths; Grand Rapids, Michigan, becomes the first community with fluoridated water
1946	Centers for Disease Control and Prevention founded; National Mental Health Act
1948	World Health Organization is founded; Donora smog incident occurs; Framingham Heart Study begins

1949	Florence Sabin reorganizes Colorado State Board of Health
1950	Korean War begins
1951	Malaria eradicated in the U.S.
1952	International Planned Parenthood founded
1953	Korean War ends with 54,246 U.S. service member deaths; James Watson and Francis Crick discover the chemical structure of DNA
1954	Richard Doll and Austin Bradford Hill publish landmark study linking smoking to lung cancer among doctors
1955	Vietnam War begins; Jonas Salk creates the polio vaccine; Cutter Incident
1956	Mercury poisoning from industrial wastewater is identified in Minamata, Japan; Min Chiu Li discovers chemotherapy for cancer
1958	Working for Volvo, Nils Bohlin invents the three-point seat belt
1961	Food and Drug Administration approves oral contraceptives
1962	Rachel Carson publishes *Silent Spring*
1964	Civil Rights Act; Surgeon General's report on *Smoking and Health*
1965	Medicare and Medicaid established; Ralph Nader publishes *Unsafe at Any Speed: The Designed-in Dangers of the American Automobile*
1966	Narcotic Addict Rehabilitation Act
1968	First heart transplant surgery
1969	*Time Magazine* reports Cuyahoga River fires
1970	Occupational Safety and Health Act
1971	Ban on tobacco advertisements on television and radio
1972	Tuskegee Syphilis Study terminated
1974	*The Belmont Report*
1975	The Indian Self-Determination and Education Act; Vietnam War ends with 90,220 U.S. service member deaths
1976	Nurses' Health Study commences
1977	Smallpox eradicated

1979	First edition of *Healthy People* published
1981	AIDS epidemic begins in the United States
1983	Amsterdam establishes the first community organized needle exchange program
1984	First seat belt law passed in New York; gas leak in Bhopal, India, kills at least 3,787 people and injures an estimated 558,125
1985	Salmonella in milk from Hillfarm Dairy, Illinois, infects 16,284 people resulting in at least two deaths
1986	Chernobyl nuclear disaster; Emergency Medical Treatment and Labor Act (EMTALA) established
1988	The Institute of Medicine releases *The Future of Public Health*
1990	Desert Storm War begins; Americans with Disabilities Act signed into law; Researchers from the National Institutes of Health use gene therapy to treat Ashanti DeSilva
1991	Desert Storm War ends with 1,948 U.S. service member deaths
1993	*E. coli* in undercooked hamburgers from Jack in the Box infects over 700 people resulting in four deaths
1996	Lead eliminated from U.S. gasoline; Dolly, the first cloned mammal, is born; Port Arthur massacre prompts Australia to outlaw automatic and semiautomatic rifles
1997	WHO declares obesity a global epidemic
1998	Five tobacco companies settle a lawsuit brought by 46 states, five U.S. territories, and the District of Columbia seeking reimbursement for health care costs resulting from smoking
2001	September 11 terrorist attacks; Anthrax attacks on U.S. Senators and news agencies; Global War on Terror begins
2003	Worldwide severe acute respiratory syndrome (SARS) outbreak; Human Genome project completed
2005	London transit bombings; Hurricane Katrina
2007	Virginia Tech shooting
2010	Affordable Care Act passed
2011	Tōhoku earthquake and tsunami; Fukushima Daiichi nuclear disaster

2012	Ebola epidemic in West Africa
2013	Boston Marathon bombing
2015	Emmanuel African Methodist Church shooting
2016	Pulse nightclub shooting

A

ACUTE ILLNESSES

Acute illnesses are a category of health problems in which symptoms come on suddenly, within hours or days, and the person recovers fairly quickly, usually within days to weeks. Examples include the common cold, ear infections, food poisoning, diarrhea, sprains, strains, animal bites, and other traumatic injuries. Most people suffer from one or more acute illnesses at some point in life. Unintentional injuries alone account for 40 million emergency room visits per year in the United States (National Center for Health Statistics, 2016). Communities that lack proper sanitation, resources, or suffer from major stressors are at higher risk for communicable disease and injury. Acute illnesses present special challenges to public health systems. Generally, public health uses population-based approaches to restore, promote, and maintain health. Disease prevention programs, such as healthy eating to prevent diabetes or cardiovascular disease, may be offered to clients at any time of year. Programs can be planned in advance, and educating in groups is cost effective. Conversely, acute illnesses require immediate or urgent, individualized health services. The person experiences symptoms, seeks medical care at a clinic, doctor's office or hospital, and timely treatment is necessary to prevent complications. This individualized care, while necessary, is resource intensive and expensive. Whereas public health strives for integrated, holistic care, acute illnesses demand unplanned, urgent treatment creating fragmented, reactionary care.

The relationship between acute and chronic illness is complex. Although many acute health problems resolve without treatment, some cases develop into more severe or chronic health problems. For example, the common childhood disease of strep throat can progress into rheumatic fever, a serious illness that causes stroke, permanent heart damage, or death. Alternatively, chronic illnesses can lead to acute problems. For someone with osteoporosis, a minor fall or traumatic blow can break bones. Early identification and treatment of acute health problems are important to prevent exacerbation to more serious problems. Health professionals must be able to accurately diagnose and treat a wide variety of nondescript illnesses. This can be a challenge. For example, the patient who presents with severe itching could have poison ivy, sunburn, allergic reactions, diabetes, or multiple sclerosis. Practitioners must be able to differentiate symptoms in order to identify the underlying cause and decide on the correct treatment. Although acute illnesses can be a challenge to public health, they do provide an entry point for holistic care. The person with undetected osteoporosis may first present with a fracture. After initial treatment, the health care provider can refer the patient to a registered dietician for nutrition education or physical therapist for balance and strength training. Acute illnesses provide an opportunity to screen and connect patients to health promotion activities.

Acute health problems are classified as communicable diseases, noncommunicable diseases, and injuries. Local, state, territorial, and federal public health systems are responsible for monitoring and investigating communicable disease outbreaks. Local and territorial health departments surveil for reportable diseases, investigate cases, develop and implement plans to control spread, provide expert advice, and disseminate health education materials. The National Notifiable Disease Surveillance System (NNDSS) is a national system listing 77 notifiable health conditions. The database enables individuals and groups to share and analyze outbreaks and trends. The CDC is responsible for providing timely and accurate information to physicians, nurses, public health professionals, epidemiologists, and other scientists by publishing the NNDSS data in *Morbidity and Mortality Weekly Reports* (*MMWR*). The NNDSS lists health problems by name, not by acute versus chronic categories. This means that we do not have clear data on the cost of acute illnesses to society.

Although the healthy person recovers rapidly from an acute illness and suffers few, if any, consequences, acute health problems create challenges to society. Acute illnesses come on suddenly and unexpectedly, requiring personalized care that is expensive and fragmented. Careful monitoring and timely treatment are critical to controlling outbreaks. Public health professionals have developed systems to remain alert for cases and act quickly when cases are detected. Although acute illnesses challenge health systems, they also provide opportunities for ongoing health promotion. The next steps are to increase systems of care within impoverished areas, measure the overall financial burden of acute illnesses on society, develop cost-effective systems, and improve integration of acute, chronic, and preventive health care.

Sally Kuykendall

See also: Chronic Illness; Disability; Disease; Epidemic; Handwashing; Health; Infectious Diseases; Influenza; Injuries; Medicine; Nutrition; Prevention

Further Reading

Centers for Disease Control and Prevention. (2015). *National Notifiable Diseases Surveillance System (NNDSS)*. Retrieved from https://wwwn.cdc.gov/nndss/history.aspx.

Hirshon, J. M., Risko, N., Calvello, E. B., Stewart de Ramirez, S., Narayan, M., Theodosis, C., & O'Neill, J. (2013). Health systems and services: The role of acute care. *Bulletin of the World Health Organization*, *91*(5), 386–388. doi:10.2471/BLT.12.112664

National Center for Health Statistics. (2016). *National Hospital Ambulatory Medical Care Survey: 2011 Emergency department summary tables*. Retrieved from http://www.cdc.gov/nchs/data/ahcd/nhamcs_emergency/2011_ed_web_tables.pdf.

ADDICTIONS

Addiction is a chronic brain disease characterized by an overwhelming desire for a specific substance or activity, such as tobacco, alcohol, drugs, or gambling. The desire escalates to such a point that other basic needs, such as eating, sleeping, and relationships, are ignored. Eventually, the individual may lose the ability to function at school, work, or home. The wide array of addictive substances, objects, and activities mean that many different individuals and their loved ones are affected.

Addictions create unique challenges to public health. According to the National Institute on Drug Abuse's (NIDA) nationwide trends research (2015), 55.8 million Americans aged 12 and older were current cigarette smokers, which constituted a total of 21.3 percent of the U.S. population in 2013. More than 24 million Americans aged 12 or older—9.4 percent of the population—have used an illicit drug in the past month. After alcohol, marijuana has the highest dependency rate of all other illicit substances. More than 4 million Americans met the clinical criteria for either substance dependence or abuse of marijuana in the past year, while 1.9 million Americans met the criteria for dependency or addiction to pain relievers. Substance abuse accounts for many cases of intentional and unintentional injuries, lung and cardiovascular diseases, stroke, cancers, and mental health disorders.

The last century witnessed a major shift in the way addictions are viewed and treated. One hundred years ago addictions were believed to be a moral flaw related to weak willpower. Today, we understand addiction as a treatable disease of the brain with psychological and social implications. Addiction research started in the 1930s; however, it was not until 1963 that the American Public Health Association published an official statement that identified alcoholism as treatable (White, 1998). Three years later, in 1966, the National Center for the Prevention and Control of Alcoholism was created as a subsection of the National Institute on Mental Health. In the same year, the Narcotic Addict Rehabilitation Act was passed. This marked a major turning point in the history of addiction treatment in the United States. For the first time, the federal government provided support to develop addiction treatment services in communities (White, 1998). One year later, in 1967, the American Medical Association recognized alcoholism as a disease (White, 1998). The National Association of Alcoholism and Drug Abuse Counselors and the National Institute on Drug Abuse (NIDA) were founded two years later, in 1972. Despite progress and efforts by public health and medical research, in 1987, President Reagan announced the nation's War on Drugs, replacing addictions treatment with punishment and incarceration (White, 1998). That same year, the American Medical Association expanded the definition of addictions by recognizing all drug dependencies as diseases and helping to legitimize addiction treatment within the medical field. In 1991, the American Society of Addiction Medicine (ASAM) published *Patient Placement Criteria for the Treatment of Psychoactive Substance Use Disorders*. These guidelines set a precedent, tailoring treatment from a single set of treatment criteria for all individuals to individualized care models (White, 1998). Despite political setbacks and continued stigma against those with addictions, public health and medical organizations have made enormous strides in the understanding and treatment of addictions.

How Addictions Begin

Public health uses the biopsychosocial model as a framework to understand diseases. According to this model, biological, psychological, and social factors all play a role in human health and wellness. Biological factors that increase likelihood of substance dependency are genetics, using addictive substances during critical periods of brain development, existing medical conditions, and mental health disorders. Addictions start as a biological process within the brain. In a healthy brain, nerves send, receive, and process information. Addictive drugs contain chemicals that disrupt brain function and structure. Disruption can happen in two ways. The first is by mimicking the brain's natural chemical messages. The structure of some drugs, for example, marijuana and heroin, are highly similar to neurotransmitters. In fact, the drugs are so similar that the brain is tricked into sending abnormal messages when these substances enter the body. The second way that drugs can disrupt brain function is by overstimulating the reward circuit. Some drugs (e.g., methamphetamine and cocaine) cause neurotransmitters to release unnaturally large amounts of dopamine. Dopamine controls motivation, emotion, movement, and pleasure. Overproduction of dopamine produces feelings of euphoria, creating a motivation for ongoing usage. Although the brain is initially rewarded for using the drug, as substance use continues, the brain becomes used to the oversupply of dopamine and compensates by decreasing its own production. The drug has less of an impact—and to experience the same high the person must use more of the substance—a condition known as tolerance. The brain adapts to using the substance, and when the person tries to stop, he or she experiences painful physical and emotional withdrawal.

The teenage brain, which is going through rapid growth and development, is particularly susceptible to physical and psychological dependence. Psychological causes and consequences of substance addiction are intrinsically related to the brain patterns described above. From a psychological perspective, drug addiction is conceptualized as a chronic disease that results in compulsive and obsessive drug seeking and use. The initial decision to take drugs is often voluntary; however, once an individual becomes addicted to drugs, the physical brain changes over time. These changes affect self-control and the ability to resist urges to take the drug. Just as there are biological and psychological factors that can predispose an individual to substance addiction, there are both social and environmental factors that do the same. For example, living in an environment where adults (e.g., parents) use illicit substances during childhood is linked to a heightened likelihood of developing substance dependence in adolescence (Swadi, 1999). Other direct social and environmental factors are poor parental monitoring, poor parental attachment, and affiliation with drug-taking peer groups (Swadi, 1999). Substance use and eventually abuse are used as a way to self-medicate for those living in harsh or disadvantaged communities. Dealing with substance addiction creates a plethora of negative social consequences, which include loneliness, familial and social rejection, poor academic achievement, unemployment, and homelessness. These devastating consequences lead, in turn, to further usage, which ultimately creates a vicious cycle.

Preventing Addictions

Public health breaks the cycle of addiction through effective, evidence-based programs. The Institute of Medicine categorizes prevention programs as universal, selected, or indicated. Universal prevention, previously referred to as primary prevention, prevents substance abuse before the behavior starts. Although people of all ages can be susceptible to developing a substance dependency—even babies still in utero—adolescents are most susceptible. According to NIDA's nationwide trends research (2015), 22.6 percent of 18- to 20-year-olds reported using an illicit drug in the past month. For this reason, adolescence, generally occurring between ages 12 and 18 years of age, is considered the most critical time for universal prevention of substance abuse. The Truth Campaign by the American Legacy Foundation is an example of an effective cigarette smoking prevention program. By deconstructing the messages embedded in cigarette advertising, the Truth Campaign has effectively reduced smoking among middle school students by 19 percent and among high school students by 8 percent (Zucker, Hopkins, Sly, Urich, Kershaw, & Solari, 2000).

Selected prevention programs work by reducing risk factors and enhancing protective factors. These programs focus on at-risk populations and are often geared toward a particular setting and audience (NIDA, 2014). The Model Adolescent Suicide Prevention Program (MASPP) was developed to reduce trauma, violence, substance abuse, and suicides among a specific tribal nation of Native Americans in New Mexico. Over the intervention period of 15 years, the program reduced self-destructive behaviors by 73 percent (May, Serna, Hurt, & DeBruyn, 2005). Indicated programs target people who are already using drugs with the goal of stopping drug use, maintaining abstinence, and controlling long-term effects of the chronic drug use. Indicated prevention programs, such as family therapy, are part of a comprehensive drug treatment program.

Treatment

The treatment of addictions is tailored to the type of drug being abused (stimulant, depressant, hallucinogen, or opioid), length of abuse, and individual biopsychosocial circumstances. People who abuse drugs experience critical moments when they recognize the need for help and actively seek treatment. Therefore, it is important that treatment centers are conveniently located within all communities and continuously accessible. These critical moments may not necessarily be voluntary.

Interventions by family members or court mandates can be just as effective as voluntary treatment. The first stage of substance abuse treatment for mind-altering substances is medical detoxification. During this stage, health professionals will support the patient through drug withdrawal, correct any malnutrition or electrolyte imbalances, and screen for additional health issues related to substance abuse, such as hepatitis B, HIV/AIDS, tuberculosis, or other infectious diseases. The length of time for detoxification varies. With some drugs, detoxification takes months, and adjunct therapies such as methadone may be used to alleviate cravings. Comprehensive drug treatment must also include the psychological and social aspects of drug use. Long-term counseling, behavioral therapy, and monitoring help the person to maintain abstinence, deal with stressors, problem solve effectively, avoid situations that might lead to relapse, establish healthy interpersonal relationships, and treat comorbid mental health problems. Because the person is learning new ways to interact in the world, the most effective treatments are long term, continuing for more than three months and including loved ones. After initial withdrawal, the challenge is to keep the person engaged in recovery and to prevent relapses. Random drug screens also help prevent relapse because a positive screen indicates the need to change or reassess therapy (NIDA, 2012).

Addictions are a chronic health problem affecting millions of Americans. Fortunately, the disease is treatable. Due to the large variety of ways substance addiction disrupts individuals' lives, effective treatment must incorporate many components. Effective treatment assists individuals to stop taking drugs, maintain sobriety, and regain productive functioning. When it comes to substance addiction prevention, shaping youth's perception about drugs is vital. Prevention programs should address all types of drug use, should be geared toward the specific type of drug use prevalent in the local community, and finally should be specific to the contextual characteristics (e.g., age, ethnicity, gender) of the population being addressed.

Ariel A. Friedman and Nadav Antebi-Gruszka

See also: Alcohol; Cancer; Collaborations; Epidemic; Hepatitis; Human Trafficking; Mental Health; National Institutes of Health; National Institute on Drug Abuse; Prescription Drugs; Prevention; Substance Abuse and Mental Health Services Administration; Syringe Service Programs; Truth Campaign, The; Wynder, Ernst Ludwig; *Controversies in Public Health:* Controversy 2

Further Reading

Dutra, L., Stathopoulou, G., Basden, S. L., Leyro, T. M., Powers, M. B., & Otto, M. W. (2008). A meta-analytic review of psychosocial interventions for substance use disorders. *The American Journal of Psychiatry*, *165*(2), 179–187.

Hawkins, J. D., Catalano, R. F., & Miller, J. Y. (1992). Risk and protective factors for alcohol and other drug problems in adolescence and early adulthood: Implications for substance abuse prevention. *Psychological Bulletin*, *112*(1), 64.

Kuss, D. J., & Griffiths, M. D. (2012). Internet gaming addiction: A systematic review of empirical research. *International Journal of Mental Health and Addiction, 10*(2), 278–296.

Macleod, J., Oakes, R., Copello, A., Crome, I., Egger, M., Hickman, M., & Smith, G. D. (2004). Psychological and social sequelae of cannabis and other illicit drug use by young people: A systematic review of longitudinal, general population studies. *The Lancet, 363*(9421), 1579–1588.

Mathers, B. M., Degenhardt, L., Phillips, B., Wiessing, L., Hickman, M., Strathdee, S. A., & Mattick, R. P. (2008). Global epidemiology of injecting drug use and HIV among people who inject drugs: A systematic review. *The Lancet, 372*(9651), 1733–1745.

May, P. A., Serna, P., Hurt, L., & DeBruyn, L. M. (2005). Outcome evaluation of a public health approach to suicide prevention in an American Indian tribal nation. *American Journal of Public Health, 95*(7), 1238–1244. doi:10.2105/AJPH.2004.040410

McLellan, A. T., Lewis, D. C., O'Brien, C. P., & Kleber, H. D. (2000). Drug dependence, a chronic medical illness: Implications for treatment, insurance, and outcomes evaluation. *Journal of the American Medical Association, 284*(13), 1689–1695.

National Institute on Drug Abuse. (2012). *Principles of drug addiction treatment: A research-based guide* (3rd ed.). Retrieved May 27, 2016, from https://www.drugabuse.gov/publications/principles-drug-addiction-treatment-research-based-guide-third-edition/principles-effective-treatment.

National Institute on Drug Abuse. (2014). *DrugFacts: Lessons from prevention research.* Retrieved January 11, 2016, from http://www.drugabuse.gov/publications/drugfacts/lessons-prevention-research.

National Institute on Drug Abuse. (2015). *DrugFacts: Nationwide trends.* Retrieved January 5, 2016, from http://www.drugabuse.gov/publications/drugfacts/nationwide-trends.

Swadi, H. (1999). Individual risk factors for adolescent substance use. *Drug and Alcohol Dependence, 55*(3), 209–224.

White, W. L. (1998). *Slaying the dragon: The history of addiction treatment and recovery in America.* Bloomington, IL: Chestnut Health Systems/Lighthouse Institute.

Zucker, D., Hopkins, R. S., Sly, D. F., Urich, J., Kershaw, J. M., & Solari, S. (2000). Florida's "truth" campaign: A counter-marketing, anti-tobacco media campaign. *Journal of Public Health Management and Practice, 6*(3), 1–6.

ADMINISTRATION, HEALTH

Health administration is a discipline that teaches individuals how to apply health care technical skills in health care systems operation and management, health system planning, human resources management, health law and regulations, health information technology, health care resource allocation and policy making, business and financial management, health care ethics, and public relations. Health administration may be applied to any specific types of health care services involving clinical and nonclinical operation. In other words, health administration involves integration and coordination of the various functions of clinical and nonclinical delivery of health services, a management decision-making process with policies and procedures that align toward achieving the health organizational goals and objectives. Health administration is a discipline that deals with legal and professional management of health care operations, health policy formulation and analysis, leadership coordination, operational processes, and implementation of policies toward the delivery of health care or health services across health systems. In health administration, health organizational goals and objectives must align with (federal, state, and local) health legislation, regulation, and constitutional provisions of the respective region. Health administration is a discipline that studies the execution of health care leadership shared decision and implementation processes of health institution organizational policies toward achieving organizational goals in the delivery of health services within the public and private sectors.

Basic Courses for Discipline and Degree

A health administration degree prepares prospective health care administrators to be equipped with knowledge in achieving and fulfilling the demands and responsibilities of health services delivery. The evolving nature of health care service delivery, the size and function of a health facility, and the evolving regulatory processes make health care administration discipline draw more knowledge from the field of business administration and management sciences (including economics, law, financial management, and organizational culture). Health administration programs are structured toward developing business competencies and planning skills, understanding core organizational management theory, and understanding the essentials of leadership ethics and communication, research analysis, and evaluation. Depending on the types of health care administration degrees, core coursework usually includes health care delivery systems, health regulation and policy, health economics, health care marketing, health care financing, health resources management, leadership theory and practice, population health and epidemiology, medical terminology, health information technology system, risk management and quality improvement, managed health care and reimbursement, health program evaluation, and global health care. At the undergraduate level, health administration core courses prepare students for leadership skills, management concepts in administration, general concepts on health administration, and health services delivery. Foundational courses on health administration are blended with basic principles of business operation and planning, accounting and financing, marketing, human resources administration, economics, law and policy, organizational leadership and culture, and basic statistical analysis.

At the graduate level, health administration courses equip students with advanced management skills and career opportunities for senior-level administrative and health leadership positions. Graduate health administration programs are structured to equip health administrators with advanced skills and competencies in health care financial management, resources management, health evaluation, health policy and regulation, strategic management and planning, risk analysis and quality improvement, health analytic research, economics of health care, epidemiology, and population health management. Health administration programs may be tailored for different concentrations that will enable health care practitioners to improve their management skills in their specialties. At the graduate level, such concentrations may include general health administration, nursing administration, long-term care administration, behavioral health administration, hospital administration, gerontology, health education, health and wellness, health and human services, health informatics, population health, and health policy administration. At the doctoral degree level, health administration programs focus on leadership, scholarship, and practice development. The doctoral level of health administration study involves solving complex administrative and research problems in the delivery of health services. These programs prepare students to be new knowledge contributors, complex health problem solvers, health policy analysts, developers of health policy decisions of the future, and health care leaders within clinical and nonclinical fields of health.

The study of health administration prepares students to become health administrators, health executives, or health leaders within nonclinical and clinical branches of health care with the intention of managing health care operations and services, managing staff, strategically planning, coordinating care, managing finance, making policy decisions, and representing their organizations. Health administrators' responsibilities may include organizing and managing health operations and businesses, preparing budgets and authorizing expenditures, strategically planning and implementing policies and procedures, ratifying contracts or authorizations for purchases, formulating and analyzing health policies, and engaging in health operations and research. Health administrators may work in all areas of health and health service delivery within public and private health care organizations. They may work in a government-owned health system, and health department, or agency. They could also work for corporate for-profit and nonprofit health organizations (such as hospitals, nursing homes, home health agencies, community health centers, and human services), health insurance and managed care organizations, the pharmaceutical industry, medical device and equipment companies, health consulting firms, health-related national associations (American Hospital Association, America Health Information Management Association, American College of Healthcare Executives), and health research institutes.

Generalists and Specialists

Health administrators work as either generalists or specialists. They use their management and leadership skills to achieve customer-focused patient care and services within a health system. The size and type of the health organization determines the function and responsibilities of health administrators. For example, a large facility may have a hierarchy of leadership from chief executive officer, senior director, director, and manager, to unit head or coordinator. On the other hand, a health administrator of a smaller facility may be directly involved in operational decision making, staffing, hiring and retention, financial management and disbursement, procurement management, and vendor contracting.

A generalist health administrator is a business-oriented manager with technical skills and vast knowledge in leading and operating an entire health facility. Generalist health administrators are expected to be experts with high efficiency in organizing quality patient medical care with the available resources, implementing the organizational mission philosophy and strategic goals set forth by the hospital board, directing and managing the day-to-day hospital business operation and administration, collaborating with interdisciplinary and multidisciplinary medical and nonmedical staff and leaders, building trust among all stakeholders, and ensuring compliance to all health policies and regulations. Health administrators involved in hospital management and administration are generalists whose responsibilities may include managing multiple departments, building trust through open communications, resolving conflicts, developing and implementing strategic goals, driving innovation and organization culture, representing the health organization, and integrating various clinical and nonclinical departmental functions in the delivery of hospital services.

Specialist health administrators are health care management experts who lead and operate specific departments, clinical units, or health care programs within a health system (health organization). Specialized health administrators may have career paths within their field. For example, they may be nurses, pharmacists, radiologists, health record administrators, or clinicians. Specialist health administrators could also be specialists, managers, or directors who have a specific knowledge about something or responsibilities to daily operations of health-specific strategic goals and objectives.

Specialist health administrators may have responsibilities in day-to-day operations, program planning and management, policy implementation, program evaluation, budgeting, staffing and retention, legal claims, public relations, risk management, and quality improvement. A specialist health administrator may become a director of various things, such as a nursing staff, ancillary administration, an outpatient facility, operations, hospital marketing, medical billing and reimbursement, human resources, residential care, behavioral health, health finance, health research outcome, an accounting department, or medical records.

Each of these specialties, units, or departments in health has strategic goals and objectives toward health care service delivery, which a specialist health administrator may be given the mandate to achieve. A health administrator with the designation of clinical manager or director has the responsibilities to coordinate and manage rehabilitation care, nursing care, surgical care, and other patient care activities in their unit. Health administrators with state licenses to practice as nursing home administrators operate the day-to-day activities across all units and departments that work toward proper delivery of patient care to their residents. Nursing home administrators implement cost containment measures, assist in human resources retention, manage compliance to labor and employment law, monitor and disburse funds for procurement and medical supplies, and ensure compliance of quality improvement to resident care and safety. Health administrators with designations as medical records managers or health information managers secure patient health records in compliance with the Health Insurance Portability and Accountability Act of 1996 (HIPAA) regulation, assist in the collection of patient health records, process medical records related to patient treatment and diagnosis, and organize patient health information about patient conditions. Medical practice administrators, managers, or directors with health administration qualifications coordinate and manage activities in a medical group practice, including patient scheduling, electronic health record use and data capture, and maintenance of patient medical records. They oversee medical billing and medical coding, supply inventory, accounting and payroll, and medical staffing and evaluation. And they ensure regulatory compliance on policy.

Godyson Orji

See also: American Public Health Association; Certified in Public Health; Code of Ethics; Council on Education for Public Health; Degrees in Public Health; Health Education; *Nation's Health, The*; Public Health in the United States, History of; Substance Abuse and Mental Health Services Administration; Veterans' Health

Further Reading

National Center for Education Statistics (NCES). (2010). *Classification of Instructional Programs Code 51.0701: Health/Health Care Administration/Management.* Retrieved from http://nces.ed.gov/IPEDS/CIPCODE/cipdetail.aspx?y=55&cipid=88761.

National Center for Education Statistics (NCES). (2010). *Classification of Instructional Programs Code 51.2211: Health Services Administration.* Retrieved from https://nces.ed.gov/ipeds/cipcode/cipdetail.aspx?y=55&cipid=87654.

ADVERSE CHILDHOOD EXPERIENCES (ACEs)

Adverse childhood experiences (ACEs) are traumatic experiences, such as abuse, neglect, or household dysfunction, which occur during the first 18 years of life. From 1995 to 1997, researchers at Kaiser Permanente health systems and the Centers for Disease Control and Prevention (CDC) surveyed 17,000 members of a health maintenance organization to investigate childhood experiences and health status (Felitti et al., 1998). The ACE study found significant relationships between distressing experiences and heart disease, cancer, diabetes, and many other health problems. Furthermore, results suggested dose-response relationships where respondents with a higher number of ACEs were more likely to report health problems. Subsequent studies expanded to other diseases and other populations. Public health experts believe that ACEs may be one of the most important determinants of health. Early traumatic experiences are believed to impact brain and social development, prompting unhealthy behaviors that result in antisocial behavior and disease. There is a need to increase public awareness of ACEs and to support and implement evidence-based prevention and intervention programs. Through trauma-informed care, public health and medical professionals explore past traumas that may have led to unhealthy behaviors. Validating adverse childhood experiences frees the individual from guilt and shame and helps him or her to understand motivations underlying unhealthy, potentially self-medicating behaviors. Treating and reducing ACEs can significantly reduce premature morbidity and mortality, demands on health care systems, and the economic impact of disease, improving the quality of life for millions of people.

The original ACE study compared three components: adverse childhood experiences, negative health behaviors, and diseases. The adverse childhood experiences chosen for the initial ACE survey included emotional abuse, physical abuse, sexual abuse, violence against the mother, parental separation or divorce, emotional or physical neglect, or living in a household with adults who were substance abusers, mentally ill, suicidal, or incarcerated. The negative health behaviors studied were smoking, obesity, physical inactivity, depressed mood, suicide attempts, alcoholism, drug abuse, and high-risk sexuality (defined as 50 or more sexual partners). Diseases selected for the survey were ischemic heart disease, cancer, stroke, chronic bronchitis, emphysema, diabetes, hepatitis, and bone fractures. One final outcome was response to the question, "Do you consider your physical health to be excellent, very good, good, fair, or poor?" The study found that almost two-thirds of participants had at least one ACE and 20 percent had at least three ACEs (CDC, 2016).

Since the original study, other research confirmed positive correlations between ACEs and adolescent pregnancy, poor academic achievement, alcoholism, anxiety, asthma, depression, diabetes, illicit drug use, intimate partner violence, obesity, sexually transmitted diseases, smoking, suicide attempts, poor work performance, quality of life, and interaction with the juvenile justice system (CDC, 2016; Huang et al., 2015; Iniguez & Stankowski, 2016). Despite the many studies of ACEs as a disease determinant, many questions remain. The ACE studies are retrospective, which means researchers ask patients to recall past experiences. Researchers cannot say that ACEs cause disease—only that ACEs and health problems exist together. Theoretically, a third unidentified factor may be present, which creates both ACEs and disease. Alternatively, people with disease have had time and reason to reflect on their life, which means they are more likely to recall ACEs in comparison to people without disease.

Studies have also revealed conflicting results. One study found an inverse relationship between ACEs and hypertension, hypercholesterolemia, myocardial infarction, and cancer (Iniguez & Stankowski, 2016). Another study of more than 39,000 participants found gender differences in number of ACEs and risk behaviors for HIV (Fang et al., 2016). Results showed a dose-response relationship between ACEs and IV drug use, sexually transmitted infections, and anal sex among males. Risk behaviors did not increase for females until they accumulated three ACEs. Schreier et al. (2015) found ethnic differences. Pregnant women with histories of physical or sexual abuse had high cortisol levels—a biological marker for stress—and the increases were more pronounced among African American women. Despite the wealth of information, more studies are needed to understand how ACEs impact health and why some people succumb to the damaging influences of childhood experiences while others appear resilient.

Experts postulate the pathways between adverse experiences, risky behavior, and disease. When dealing with a stressful experience, the body reacts with the sympathetic-parasympathetic response. Behaviors associated with traumatic experiences are violence (fight), truancy and running away (flight), or withdraw, depression, and self-medication (freeze). The adolescent living in a household with domestic violence may initially use smoking to self-medicate, and as the stress becomes more severe or tolerance to nicotine develops she may turn to other illicit drugs or risky sexual behaviors. Smoking increases risk for lung cancer or chronic obstructive pulmonary disease, and illicit drug use and high-risk sexuality would increase risk of hepatitis or HIV/AIDS. Reluctance to seek medical care exacerbates health problems. Alcalá, Mitchell, and Keim-Malpass (2016) found that women with a history of physical or sexual abuse were less likely to get a Pap test. Failure to obtain routine screening or medical care increases risk for cervical cancer.

One pathway to disease currently under investigation is early brain development. During childhood, the human brain is constantly developing. Environmental stresses create *downstream* consequences. De Brito et al. (2013) used MRI to compare the brains of children with and without histories of maltreatment. The maltreated children had decreased gray matter in the regions of the brain that regulate emotions, decision making, and memory. The researchers propose that physiological changes in the orbitofrontal cortex may lead to social impairment and increased risk-taking. Changes in the middle temporal gyrus may contribute to depression and PTSD. Edmiston et al. (2011) examined the effects of childhood maltreatment on limbic brain structures in adolescents with no psychiatric diagnoses. Limbic structures are involved with emotion, stress, learning, and memory. They found higher scores on a maltreatment questionnaire were negatively correlated with gray matter volumes in many brain regions, including the prefrontal cortex, striatum, amygdala, sensory association cortices, and cerebellum. Different types of abuse were associated with changes in different regions of the brain. Interestingly, females had more changes in emotional regulatory regions while males had more changes in impulse control regions. This study showed that, even in adolescents not suffering from psychiatric disorders, there are still changes that take place in the brain because of ACEs that increase risk for behavioral problems. Poletti et al. (2015) suggest that brain alterations may influence development of schizophrenia. The evidence that ACEs create physiological changes to the brain that can influence later behavior raises the question of whether such changes are irreversible. If someone is exposed to traumatic experiences during childhood, can the brain be rewired toward healthy, prosocial behaviors?

Intervention and prevention are key to overcoming ACEs. Public health professionals use selected, indicated, and universal prevention mechanisms to prevent

ACEs and to create positive coping mechanisms among people who are already living with ACEs (Black, Davis, & Dempsey, 2010). Universal prevention focuses on preventing ACEs within the general population, regardless of risk. Ways to prevent ACEs include early childhood education programs, public service announcements, parenting education, dating violence prevention programs, and job training. Selected prevention focuses on vulnerable populations and is achieved by educating health care providers and community leaders on the effects of ACEs, screening for ACEs during medical visits, and early referral to community resources. Indicated prevention focuses on controlling the negative sequelae of ACEs among individuals who are already experiencing or have experienced ACEs. Intervention includes counseling to understand and change negative behaviors. A critical aspect of indicated prevention is that individuals exposed to ACEs have unique personality characteristics that make them resistant to treatment. People with ACEs have higher rates of neuroticism, hopelessness, rumination, and loss of control than those who have not experienced ACEs. They are less resilient when faced with anxiety or depression and are more likely to have lower levels of education and income. Indicated prevention requires long-term commitment to change by the individual, family members, and caregivers.

ACEs are complex social and medical problems that significantly impact morbidity, mortality, and quality of life. By integrating ACE screening and awareness into health care practices, public health professionals are developing new ways to educate parents and communities on the impact of childhood experiences. For some adult survivors of ACEs, recognizing and validating past traumas and helping the person to draw connections between past experiences and current behaviors can be enough to help him or her move beyond the trauma. For others, counseling with long-term follow-up may be needed. Primary prevention by educating today's parents, grandparents, and community leaders on child brain development can prevent ACEs. Efforts will require larger, systematic approaches by medical professionals, counselors, policy makers, educators, criminal justice systems, and the larger community.

Sarah R. Green and Maria DiGiorgio McColgan

See also: Behavioral Health; Child Maltreatment; Intimate Partner Violence; Mental Illness; Prevention; Social Determinants of Health; *Controversies in Public Health:* Controversy 2

Further Reading

Alcalá, H. E., Mitchell, E., & Keim-Malpass, J. (2016). Adverse childhood experiences and cervical cancer screening. *Journal of Women's Health, 26*(1), 58–63.

Black, S., Davis, M. B., & Dempsey, S. H. (2010). Practitioner recommended practices for children exposed to domestic violence. *Health Promotion Practice, 11*(6), 900–907.

Centers for Disease Control and Prevention. (2016). *About the CDC-Kaiser ACE Study.* Retrieved from https://www.cdc.gov/violenceprevention/acestudy/about.html.

De Brito, S., Viding, E., Sebastian, C., Kelly, P., Mechelli, A., Maris, H., & McCrory, E. (2013). Reduced orbitofrontal and temporal grey matter in a community sample of maltreated children. *Journal of Child Psychology and Psychiatry*, *54*(1), 105–112.

Edmiston, E., Wang, F., Mazure, C., Guiney, J., Sinha, R., Mayes, L., & Blumberg, H. (2011). Corticostriatal-limbic gray matter morphology in adolescents with self-reported exposure to childhood maltreatment. *Archives of Pediatrics & Adolescent Medicine*, *165*(12), 1069–1077.

Fang, L., Chuang, D., & Lee, Y. (2016). Adverse childhood experiences, gender, and HIV risk behaviors: Results from a population-based sample. *Preventive Medicine Reports*, *4*, 113–120.

Felitti, V., Anda, R. F., Nordenberg, D., Williamson, D., Spitz, A. M., Edwards, V., Koss, M., & Marks, J. S. (1998). Relationship of childhood abuse and household dysfunction to many of the leading causes of death in adults: The Adverse Childhood Experiences (ACE) Study. *American Journal of Preventive Medicine, 14*(4), 245–258.

Huang, H., Yan, P., Shan, Z., Chen, S., Li, M., Luo, C., & . . . Liu, L. (2015). Adverse childhood experiences and risk of type 2 diabetes: A systematic review and meta-analysis. *Metabolism*, *64*, 1408–1418.

Iniguez, K. C., & Stankowski, R. V. (2016). Adverse child experiences and health in adulthood in a rural population-based sample. *Clinical Medicine & Research, 14*(3–4), 126–137.

Poletti, S., Mazza, E., Bollettini, I., Locatelli, C., Cavallaro, R., Smeraldi, E., & Benedetti, F. (2015). Adverse childhood experiences influence white matter microstructure in patients with schizophrenia. *Psychiatry Research: Neuroimaging*, *234*, 35–43.

Robert Wood Johnson Foundation. (n.d.). *Adverse childhood experiences: A collection of news, perspectives, and other resources to help raise awareness, prevent ACEs and improve resiliency.* Retrieved from http://www.rwjf.org/en/library/collections/aces.html.

Schreier, H. C., Enlow, M. B., Ritz, T., Gennings, C., & Wright, R. J. (2015). Childhood abuse is associated with increased hair cortisol levels among urban pregnant women. *Journal of Epidemiology and Community Health*, *69*(12), 1169–1174.

AFFORDABLE CARE ACT (ACA)

The Patient Protection and Affordable Care Act, often referred to only as the Affordable Care Act (ACA), was instituted on March 30, 2010, and sustained by the United States Supreme Court on June 28, 2012. The law was created to allow individuals and businesses to be the primary decision makers in their health care, enabling participants to choose a health care plan that fit within their budget while also making the insurance marketplace more competitive. Under the ACA, employers and individuals are eligible for tax credits to assist in covering the costs of their chosen health plan. The ACA expands Medicaid eligibility and streamlines the application process for the Children's Health Insurance Plan (CHIP). HHS.gov states that the ACA "gives flexibility to States to adopt innovative strategies to improve care and the coordination of services for Medicare and Medicaid beneficiaries. And it saves taxpayer money by reducing prescription drug costs and payments to subsidize care for uninsured Americans, as more Americans gain insurance under reform" (U.S. Department of Health and Human Services, 2015).

Any nation's health system is a unique product of its history, politics, and national values. Canada, for instance, has a national health insurance model whereby the government pays for health services for Canadian citizens; this is known as a single-payer model. In contrast, the United States is primarily a private health system whereby employers and employees pay the costs of private health insurance. Veterans and Native Americans are covered by Veterans Affairs and the Indian Health Service, respectively, wherein the U.S. federal government pays for these separate health care systems. Finally, citizens and permanent residents 65 years and older are covered by Medicare, and citizens and lawfully present immigrants who are financially eligible for Medicaid receive health care comparable to Canada's model. Compared to Canada, the United States has a far more complex health system because different groups in the population access health care in different ways.

Health care in the United States relies on costly, technologically advanced medicine. Yet the U.S. health system has a long history of denying access to people who are unemployed or cannot afford health insurance on their own. In 2010 it was estimated that 50 million Americans, or 16 percent of the population, did not have health insurance (U.S. Census Bureau, 2011). The past century has seen repeated efforts to expand health insurance to uninsured populations, but these efforts have been resisted by private stakeholders. Two of the most powerful groups are

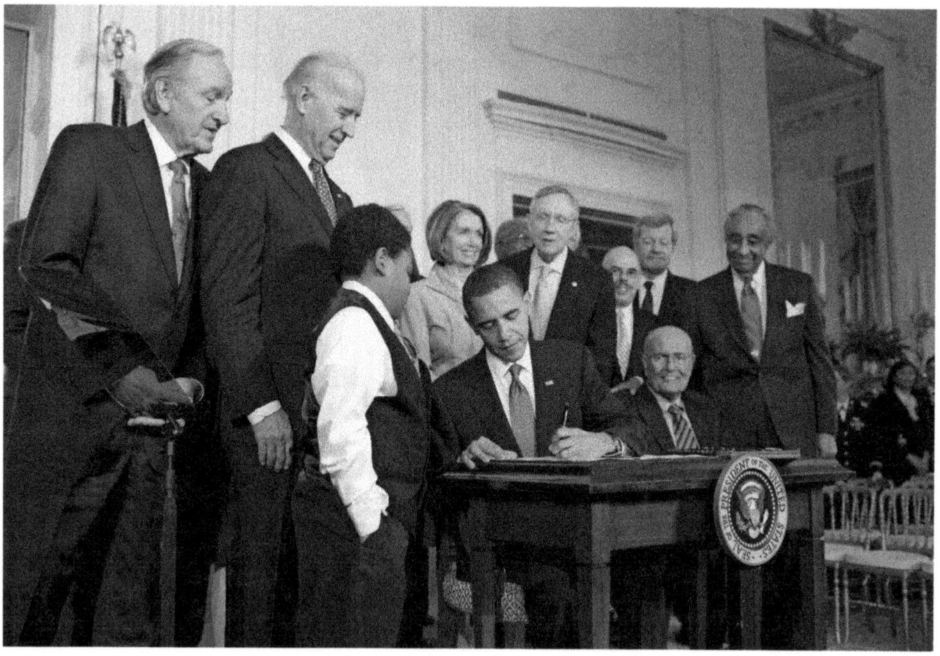

Eleven-year-old Marcelas Owens watches as President Obama signs the Patient Protection and Affordable Care Act. Marcelas's mother died when she was unable to afford medical care. The Affordable Care Act expanded access to health services for 50 million Americans. (The White House/Pete Souza)

physicians represented by the American Medical Association (AMA) and the health insurance industry. The AMA's concern has been that expanded health insurance would shift power from physicians to other groups in the health system including hospitals, the health insurance industry, and the government. The health insurance industry has been concerned universal health insurance would have a negative impact on the industry's profit margins.

Successive attempts to provide health insurance to all American citizens have failed because of "path dependence" (Starr, 1982, p. 7): the present health system is a product of historical decisions that have instituted a mode of delivery resistant to change. A century of struggle to reform health care finally succeeded, however, with the passage of the Affordable Care Act (ACA) in 2010. Cognizant of path dependence, President Barack Obama's administration carefully attended to the history of failed attempts to introduce comprehensive insurance coverage in the United States and so meticulously consulted stakeholders such as the health insurance industry and the AMA in their health policy proposals. Continued opposition to the ACA years after its passage reflects the complexity of health care reform wherein politics and historical precedent play a major role in influencing policy design.

The ACA assigns the responsibility of health care to the individual. It eliminates copays for preventive care. Individuals can now choose their preferred provider that is available within their insurance network, and women can visit their OB-GYN without preauthorization or referral. Parents have the ability to cover their dependent child until 26 years of age without exclusion of life events such as marriage or employment. An insurance carrier can no longer preclude a person or increase the cost of premiums for a person with a preexisting condition such as diabetes or HIV. Health insurance plans are required to eradicate their previously imposed lifetime and annual limits for covered nonessential services (U.S. Department of Health and Human Services, 2015). Companies are banned from increasing copays or coinsurance amounts for emergency services or canceling a policy due to an honest error made on the initial application. Plan summaries must be written in laymen's terms that are easily understood. Members can appeal their insurance decision to deny services.

Since its passage in 2010, the ACA is beginning to deliver the benefits of expanded health care coverage and lower costs. The latest estimates indicate substantial gains in enrollment after enactment of the ACA, with the number of persons uninsured having dropped to 33 million, or 10.4 percent of the population (U.S. Census Bureau, 2014). However, the United States continues to be a global outlier in health spending, with limited return on health quality or population health. U.S. health expenditures in 2011, for example, were $8,500 per person, in comparison with Canada, which spends approximately $4,000 per person on health. Despite its expenditure, the United States performs the poorest across a range of indicators of health care quality and population health in comparison with other Western countries (Davis, Stremikis, Squires, & Schoen, 2014, p. 11). The ACA has made significant improvements in broadening access to health care, yet comparisons among Western countries show that further reform is needed. The lessons from the past as well as analysis of the current political climate are important considerations in analyzing health policy reform.

Catherine van de Ruit and Leapolda Figueroa

See also: Care, Access to; Centers for Medicare and Medicaid Services; Children's Health; Health Policy; Immigrant Health; Medicaid; Medicare; Public Health Law; School Health; *Controversies in Public Health:* Controversy 5

Further Reading

Davis, K., Stremikis, K., Squires, D., & Schoen, C. (2014). *Mirror, mirror on the wall mirror: How the performance of the U.S. health care system compares internationally*. New York: The Commonwealth Fund. Retrieved from http://www.commonwealthfund.org/~/media/files/publications/fund-report/2014/jun/1755_davis_mirror_mirror_2014.pdf.

Starr, P. (1982). *The social transformation of American medicine*. New York: Basic Books.

U.S. Census Bureau. (2011). *Income poverty and health insurance coverage in the United States: 2010*. Washington, DC: U.S. Government Printing Office.

U.S. Census Bureau. (2014). *2013 and 2014 current population survey reports*. Washington, DC: U.S. Government Printing Office.

U.S. Department of Health and Human Services. (2015). Health care. *About the law: The Affordable Care Act section by section*. Retrieved from http://www.hhs.gov/healthcare/about-the-law/read-the-law/.

AGING

The many public health advancements of the 20th century allow people to live longer, healthier lives. However, more people living longer can prevent challenges for public health. Aging involves changes that occur within organisms that lead to physical maturation and an eventual reduction in the ability of the body to function. With humans, physical maturation typically stops after age 30. Subsequently, senescence, the process of growing older, occurs. Systems that allow the body to survive become increasingly vulnerable to physical breakdown and disease. This deterioration eventually results in death. Though biological changes are the most visible signs of senescence, aging also involves psychological and sociological aspects. As the baby-boomer population ages, senior citizens may quickly outnumber younger people. This demographic shift presents unique challenges. If the elderly, who often suffer from chronic diseases or disabilities at greater rates than others in the general population, require more health care and social services than the workforce can provide, the nation will face a crisis in health care services. Public health offers one mechanism for filling the disconnect between supply and demand. Invested development of public health systems, such as home health care and visiting nurses, can enable the elderly to remain in their homes and to actively contribute to society. Promoting health throughout the life span and supporting people as they age supports healthy, diverse communities. Senior citizens have much to offer youth. Daily or regular interaction and communication between different generations allows for healthy discourse. Exposing youth to the elders of the society ensures that cultural traditions and values, the roots of the community, are carried on into future generations.

No single theory explains biological aging. A variety of theories exist that attempt to clarify the process. The *wear and tear* perspective implies that the body breaks down as a result of use. Every species has a predetermined life span, or maximum age of survival. Depending on how the body is used, the body will simply wear out while moving toward the end of life. With more specificity, *cellular aging theory* argues that cells, the smallest structural unit of an organism, replicate slower as an organism moves toward death. Some cells in parts of the body only have a finite number of replications. Consider T cells, which aid in the ability of the immune system to fight disease. These cells lose their capacity to reproduce, and this reduces the ability of the human body to combat illnesses in later life. Some cells do not replicate at all. This includes certain nerve, brain, and muscle cells. After maturation, any irregularities in these areas are irreversible and permanent, though certain surgical interventions may create functionality in some cases. *Telomere theory* states that every time a cell divides, structures called telomeres at the end of DNA, shorten. Telomeres can act as a biomarker for health status. Elderly individuals with shorter telomeres have higher rates of cirrhosis of the liver and colon cancer. Analogous to the rusting process in metals, *free radical theory* implies oxidative stress creates aging. Atoms and molecules typically have paired electrons. After exposure to oxygen through metabolic processes, damage occurs within cells and some end up with free radicals. These are atoms or molecules with unpaired electrons that represent oxidative damage. The accumulation of oxidative damage throughout life triggers age-related biological decline. No one theory describes all aspects of aging. Combined, the theories provide some explanation and understanding of the biological aging process.

Advancements in medical technology and public health have significantly increased average life span. As a greater number of people enter and experience aging, techniques used to manage the aging process become more popular. Though the success of such initiatives is limited, more people than ever are trying these different therapies. Enzyme therapy has the potential to lengthen telomeres, but side effects related to genetic mutations create tumors and currently limit widespread use. Free radical therapy involves the implementation of antioxidants. Antioxidants are compounds that donate electrons to free radicals and create balance within a cell. Though synthetic antioxidants exist, there are high levels of antioxidants in natural food sources such as legumes, fruits, and vegetables, with the highest presence in beans, berries, apples, and artichokes. Caloric restriction, predominantly through the reduction of fat and carbohydrates, is another technique used to counter aging. Extreme variations focus on limiting all calories and encourage a perpetual feeling of hunger for successful anti-aging results. Growth hormone therapy is another procedure. One of the most common substances related to this is dehydroepiandrosterone (DHEA). The brain and adrenal glands produce DHEA. The body then converts it to estrogen and testosterone. DHEA is the most abundant steroid in the human body. Its production peaks in early adulthood and declines significantly afterward. Older adults can take DHEA orally or through injections. The treatment is effective in increasing skin thickness, but has limited impact in areas such as brain functioning. Human growth hormone (HGH) treatments are also available. HGH successfully improves muscle mass and bone density. Adverse effects occur with prolonged use including joint pain and an elevated risk of diabetes.

Psychological aging involves both cognitive and personality changes. With cognition, normal aging results in a natural decline in some aspects of intelligence and memory. The two primary forms of intelligence are fluid and crystallized (Horn & Cattell, 1966). Fluid intelligence concerns biologically related aptitude, independent of personal experience. Commonly referred to as street smarts, fluid intelligence is the ability to recognize and solve problems using natural intuition. Crystallized intelligence involves the abilities and knowledge a person develops throughout life, including book smarts. In the classic aging pattern, fluid intelligence declines as crystallized intelligence becomes stronger. Elderly people do worse on performance-based tests related to fluid intelligence. This may be because many tests have time limits. The aged person, with slower reaction times related to age-related neurological declines, has the right answers, but cannot respond fast enough. Timed tests also elevate the anxiety, interfering with the tests. Tests on spatial orientation and reasoning also show a lower performance, regardless of time limits. Intelligence in the aged person is related to educational attainment, occupational experiences, reaction times, hearing, and vision.

As the brain ages, significant changes occur in working and long-term memory. Working memory, referred to as short-term or primary memory, declines with age. The decline is especially prevalent if an older person attempts to manage multiple pieces of information at the same time. Decreased attention spans that occur in aging challenge the brain's ability to navigate complex tasks or systems. Aside from memory linked to verbal knowledge and performance memory related to carrying out specific tasks, long-term memory is worsened for the aged. Accurately recalling information from a distant time is difficult, unless the event had a significant impact on the person. There are a number of techniques that older adults can use to improve, sustain, or trigger memory. Mediators, such as acronyms, help with information recall. For example, the American Cancer Society used the acronym CAUTION to remind people of the warning signs of various forms of cancer. CAUTION stands for "Change in bowel or bladder habits; A sore that does not heal; Unusual bleeding or discharge; Thickening or lump in the breast, testicles, or elsewhere; Indigestion or difficulty swallowing; Obvious change in size, color, or shape of a wart, mole, or mouth sore; and Nagging cough or hoarseness." Other external memory aids, such as written lists, are also helpful in maintaining adequate psychological functionality for activities of daily living.

Stage theories propose that as people age, they move through different psychological phases. These stages may be displayed through personality and actions. For example, compared to younger people, the elderly are more likely to have a greater sense of purpose, as well as a greater sense of self. Elders may say or do things that they did not have the confidence to say or do when they were younger. When used to improve families, communities, and society, this increased sense of self can create many positive results. However, patterns of interaction and cognitive impairments may also be exhibited as negative personality traits. Life disruptions such as divorce, death of a spouse, retirement, physical disability, or dementia may trigger feelings of grief, remorse, sorrow, or depression. The resulting stress of these life events not only impacts psychological well-being but also produces physical changes. Telomere length is shortened lowering life expectancy—the statistical measure of how long a person will live given his or her year of birth.

Sociological aging relates to the impact of social networks, institutions, and culture on the elderly. In many societies, the elderly maintain traditions and pass important cultural values to the next generation. *Continuity theory* argues that the more a person can maintain former roles through the aging process, the more positive the aging experience will be. This could include family caregiving, part-time paid positions, or volunteer work. *Activity theory* implies sustaining social ties through any form of interaction, new roles or old, leads to higher levels of life satisfaction. Active social involvement can stabilize or elevate self-esteem as a person ages. Maintaining positive support networks helps to counteract some of the negative emotional effects of aging. It can be difficult to maintain those networks when, for example, employers push for premature retirements. *Disengagement theory* implies that some cultures devalue the elderly. Institutional living drives senior citizens away from valued social networks. This isolation hinders successful aging. Areas known as *blue zones* exist throughout the world. Specific areas of Italy, Greece, Japan, and Costa Rica have relatively high numbers of centenarians, people 100 and older. Researchers identified similarities in cultural behavior patterns and found commonalities in types of food eaten (semi-vegetarian), physical activity, and social integration (Buettner, 2010). Aging is influenced by biological and psychological dynamics on top of sociocultural foundations. The ethical dimensions related to encouraging or discouraging behaviors known to increase positive aging and prolong life are currently being explored by public health professionals and researchers.

Aging is and will continue to be an important issue for years to come. An increased understanding of the principles of biological, psychological, and sociological aging is critical to promoting quality of life throughout the life span. With the baby-boomer generation's ongoing shift into old age, more adults will provide care for aged loved ones and more health care workers will be dedicated to elder care. These caregivers will need knowledge of best practices in elder care for those they care for and to navigate their own aging processes.

Jason S. Ulsperger

See also: Affordable Care Act; Alzheimer's Disease; Chronic Illness; Community Health; Disability; Elder Maltreatment; Medicaid; Men's Health; Motor Vehicle Safety; Prevention; Social Security Act; Women's Health

Further Reading

Bensadon, B. A. (2015). *Psychology and geriatrics: Integrated care for an aging population*. London: Academic Press.

Buettner, D. (2010). *The blue zones: Lessons for living longer from the people who've lived the longest*. Washington, DC: National Geographic.

Calado, R. T. (2014). *Telomeres in health and disease*. Waltham, MA: Academic Press.

Horn, J. L., & Cattell, R. B. (1966). Refinement and test of the theory of fluid and crystallized general intelligences. *Journal of Educational Psychology, 57*, 253–270.

Epel, E. S., Blackburn, E. H., Lin, J., Dhabhar, F. S., Adler, N. E., Morrow, J. D., & Cawthon, R. M. (2004). Accelerated telomere shortening in response to life stress. *Proceedings of the National Academy of Sciences, 101*, 17312–17315.

Hooyman, N., & Asuman Kiyak, H. (2014). *Social gerontology: A multidisciplinary perspective*. Harlow, Essex: Pearson.

McDonald, R. B. (2014). *Biology of aging*. New York: Garland Science.

Merrill, G. F. (2015). *Our aging bodies*. New Brunswick, NJ: Rutgers University Press.

Verhaeghen, P. (2014). *The elements of cognitive aging: Meta-analyses of age-related differences in processing speed and their consequences*. New York: Oxford University Press.

AGRICULTURAL SAFETY

Farming, ranching, and agricultural management are among the most dangerous jobs in the nation. Agricultural workers die at a rate of 24.7 per 100,000 full-time equivalent (FTE) workers, almost double the rate of police deaths, 13.5 per 100,000 FTE workers (U.S. Bureau of Labor Statistics, 2016). Farm laborers are vulnerable to injuries through handling large, dangerous machinery, falls, extreme heat and cold, heavy lifting and repetitive forceful body motions as well as working in unsanitary conditions where they are exposed to pesticides, harsh chemicals, air contaminants, zoonotic infections, and loud noises. The nature of farm work is difficult, grueling work, which puts great physical strain on the body. The digging, cutting, chopping, and grinding necessary to grow the nation's food is performed using sharp, powerful tools and machinery. Because many farms are family operated, children frequently participate in dangerous tasks. Consider that when a farmer plows the fields, it seems easier and more efficient to put young children on the back of a tractor rather than driving 20 miles to drop the child off at the local day care center. Farm-associated injuries among youth cost an estimated $1 billion annually (Zaloshnja, Miller, & Lee, 2011). Public health's goal is to reduce work-related deaths among farmers, fishers, and hunters by 10 percent over 10 years (Office of Disease Prevention and Health Promotion, 2016). The U.S. Department of Labor, National Institute for Occupational Safety and Health (NIOSH), and Centers for Disease Control and Prevention (CDC) offer multiple initiatives, training programs, grants, and publications to gather information on the dangers of farming and implement programs and policies to reduce agriculture-related injuries, diseases, and deaths. The National Children's Center for Rural Agricultural Health and Safety established guidelines encouraging parents to match farm chores with children's age and developmental abilities. To date, efforts indicate some signs of success. NIOSH reports a 56 percent reduction in farm-related injury rates among youth between 1998 and 2009 (Ten Great Public Health Achievements—United States, 2001–2010, 2011). However, the nature of agricultural workers as independent contractors, many of whom are poor, migrant workers, and the values of farmers as autonomous agents, operating free from bureaucratic oversight, presents obstacles in creating safe workplaces for workers, farm managers, and farm families.

The health of agricultural workers lags behind other industries. Early efforts to protect the U.S. workforce focused on miners, railroad workers, and steelworkers. As independent self-employed workers, agricultural workers were not part of organized labor unions advocating for safe working conditions. In the United States, farm safety traces back to the First Cooperative Safety Congress in Milwaukee, Wisconsin (1912). The Safety Congress evolved into the National Safety Council (1913) and over time, a network of farm safety specialists evolved. In 1937, the National Safety Council formally addressed the problem by creating a national plan for farm safety. Today, the National Safety Council, U.S. Department of Agriculture (USDA), state extension services, the 4H chapters, Future Farmers of America (FFA), and Bureau of Labor Standards create a network promoting agricultural worker safety.

Approximately half of all farm fatalities are the result of injury by motor vehicle. Although no national data were collected on farm injuries prior to the invention of the tractor, early safety experts claimed that the transition from horsepower to gas-powered vehicles greatly increased the number and severity of injuries. A survey of more than 6,000 farms in Kentucky found that 1 out of 10 farms experience a tractor rollover and operators without rollover protective structures (ROPs) lose an average of 98 workdays during recovery while operators with ROPs and seatbelts lose an average of 22 workdays (Cole, Myers, & Westneat, 2006). Other vehicular hazards are getting loose clothing or hair caught in an operating machine, damaged or missing protective shields, carbon monoxide poisoning, sudden and unanticipated changes in vehicular balance due to towed harvesting equipment, and all-terrain vehicles. To prevent injuries, OSHA recommends using approved safety equipment, following the manufacturer's recommendations regarding use and safety, shutting off the engine and removing keys from the ignition when the vehicle is not in use, and storing fuel in a separate location from the equipment.

While working in the summer and winter, agricultural workers are exposed to extremes in heat and cold. Prolonged exposure to heat can result in heat exhaustion, heat cramps, heat stroke, and death. As the body attempts to cool itself through sweating, water and salt are excreted. Initially, the person may experience symptoms of dehydration, thirst, irritability, dizziness, or confusion. Excessive sweating can lead to severe fluid and electrolyte imbalances with fainting, seizures, muscle spasms, or death. Individuals with underlying health conditions of diabetes or alcoholism and the young or old are at highest risk for heat-related illnesses. OSHA recommends knowing the signs of heat-related illnesses, drinking water every 15 minutes regardless of thirst, wearing light clothing for protection from the sun, resting in the shade, and using a buddy system to monitor the health of coworkers.

The rate of falls among agricultural workers (48.2 per 100,000 workers) is higher than other hazardous industries (OSHA, n.d.). Falls occur while working on slippery or unstable surfaces, at high elevations, or near unprotected shafts or manure pits. Incidents can be prevented by identifying risky situations in advance, eliminating the risk, installing fall prevention devices, and using safety nets, catch platforms, or safety harnesses. Falls into silos or grain bins are a concern. Filling the grain bin is a particularly high-risk agricultural task. The farmer loads grain through high speed conveyors at the top of the silo and an auger pulls the grain from the bottom. Many things can go wrong. The shafts can become blocked; pockets of air or bridges of forage can form within the silo or methane gas buildup, resulting in fire or asphyxiation. If the worker enters the grain bin while the auger is operating, the grain acts like quicksand. The person can be trapped within 4 to 5 seconds, pulled under the pile of grain and suffocate within 22 seconds. An operator should never enter the storage bin to clear or check the grain flow. OSHA provides specific safety and health information on grain handling.

The physical labor of farming requires lifting, bending, twisting, and kneeling. Forceful and repetitive motions cause work-related backache or pain in the shoulders, arms, or hands. In California, the annual cost of farm workers' compensation for back injuries is estimated at $22 million (Baron, Estill, Steege, & Lalich, 2001). Although technology can decrease some bodily strain, the task of handling heavy vibrating machinery or poorly designed tools can create other ergonomic problems. The Centers for Disease Control and Prevention and NIOSH offer *Simple Solutions* to reduce work-related musculoskeletal disorders recommending inexpensive tools and collaborations between management and workers to improve work processes (Baron, Estill, Steege, & Lalich, 2001).

Tractor rollovers, heat stroke, falls, dangerous gases, zoonotic infections, and musculoskeletal disorders create a hazardous environment for the millions of agricultural workers who grow and harvest the food that we eat. Despite the slow progression of health and safety measures on farms, many groups are now working to address the health and safety of farm workers. Partnering with community-based groups, federal, state, and local organizations balance sharing best practices in farm safety with the autonomous nature of farming.

Sally Kuykendall

See also: Health Resources and Services Administration; Rural Health; U.S. Department of Agriculture; State, Local, and Territorial Health Departments

Further Reading

Baron, S., Estill, C.F., Steege, A., & Lalich, N. (2001). *Simple solutions: Ergonomics for farm workers.* U.S. Department of Health and Human Services, Public Health Service, Centers for Disease Control and Prevention, National Institute for Occupational Safety and Health. Retrieved from https://www.cdc.gov/niosh/docs/2007-122/.

Cole, H. P., Myers, M. L., & Westneat, S. C. (2006). Frequency and severity of injuries to operators during overturns of farm tractors. *Journal of Agricultural Safety and Health, 12*(2), 127–138.

International Society for Agricultural Safety and Health. (n.d.). Retrieved from https://isash.org/.

National Institute for Occupational Safety and Health Division of Safety Research. (2014). *Agricultural safety.* Retrieved from https://www.cdc.gov/niosh/topics/aginjury/.

Occupational Safety and Health Administration (OSHA). (n.d.). *Agricultural operations.* U.S. Department of Labor. Retrieved from https://www.osha.gov/dsg/topics/agriculturaloperations/.

Office of Disease Prevention and Health Promotion. (2016). *Healthy people 2020.* Retrieved from https://www.healthypeople.gov/2020/topics-objectives/objective/osh-15.

Ten Great Public Health Achievements—United States, 2001–2010. (2011). *Morbidity and Mortality Weekly Report, 60(19)*, 619.

U.S. Bureau of Labor Statistics. (2016). Current Population Survey, Census of Fatal Occupational Injuries. Retrieved from http://www.bls.gov/iif/oshwc/cfoi/cfoi_rates_2014hb.pdf.

Zaloshnja, E., Miller, T., & Lee, B. (2011). Incidence and cost of nonfatal farm youth injury, United States, 2001–2006. *Journal of Agromedicine, 16*(1), 6–18.

AIR POLLUTION

Air pollution is "a mixture of natural and man-made substances in the air we breathe" (National Institute of Environmental Health Sciences, 2017). Outdoor air pollution consists of noxious gases, ozone, and fine particles released by burning fossil fuels. Indoor air pollution consists of noxious gases, household products, building materials, tobacco smoke, allergens, mold, and pollen. The direct health effects of air pollution are asthma, birth defects, cancer, carbon monoxide poisoning, developmental disabilities, heart disease, heat stress, and reproductive problems. Some of the same human activities that create air pollution warm the air creating climate change. Global warming raises air temperature and impacts water temperature, air quality, plant growth, and pathogens. Diseases related to global warming such as asthma, malaria, and malnutrition are on the rise. Public health professionals attempt to reduce the health hazards caused by air pollution by monitoring the environment and environmental health, responding to weather-related disasters, and educating the public on ways to reduce detrimental impact on the environment. Environmental health scientists monitor and report Air Quality Index (AQI) to assist individuals and communities in reducing harmful daily exposure.

The idea that our environment influences health traces back to the fourth century BC when Hippocrates countered the belief that illnesses were punishment from the

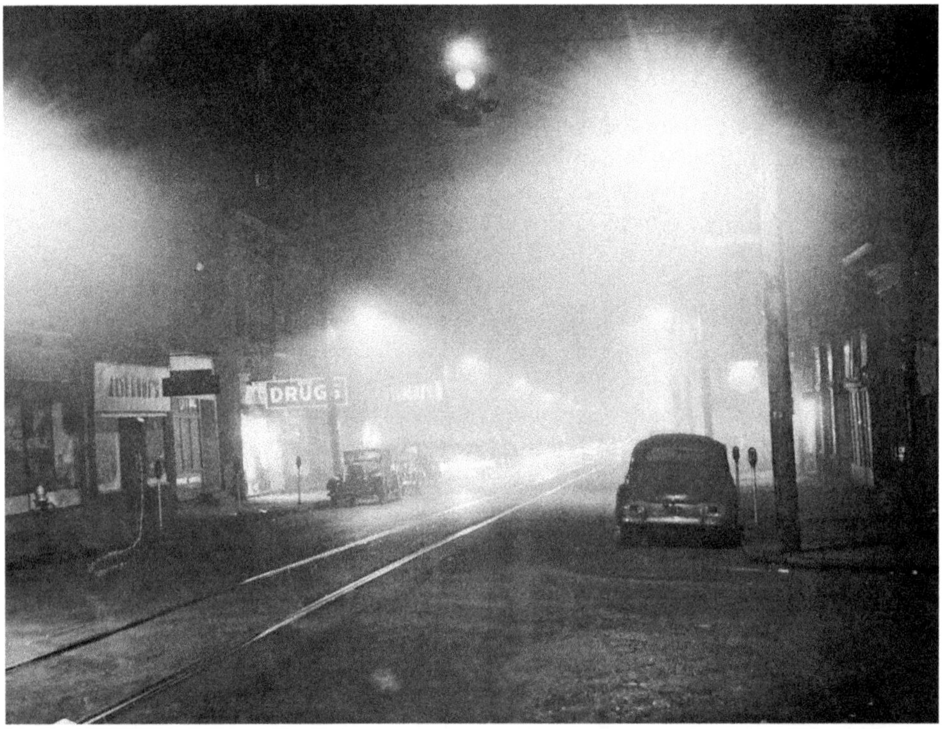

Noon in the steel mill town of Donora, Pennsylvania, on October 29, 1948. As thick, corrosive air pollution hung over the valley of the Monongahela River, residents struggled to breathe. (Bettmann/Getty Images)

gods and encouraged physicians to examine the patient's diet, personal behaviors, and environment. In the United States, official recognition of air pollution as a health hazard started with the Donora smog incident of 1948. Donora was a booming mill town toiling to meet the nation's post–World War II demand for steel and zinc products. Located in a valley on the Monongahela River, residents were accustomed to morning fog. On October 26, smoke from the mills combined with thick fog to form smog. The smog contained particulate pollution, ozone, and sulfuric acid. Initially, residents went about their daily business, expecting the smog to lift. However, a temperature inversion acted like a cap over the valley, holding the yellow, acrid smog in place. An estimated 5,000 to 7,000 workers and residents struggled to breathe through the corrosive air. Four hundred people were hospitalized and 20 people died. Local doctors warned those who could get out of town to leave. Although the mill owners did not believe the mills were the problem, they slowed down production as a safeguard. On October 31, the toxic fumes dissipated as a cold front moved in and rain cleaned the air. The Donora incident was investigated by the Pennsylvania Department of Health, United Steelworkers, Donora Borough Council, and the Division of Industrial Hygiene of the Public Health Service, and Donora became the first official investigation of air pollution in the United States.

In 1955, Congress passed the Air Pollution Control Act supporting research and prevention. The act was followed by the Clean Air Acts of 1963, 1970, and 1990.

Physiologically, the body needs oxygen to convert carbohydrates and fats into energy in order to fuel body functions. Oxygen enters the body via the nasotracheal pathways, travels through the bronchi and bronchioles, and into the microscopic alveoli where oxygen is exchanged with carbon dioxide from the blood. Air pollution damages the body in two ways, either by irritating sensitive respiratory tissue or by functioning as an inhaled poison. Smoking and pollutants irritate the airways causing inflammation, spasms, and shortness of breath. The irritation and bronchospasms make it difficult for the person to inhale oxygen and to exhale carbon dioxide resulting in classic symptoms of coughing, wheezing, and difficulty breathing. Continued exposure to pollutants hardens or scars the respiratory tissue, permanently reducing the body's ability to exchange gases. Diseases associated with continued exposure are chronic obstructive pulmonary disease (COPD), emphysema, chronic bronchitis, asthma, lung cancer, and pneumonitis. Toxic air pollutants act as poisons, introduced into the body through the lungs. Air toxics include benzene (found in gasoline), perchloroethylene (emitted by dry cleaning), methylene chloride (a solvent and paint stripper), asbestos, toluene, cadmium mercury, chromium, and lead. Exposure to air toxics can cause cancer, reproductive problems, and birth defects. Air pollution is an insidious killer. In many cases, disease, symptoms, and death may not occur for a decade after exposure or may be disguised as other health problems. The World Health Organization (2014) estimates 7 million premature deaths each year due to air pollution and identifies the most common air pollution–related diseases as ischemic heart disease, stroke, COPD, lower respiratory infections in children, and lung cancer. Researchers at Massachusetts Institute of Technology (MIT) estimate that combustion emissions account for 200,000 premature deaths per year in the United States and changes in ozone account for 10,000 deaths. The highest numbers of deaths are related to black carbon emissions from road transportation and sulfur dioxide emissions from power generation (Caiazzo, Ashok, Waitz, Yim, & Barrett, 2013).

Ozone (O_3) is a powerful oxidizing agent found in two layers of the earth's atmosphere. In the upper atmosphere, ozone creates a protective layer, screening people, animals, and plants from the sun's damaging ultraviolet rays. At the ground level, ozone forms when vehicle exhaust and by-products from manufacturing interact with sunlight. The oxidizing agent irritates the respiratory system and causes coughing, pain on inhalation, wheezing, and difficulty breathing. People with preexisting respiratory problems, older adults, babies, children, and people who work outside are particularly vulnerable to high ozone levels. In addition to the problem of ground level ozone, burning fossil fuels and other human activities increase the buildup of carbon dioxide, methane, and other gases. This process warms the environment and upsets the balance of nature. Climate change increases the frequency and severity of heat waves, floods, and other extreme weather events; expands the geographic regions of disease-carrying vectors (mosquitos and ticks); lengthens the seasons for mold, plant allergen, and pollen growth; and raises sea levels contaminating water and food supplies. All of these problems increase public demand for health care, stressing current health care systems. Additionally, the loss of property, loved ones, and community caused by flooding, drought, or wildfires causes trauma that impacts mental health.

Public health addresses air pollution and climate change through macro-, meso-, and micro-level interventions. Macro-level interventions are laws, regulations, and policies designed to achieve large-scale changes. The U.S. Environmental Protection Agency (EPA) guides national efforts to reduce environmental risks, establishes environmental policy, works to protect the home, work, school and community environments, and works with other countries to protect the environment. The National Institute of Environmental Health Sciences (NIEHS) works to increase public awareness of how the environment influences health and supports environmental health research. The American Lung Association educates, advocates, and supports research to prevent lung disease and assists people affected by lung disease. The Air Pollution and Respiratory Health Branch (APRHB) of the Centers for Disease Control and Prevention performs surveillance, implements evidence-based programs, and supports partnerships to prevent and reduce environmental-related respiratory illnesses. AirNow is a group of federal, tribal, state, and local agencies that provide the public with real-time air quality data. The Air Quality Index (AQI) is a composite measure of ground-level ozone, particle pollution, carbon monoxide, sulfur dioxide, and nitrogen dioxide. AQI ranks the quality of air locally on a scale of 0 to 500 where 0 to 50 is good quality air and 301 to 500 is hazardous. People with existing lung conditions or those vulnerable to air pollution are advised to monitor air quality when planning outdoor activities and avoid hazardous conditions.

Meso-level interventions are organizational level changes. In anticipation of the 1996 summer Olympics, the city of Atlanta converted public transportation vehicles from diesel to natural gas. As a result, acute asthma attacks decreased 44 percent and peak ozone concentrations decreased 28 percent (Friedman, Powell, Hutwagner, Graham, & Teague, 2001). Micro-level interventions are designed to impact individual or community-level changes. Individuals can reduce their exposure and generation of air pollution by following these recommendations:

- Don't smoke or allow others to smoke in your home or workplace.
- Check air quality daily and plan outdoor activities based on personal health status. Avoid outdoor exercise when air quality is poor, and avoid exercising near heavy traffic.
- Reduce home energy use by turning off unused lights and electronics, use shades and blinds to heat or cool your home, naturally, adjust the thermostat, and buy electronics with the energy star label.
- Use environmentally safe paints and cleaning products.
- Opt for clean forms of transportation—walk, bicycle, carpool, public transportation, ride share, or drive a green vehicle.

- Reduce trips by planning shopping routes and combining errands.
- Refuel vehicles according to instructions and refuel after dusk to reduce emissions.
- Don't burn leaves, firewood, or trash.
- Use hand-powered or electric yard tools.

Small, step-wise changes can make an enormous difference to the environment and population health.

Air pollution is an environmental issue that impacts public health directly and indirectly. Although children and those with impaired respiratory systems are at highest risk, the effects of global warming with severe weather events, elevated sea levels, increased humidity, and drought affect everyone throughout the world. It is imperative that individuals and communities recognize and reduce human activities that impact the environment. Government agencies designed to protect the environment and public health provide numerous, science-based resources and suggestions to understanding and alleviating this complex problem.

Sally Kuykendall

See also: Behavioral Health; Cancer; Centers for Disease Control and Prevention; Environmental Health; Environmental Protection Agency; Global Health; Healthy Places; Maternal Health; Motor Vehicle Safety; Physical Activity; World Health Organization

Further Reading

AirNow. (2017). Retrieved from https://airnow.gov/index.cfm?action=airnow.main.

American Lung Association. (2017). *10 Tips to protect yourself from unhealthy air.* Retrieved from http://www.lung.org/our-initiatives/healthy-air/outdoor/air-pollution/10-tips-to-protect-yourself.html.

Caiazzo, F., Ashok, A., Waitz, I. A., Yim, S. H., & Barrett, S. R. (2013). Air pollution and early deaths in the United States. Part I: Quantifying the impact of major sectors in 2005. *Atmospheric Environment, 79,* 198–208. doi:10.1016/j.atmosenv.2013.05.081

Davis, D. L. (2002). *When smoke ran like water: Tales of environmental deception and the battle against pollution.* New York: Basic Books.

Friedman, M., Powell, K., Hutwagner, L., Graham, L., & Teague, W. (2001). Impact of changes in transportation and commuting behaviors during the 1996 Summer Olympic Games in Atlanta on air quality and childhood asthma. *Journal of the American Medical Association, 285*(7), 897–905.

Helfand, W. H., Lazarus, J., & Theerman, P. (2001). Donora, Pennsylvania: An environmental disaster of the 20th century. *American Journal of Public Health, 91*(4), 553.

National Institute of Environmental Health Sciences. (2017). *Air pollution.* Retrieved from https://www.niehs.nih.gov/health/topics/agents/air-pollution/index.cfm.

U.S. Environmental Protection Agency. Retrieved from https://www.epa.gov/.

U.S. Global Change Research Program. (2016). *The impacts of climate change on human health in the United States: A scientific assessment.* A. Crimmins, J. Balbus, J. L. Gamble, C. B. Beard, J. E. Bell, D. Dodgen, R. J. Eisen, N. Fann, M. D. Hawkins, S. C. Herring,

L. Jantarasami, D. M. Mills, S. Saha, M. C. Sarofim, J. Trtanj, & L. Ziska (Eds.). U.S. Global Change Research Program, Washington, DC, 312 pp. Retrieved from https://health2016.globalchange.gov/.

World Health Organization. (2014). *7 Million premature deaths annually linked to air pollution.* Retrieved from http://www.who.int/mediacentre/news/releases/2014/air-pollution/en/.

ALCOHOL

The consumption of alcoholic beverages and its consequences are of urgent concern to public health. In the United States, alcohol is the third leading preventable cause of death, causing the premature death of thousands of people as well as causing illness and injury. The field of public health seeks to understand alcohol use as well as to curb its negative health impacts, in contrast to its very different picture in popular culture.

Alcohol's role in global public health is summarized in the following key facts (WHO, 2014):

- Worldwide, 3.3 million people die every year due to harmful use of alcohol, which represents 5.9 percent of all deaths.
- The harmful use of alcohol is a causal factor in more than 200 disease and injury conditions.
- Overall 5.1 percent of the global burden of disease and injury is attributable to alcohol.
- Alcohol consumption causes death and disability relatively early in life. In the age group 20 to 39 years approximately 25 percent of the total deaths are attributed to alcohol.

In 2013 in the United States, roughly half (52.2 percent) of those 12 years old or greater are drinkers of alcohol, according to the National Survey on Drug Use and Health. Nearly one-fourth (22.9 percent) of those 12 and older were binge drinkers (sometimes called heavy episodic drinkers). Binge drinking is usually defined for females as consuming four or more drinks in a row, and for males as consuming five or more drinks, at least once in 30 days. Rates of current drinking among youth aged 18 to 25 are 11.6 percent in 2013, with 6.2 percent of youth binge drinking.

Harm to individual health from alcohol use includes its role as a human carcinogen (a cause of cancer). A substantial portion of liver cancer; cancers of the throat, mouth, and esophagus; and breast cancer in women are attributable to alcohol use. Many instances of liver cirrhosis are attributable to alcohol. Alcohol use by pregnant women poses a risk to the healthy development of the fetus. Many cases of heart disease and hemorrhagic stroke are alcohol-attributable, though alcohol in modest or small amounts is protective of heart disease and stroke. A pattern of binge or heavy episodic drinking appears to carry increased risk for some cardiovascular problems such as stroke and sudden cardiac death. Alcohol intoxication plays a significant role in unintentional injury, including motor vehicle accidents, falls, drownings, and poisonings. As for intentional injuries, homicides, suicides, and self-inflicted injuries are linked to alcohol use. Alcohol is often a primary component of sexual assault and rape.

A major public health issue is driving a car under the influence of alcohol. In 2013, 1 in 10 Americans 12 or older drove under the influence, with the highest rates among those in their twenties. Traffic accidents remain the single greatest cause of death for young Americans. But the minimum drinking age of 21, along with other reforms such as random breath testing and increased drunk driving penalties, has led to a substantial drop in the death rate in this area.

Of particular concern for individual health is establishing whether an individual has a continuing problem with alcohol. Earlier concepts such as alcoholism and alcohol abuse and dependence have given way to the phrase "alcohol use disorder" or AUD. An AUD is defined by the presence in an individual of at least two symptoms such as unsuccessful efforts to cut down use, craving, use despite problems, hazardous use, and tolerance. The AUD is classified as either mild (with two to three symptoms), moderate (with four to five), or severe (with six or more symptoms). Using these criteria, roughly 7.2 percent of Americans between the ages of 18 and older had an AUD in 2012 (9.9 percent of men and 4.6 percent of women). But only 8.4 percent of adults with an AUD received treatment. Of youth aged 12 to 17, 3.4 percent had an AUD, with only 8.9 percent of them receiving treatment.

Treatment for alcohol use disorders can range from inpatient care using pharmaceuticals to many varieties of outpatient care, including psychotherapy and group treatment. Many millions of problem drinkers have found that participation in Alcoholics Anonymous and its 12-step program is helpful in seeking sobriety.

The U.S. Community Preventive Services Task Force suggests the following strategies to reduce the harmful effects of alcohol: regulating of the density of alcohol outlets, dram shop liability (making those who sell alcohol liable for serving intoxicated patrons), increasing taxes on alcohol, monitoring the days and hours of the sale of alcohol, electronic screening and brief interventions, and enhancing the enforcement of laws that prohibit sales to minors.

There is a large gap between the costs of excessive alcohol consumption to society and how much revenue alcohol taxes generate. In 2006, excessive drinking cost an estimated $224 billion dollars or $1.90 per alcoholic drink (Bouchery, Harwood, Sacks, Simon, & Brewer, 2011). Binge drinking cost an estimated $171 billion, underage drinking cost an estimated $25 billion, and drinking during pregnancy cost an estimated $5 billion. The estimated costs are calculated by examining the major social factors impacted by alcohol use and abuse. When someone drinks alcohol, this may have implications on work productivity, health status, or legal ramifications. In the workplace, excessive alcohol can lead to illnesses, disability, premature death, or absenteeism related to addiction treatment, alcohol-related diseases, court appearances, or incarceration. Health care costs increase for those who drink because alcohol is a toxin that damages the heart, brain, liver, and other gastrointestinal organs. Alcohol impairs decision making, which increases risk of motor vehicle crashes, sexually transmitted diseases, and intentional and unintentional injuries. Drinking during pregnancy can lead to fetal alcohol syndrome (FAS), spontaneous abortion, prematurity, and low birth weight. Alcohol is a major factor behind many crimes. In 2006, criminal justice expenses related to alcohol were estimated at $73 billion (Bouchery et al., 2011). Criminal justice costs result from property damage, medical care, policing, court costs, incarceration, and lost productivity. Overall, alcohol costs an average to $746 per person in the United States. Although everyone bears the cost of excessive drinking, the federal, state, and local governments bear the largest cost, paying $94 billion or 80 cents per alcoholic drink. In comparison, federal and state taxes amount to only 14 cents per drink, leaving a gap between tax and cost.

In summary, harmful alcohol use poses a major challenge to public health, but public health, in spite of financial and cultural challenges, has made considerable advances in understanding alcohol and in creating responses that can limit its harm.

George W. Dowdall

See also: Addictions; Adverse Childhood Experiences; Behavioral Health; Birth Defects; Cancer; Heart Disease; Hepatitis; Infant Mortality; Injuries; Leading Health Indicators; Men's Health; Mental Health; Mental Illness; Motor Vehicle Safety; National Institute on Drug Abuse; National Institutes of Health; Prevention; Public Health in the United States, History of; Substance Abuse and Mental Health Services Administration; Violence; *Controversies in Public Health:* Controversy 2

Further Reading

Bouchery, E. E., Harwood, H. J., Sacks, J. J., Simon, C. J., & Brewer, R. D. (2011). Economic costs of excessive alcohol consumption in the U.S., 2006. *American Journal of Preventive Medicine*, *41*(5), 516–524.

Bouchery, E. E., Harwood, H. J., Sacks, J. J., Simon, C. J., & Brewer, R. D. (2013). Correction: Economic costs of excessive alcohol consumption in the U.S., 2006. *American Journal of Preventive Medicine*, *44*(2), 198.

Naimi, T. S. (2011). The cost of alcohol and its corresponding taxes in the US: A massive public subsidy of excessive drinking and alcohol industries. *American Journal of Preventive Medicine*, *41*, 546–547.

National Institute on Alcohol Abuse and Alcoholism. (2013). *Alcohol use disorder: A comparison between DSM-IV and DSM-5.* Bethesda, MD: National Institute on Alcohol Abuse and Alcoholism.

National Institute on Alcohol Abuse and Alcoholism. (2014). *Alcohol facts and statistics.* Retrieved from http://pubs.niaaa.nih.gov/publications/AlcoholFacts&Stats/AlcoholFacts&Stats.pdf.

National Institute on Alcohol Abuse and Alcoholism. (2014). *Rethinking drinking: Alcohol and your health.* Retrieved from http://rethinkingdrinking.niaaa.nih.gov.

Room, R., Babor, T., & Rehm, J. (2005). Alcohol and public health. *The Lancet*, *365*, 519–530.

Substance Abuse and Mental Health Services Administration. (2014). *Results from the 2013 National Survey on Drug Use and Health: Summary of national findings.* NSDUH Series H-48, HHS Publication No. (SMA) 14-4863. Rockville, MD: Substance Abuse and Mental Health Services Administration.

U.S. Centers for Disease Control and Prevention. (2014). *Alcohol and public health home page.* Retrieved from http://www.cdc.gov/alcohol/.

World Health Organization. (2014). *Alcohol fact sheet.* Retrieved from http:www.who.int /mediacentre/factsheets/fs349/en/.

ALZHEIMER'S DISEASE (AD)

More than 5.3 million Americans suffer from Alzheimer's disease (AD), a chronic disease characterized by gradual mental and physical deterioration (Alzheimer's Association, 2015c). AD is a form of dementia that mostly affects people over the age of 65. On any given day, normal, healthy, and alert individuals may forget the name of someone they just met or where they placed their house keys. But with AD, memory loss is more severe. People with AD may not remember the name or face of a close family member, the tasks of common jobs that they worked at for 20 to 30 years, or familiar activities, such as driving. In the United States, AD is currently the sixth leading cause of death, and while the disease primarily affects people over 65, adults may succumb to AD at younger ages (Alzheimer's Association, 2015a; Hebert et al., 2013). The gradual physical and cognitive decline of AD places enormous burdens on family caregivers, public health systems, and long-term care institutions. The person with AD needs close supervision and help with normal daily activities, such as dressing, bathing, and eating. As life expectancy increases and the baby-boomer generation ages, public health researchers are challenged with finding ways to improve early diagnosis and support long-term care for those affected by AD. Support of family caregivers is particularly important with AD, and the lessons learned by improving social support could have application to caring for people with other chronic, degenerative diseases.

AD was first identified by Dr. Aloysius "Alois" Alzheimer (1864–1915). Alzheimer was a German doctor specializing in psychiatry. At the time that Alzheimer practiced medicine, little was known about mental illnesses or neurological diseases. While diagnosing and treating patients with mental disorders, Alzheimer noticed differences and similarities between the symptoms and disease progression exhibited among his patients. The variety of diseases and how the diseases represented in the body and the mind puzzled Alzheimer. It is difficult to study the brain because, unlike other organs and tissues, doctors cannot simply cut open the brain to see how it works. We learn how various parts of the brain work when people undergo insult to specific regions of the brain through traumatic brain injuries, strokes, or tumors. But Alzheimer was in a unique position to observe various disorders related to the brain, and he quickly became involved in the field of neuropathology, the study of diseases of the nervous system. In 1901, Alzheimer met Frau Auguste Deter, a 51-year-old woman with unique symptoms of early memory loss. Her young age and rapid neurological deterioration perplexed Alzheimer. For the next five years, he directly and indirectly followed Deter's progress. Her symptoms and neurological deterioration were carefully documented by doctors and nurses until her death in April 1906.

In an effort to understand her disease process, Alzheimer obtained Deter's brain tissue and her medical records. He intended to visually examine the tissue—a technique that would have had limited application. Coincidentally, a colleague of Alzheimer's—Dr. Franz Nissl—had recently refined a technique called silver staining, which allowed scientists to visualize brain tissue under the microscope. Using Nissl's silver staining technique, Alzheimer could more clearly study Deter's brain tissue. The examination revealed two abnormal structures. Areas within the nerve cells that should have been straight were tangled, and areas between nerve cells that should have been clear contained sticky clusters. These abnormalities were aptly named "tangles" and "plaques" (Engelhardt & da Mota Gomes, 2015). Alzheimer's studies were groundbreaking because it was the first time that samples of brain tissue were matched with the clinical history of a patient. He continued his research of neurological diseases until his death at the age of 51.

In individuals affected by AD, beta-amyloid proteins misfold and cause blockage in the brain's vessels, called plaques. Tangles, likewise, are caused by tau proteins that become twisted into fibers. These strange structures block blood vessels and interfere with nutrients reaching the brain cells. Signals in and to the brain are no longer able to function properly. With continued malnourishment, the brain matter and neurons eventually die, and connections in the brain are lost. The vessels that create and recall new memory are affected first. And as memory continues to deteriorate, individuals struggle with long-term information. Plaques and tangles develop as a part of aging, but they develop at a much higher rate in those affected by AD.

In public health, early diagnosis of the disease is important because it expands the choice of available treatment options, makes it easier to prevent complications, and increases ability to access support systems. Once the disease has progressed, treatment options may be limited. Early diagnosis of AD is challenging, though, because diagnosis is made based on symptoms reported by the patient or caregivers, and the patient or family caregiver may focus on what seems to be more pressing health issues. Minor symptoms of forgetfulness may not be considered important at the time of the medical appointment. The Behavioral Risk Factor Surveillance System estimates that one out of eight adults over the age of 45 experiences some memory loss, yet 77 percent have never reported the problem to their health care provider.

AD progresses in three stages. The *presymptomatic or preclinical phase* occurs as the plaques and tangles are initially forming. This stage can last several years and is frequently undiagnosed. The person appears to have no noticeable symptoms. In the *predementia phase,* early memory and functional impairment is mild but present and visible to others. The person may exhibit psychological changes and some mild forgetfulness, such as having trouble remembering something that they were just told, or they may forget someone's name or have difficulty with planning. Both the individual and family members may experience frustration with the repeated forgetfulness. Mild symptoms may go unreported unless the health care professional anticipates AD and screens for symptoms, using specific questions. During the third phase of *clinical dementia*, cognitive and functional deficiencies are clearly present and easily diagnosed. At this point, large amounts of plaques and tangles can be detected in the vessels of the brain (De-Paula et al., 2012). Individuals may forget important events in their life, such as where they went to school. They may have trouble expressing themselves verbally, they may need help in getting dressed, or they may have loss of bowel and bladder control. Sufferers often reverse day and night activities, such as sleeping during the day and staying awake at night. Personality changes appear. The person may feel confused, frustrated, or suspicious and may withdraw, wander off, or engage in compulsive behaviors, such as wringing of the hands or shredding tissues. In later stages of AD, people lose the ability to care for themselves. They have difficulty communicating, walking, and performing personal hygiene. Eventually, the person has difficulty swallowing, and the body is at increased risk for malnutrition and infections. The body will eventually succumb to the physical deterioration of AD.

Increased awareness, research, and changes in practice are improving early diagnosis and treatment. Health practitioners are refining ways to screen for and diagnose AD. Rather than asking patients if they experience forgetfulness or difficulty planning, the health care provider asks patients how their memory compares to the past. This allows health care providers to use the individual's own experiences as a baseline for comparison. The term "subjective cognitive decline" is used to describe this memory loss (Reisberg et al., 2010), and focuses on using the patient's own experiences of memory and cognition to diagnose early AD, rather than comparing the patient to others. Although there is no cure for AD, pharmacologic treatments are available to ease disease-related symptoms (such as agitation and anxiety) and slow its progression.

Currently on the market are four medications thought to help slow the progression of AD called acetylcholinesterase inhibitors (AChEIs). These include tacrine, donepezil, rivastigmine, and galantamine. Another medication is memantine, which works against the nerve cell receptor N-methyl-D-aspartate (NMDA) to help reduce abnormal activity in the brain. Although medications may ease some of these symptoms and potentially relieve caregiver burden, these medications contain side effects such as nausea, vomiting, diarrhea, increased confusion, and dizziness (National Institute on Aging, 2015). Current research seeks to identify the best combination of drugs that will provide optimal benefit for patients (Shao, 2015).

As AD gradually robs the victim of personality, independence, and abilities, family and other loved ones struggle to provide safety and around the clock care. Most families must make the difficult decision of placing the individual in long-term care or caring for the person at home. The continued loss of memory and the inability to perform basic daily activities places great demands on spouses, partners, family members, and friends. Depression and anxiety are common among those taking care of people affected by the disease (Gallagher et al., 2011). Additionally, the caregiver may be experiencing his or her own issues related to physical aging and changing social demands. Supporting caregivers and finding ways to improve caregiver coping mechanisms have become a focus of current research.

As the numbers of people suffering from AD and dementia continue to grow, public health focuses on early diagnosis, improved quality of life, preventing complications, unnecessary hospitalizations, and reducing the financial and emotional cost of care. It is believed that if we can determine AD at an earlier age, more supportive measures can be put into place to help the patient, caregivers, and family members. New tests are being developed to identify AD earlier and to identify if a person is at risk for development of AD. Pharmaceutical researchers will continue to identify new medications and possible cures for AD. Caregivers play a vital role in helping the individual stay healthy and safe for as long as possible. And while family and community caregivers provide a valuable resource, serving the needs of those with AD and reducing the financial cost, it is important that society takes responsibility to support the caregiver. The information learned from this unique brain disease and the systems developed to support those with AD may be used to help other people struggling with other chronic, degenerative diseases.

Eileen L. Sullivan and Sally Kuykendall

See also: Aging; Chronic Illness; Genetics; Mental Health; National Institutes of Health; Social Determinants of Health

Further Reading

Alzheimer's Association. (2015a). *Alzheimer's disease and dementia.* Retrieved from http://www.alz.org/.

Alzheimer's Association. (2015b). *Public health Alzheimer's Resource Center.* Retrieved from http://www.alz.org/publichealth/data-collection.asp.

Alzheimer's Association. (2015c). 2015 Alzheimer's disease facts and figures. *Alzheimer's & Dementia: The Journal of the Alzheimer's Association, 11*(3), 332–384.

Alzheimer's Foundation of America. (2015). *Alzheimer's disease and caregiving support.* Retrieved from http://www.alzfdn.org/.

De-Paula, V. J., Radanovic, M., Diniz, B. S., & Forlenza, O. V. (2012). Alzheimer's disease. *Sub-Cellular Biochemistry, 65*, 329–352.

Engelhardt, E., & da Mota Gomes, M. (2015, February). Alzheimer's 100th anniversary of death and his contribution to a better understanding of senile dementia. *Arquivos de Neuro-Psiquiatria, 73*(2), 159–162.

Gallagher, D., Ni Mhaolain, A., Crosby, L., Ryan, D., Lacey, L., Coen, R. F., & . . . Lawlor, B. A. (2011). Self-efficacy for managing dementia may protect against burden and depression in Alzheimer's caregivers. *Aging & Mental Health, 15*(6), 663–670.

Hebert, L. E., Weuve, J., Scherr, P. A., & Evans, D. A. (2013, May 7). Alzheimer disease in the United States (2010–2050) Estimated Using the 2010 Census. *Neurology, 80*(19), 1778–1783.

Maurer, K., & Maurer, U. (2003). *Alzheimer: The life of a physician and career of a disease.* New York: Columbia University Press.

National Institute on Aging. (2015, June). *Alzheimer's disease medications fact sheet.* Retrieved from https://www.nia.nih.gov/alzheimers/publication/alzheimers-disease-medications.

Reisberg, B., Shulman, M. B., Torossian, C., Leng, L., & Zhu, W. (2010, January). Outcome over seven years of healthy adults with and without subjective cognitive impairment. *Alzheimer's & Dementia: The Journal of the Alzheimer's Association*, 6(1), 11–24.

Shao, Z.-Q. (2015). Comparison of the efficacy of four cholinesterase inhibitors in combination with memantine for the treatment of Alzheimer's disease. *International Journal of Clinical and Experimental Medicine*, 8(8), 2944–2948.

AMERICAN JOURNAL OF PUBLIC HEALTH (AJPH)

The *American Journal of Public Health* (*AJPH*) is the official journal of the American Public Health Association. First published in 1911, the journal is considered public health's premier journal. Professional journals allow researchers and practitioners to share information quickly and effectively in order to advance the field and improve practice. *AJPH* presents current issues in public health, law and policy, new research, and job postings. The mission of the journal is "to advance public health research, policy, practice, and education" (*AJPH*).

Public health professionals are expected to stay current in the field so that they can provide the best possible care to patients and communities. The *AJPH* supports professional competency through regular features in best clinical practices, research, program evaluation, case studies, history, and commentary of old and new problems. Journals have an advantage over books in that they have a shorter publication time. Health information changes rapidly. Books may take several years from writing to publication, whereas journal articles may be reviewed and published within months. The faster turnaround time makes professional journals the ideal first venue for emerging health problems or critical research findings.

Submissions to the *AJPH* are reviewed by three peer reviewers, associate editor, deputy editor, and editor in chief. Each reviewer critically evaluates the article to ensure that the information has scientific foundation, is not exaggerating findings, and follows ethical standards in research and public health. Fewer than one in five articles submitted are accepted for publication. More recently, Kevin Smith, director of Office of Copyright and Scholarly Communications at Duke University, criticized the *AJPH* extending limitations on public access to published articles. When authors submit an article for publication, they transfer copyright to the publisher. Transferring copyright ensures that the author does not publish the same work in multiple venues, protecting the publisher's financial investment in reviewing and editing the article. Previously, the *AJPH* restricted public access to articles for an embargo period of two years. Only people who paid for the journal or had access through library databases could access articles published within the last two years. Authors could opt for their article to be freely accessible by compensating the publisher. In 2013, *AJPH* extended the embargo period to 10 years and increased the author fee for open access to $2,500. Smith notes that a 10-year embargo period seems excessive given the critical nature of public health information and the fact that the *AJPH* frequently reports findings from taxpayer-funded research. Research funded by taxpayers should be freely available under the public access to government data laws.

Professional journals are critically important to health professionals and the general public because they ensure that current practices are based on good science.

Sally Kuykendall

See also: American Public Health Association; Core Competencies in Public Health; Winslow, Charles-Edward Amory

Further Reading

American Journal of Public Health. Retrieved from http://ajph.aphapublications.org.

Smith, K. L. (2013). Of predators and public health: Peer to peer review. *Library Journal.* Retrieved from http://lj.libraryjournal.com/2013/05/opinion/peer-to-peer-review/of-predators-and-public-health-peer-to-peer-review/#.

AMERICAN MEDICAL ASSOCIATION (AMA)

The American Medical Association (AMA) is the largest national professional organization of medical residents, physicians, and medical students in the United States. It was founded in 1847 and supports excellence in medical education and physician practice with the overall goal of promoting health among all people in the nation.

The AMA was founded by Nathan Smith Davis (1817–1904). Davis's experiences in early life greatly influenced his attitudes and values toward medical training and the medical profession. Growing up in a log cabin in upstate New York, Davis found value and reward in hard labor (Johnson, 1904). In summers, he tended the family farm, and in winter he attended school. He started medical training at the age of 17 and, soon after turning 20, graduated from the College of Physicians and Surgeons of New York. In his early medical career, Davis worked tirelessly on behalf of his patients and advocated for rigorous medical training to ensure that others practicing medicine were competent.

Recognizing the need to change medical training from within the academic system, Davis became a professor at the College of Physicians and Surgeons of New York. He later moved to Lind University in Chicago, now known as Northwestern University. The AMA originated in 1845 when Davis chaired a committee to organize the first national convention of medical societies and medical schools. This event served as the foundation for the AMA. A prolific writer and editor of several notable medical journals, Davis also served as the founding editor of the *Journal of the American Medical Association* (*JAMA*), which is still one of the most prestigious medical journals in the world. Davis made a tremendous impact on the field of medicine as a profession. Much of his stamina, efficiency, organization, and high standards had been a direct result of his farming work ethic.

The AMA currently serves approximately 225,000 members, representing about one-fourth of the physicians in the United States. Its primary goals are to reduce disease and improve public health, support and advance medical education, and support doctors as independent practitioners and sources of credible medical information. The AMA is important to public health in that the organization defines standards for physician practices. Naming and sharing best practices with doctors ensures that patients receive the best possible medical care and that communities are well informed of potential health hazards and ways to minimize hazards. The AMA provides members with many benefits, including continuing education, information on best practices in medicine and patient safety office administration and management, discounted insurance and other products, opportunities for professional networking, forums on health policy, and political advocacy. The AMA also publishes several medical journals, including *JAMA*. To achieve healthy communities, the organization offers grants to promote healthy living, healthy communities, and health literacy; scholarships to train future physicians; and presents awards to medical students, residents, and physicians who advance the stature of the profession through volunteering, leadership, or professionalism. Criticisms of the AMA center on past and current political activities. Historically, the AMA resisted government involvement in health care programs, such as Medicare and health care reform, and advocated for limits to medical malpractice lawsuits. In order to achieve the goals of improving public health and advocating for physician members, the AMA must carefully balance responsibility to the public with responsibility to physicians.

In private practice, health professionals work independently. This means that personal values, experiences, and priorities can influence patient care. The caregiver may not consciously recognize the influence or may have difficulty with differing points of view. For example, the pharmaceutical sales representative who visits physicians in their office and encourages them to prescribe specific medicine has the opportunity to unduly influence patient care. To help guide patients, doctors, residents, and medical students, the AMA has a medical ethics division. The group reviews the latest research in different areas, identifies ethical challenges, and develops guidelines for practice. The guidelines are directed by the core values of professionalism, honor, compassion, and respect. The guidelines are described in the AMA Code of Medical Ethics and cover topics such as social issues, professional relations, advertising, fees, patient records, and professional rights and responsibilities. But these guidelines are guides, not laws or policies. By advocating for doctors to act as competent, professional, and knowledgeable caregivers, the AMA ensures patients receive the best care possible.

Sally Kuykendall

See also: Code of Ethics; Core Competencies in Public Health; Ethics in Public Health and Population Health; Health Insurance Portability and Accountability Act of 1996; Health Resources and Services Administration

Further Reading

American Medical Association. (2014). *Code of medical ethics of the American Medical Association, 2014–2015: Current opinions with annotations.* Chicago, IL: American Medical Association Press.

American Medical Association. (2015). *About AMA.* Retrieved from http://www.ama-assn.org/ama.

Danforth, I. N. (1907). *The life of Nathan Smith Davis, A.M., M.D., LL.D., 1817–1904.* Cleveland: Cleveland Press. Retrieved from https://books.google.com/books?id=HRUJAAAAIAAJ&pg=PA20&lpg=PA20&dq=the+life+of+nathan+smith+davis&source=bl&ots=v3UxFIsG-8&sig=gSiVuHstGuKdZXTFG2jRrfVWRio&hl=en&sa=X&ved=0ahUKEwiLvqOZm4XNAhVCJFIKHaLSAGIQ6AEIUDAN#v=onepage&q=the%20life%20of%20nathan%20smith%20davis&f=false.

Johnson, F. S. (1904). Nathan Smith Davis. *Science, 20,* 237–240.

Jonsen, A. R. (2008). *A short history of medical ethics.* New York: Oxford University Press.

AMERICAN PUBLIC HEALTH ASSOCIATION (APHA)

The American Public Health Association (APHA) is the primary professional organization of public health practitioners, administrators, researchers, and educators in the United States. The organizational mission of the APHA is to "improve the health of the public and achieve equity in health status" (APHA, 2017). Strategically, this mission is achieved by (1) building a public health movement that sustains and advances core functions; (2) strengthening public health practice through cross-cultural, interdisciplinary teams; and (3) aligning organizational capacity and infrastructure. To promote advances within the major public health disciplines, APHA members can chose from 31 different member sections. Examples of sections include alcohol, tobacco, and other drugs; epidemiology; environment; food and nutrition; health administration; injury control and emergency health services; mental health; occupational safety and health; oral health; public health social work; and vision care. Special Interest Groups (SPIGs) in pharmacy and veterinary public health bring together members of common occupations with unique perspectives. The Student Assembly (APHA-SA) connects students who are interested in working together on public health-related issues. And while APHA provides discipline-specific sections and SPIGs, anyone who is interested in public health is welcome and eligible to join the organization. APHA recognizes that advancing the health of the nation requires many different skills, diverse expertise, and cultures. APHA seeks to join skills and perspectives optimizing available talent and promoting public health.

APHA member benefits include access to news, professional development, networking, and other resources. APHA offers several news outlets and professional journals. Available in both hard copy and electronic format, the *American Journal of Public Health* (*AJPH*) is a monthly, peer-reviewed professional journal that covers the latest research and evidence-based practices as well as editorial, historical, and special reports. *The Nation's Health* is published 10 times per year. *The Nation's Health* features the latest public health news and policies presented in a newspaper format. APHA Press publishes books and periodicals on public health topics. *Inside Public Health* is APHA's monthly newsletter covering public health news and professional events.

Members have an opportunity to network with other public health professionals through APHA's professional communities, committees, forums, and assemblies. APHA's Annual Meeting and Expo is the world's largest gathering of public health professionals. Each year, more than 12,500 professionals gather to share ideas, concerns, and evidence-based practices, acquire new information, peruse the latest resources and publications and to support one another. The Public Health CareerMart lists jobs for public health professionals. The Career Development Center provides discounted professional career services, such as résumé review and career coaching. APHA supports student members and early career professionals with discounted membership rates and specialized resources.

The APHA supports public health practitioners by communicating science, policies, news, concerns, and advancements related to public health practice. In supporting public health professionals, the organization plays a key role in improving health of current and future generations of Americans.

Sally Kuykendall

See also: American Journal of Public Health; Certified in Public Health; Code of Ethics; Core Competencies in Public Health; Cornely, Paul B.; Eliot, Martha May; *Nation's Health, The*; Public Health in the United States, History of; Society of Public Health Education; Wegman, Myron Ezra; Winslow, Charles-Edward Amory

Further Reading

American Public Health Association. (2017). Retrieved from https://www.apha.org/.

AMERICANS WITH DISABILITIES ACT (ADA)

The Americans with Disabilities Act (ADA) was passed into law by George H. W. Bush on July 26, 1990. The act specifically prohibits discrimination to an individual with a qualified disability by employers; this includes federal, state, and local government agencies. The ADA defines a covered employer as one who employs 15 or more workers. The ADA was molded after the Civil Rights Act of 1964 and section 504 of the Rehabilitation Act of 1973. The ADA guarantees that people with disabilities are provided the same opportunities as all others who "purchase goods and services, as well as participate in state and local government programs and services" (Department of Justice, 2017). The ADA is relevant to public health in that it ensures that people with disabilities have the same rights and privileges in seeking, attaining, and maintaining employment as abled-bodied people. The ability to engage in meaningful employment is a critical aspect of mental and physical health.

A disabled person is defined as one who has a "physical or mental impairment that affects one or more major life activity, the impairment is recorded, or is regarded as having such impairment" (Equal Employment Opportunity Commission, 2017). A person (employee or applicant) who encompasses any of the above is one, who with or without satisfactory accommodation can properly perform the fundamentals of his or her job descriptions. Satisfactory accommodations are making the workplace accessible, offering alternative work schedules, reassessment of job duties, offering another unfilled position, modifying work equipment, or having training resources available in braille or through interpreters.

The employer is required to make the appropriate adjustments so long as it does not cause any difficulty on the employer's business. According to the ADA, "a hardship is defined as an action requiring significant difficulty or expense in relation to the size of the organization, financial resources, or the nature and structure of the organization" (Equal Employment Opportunity Commission, 2017). Furthermore, the employer does not have to provide any of the above changes unless

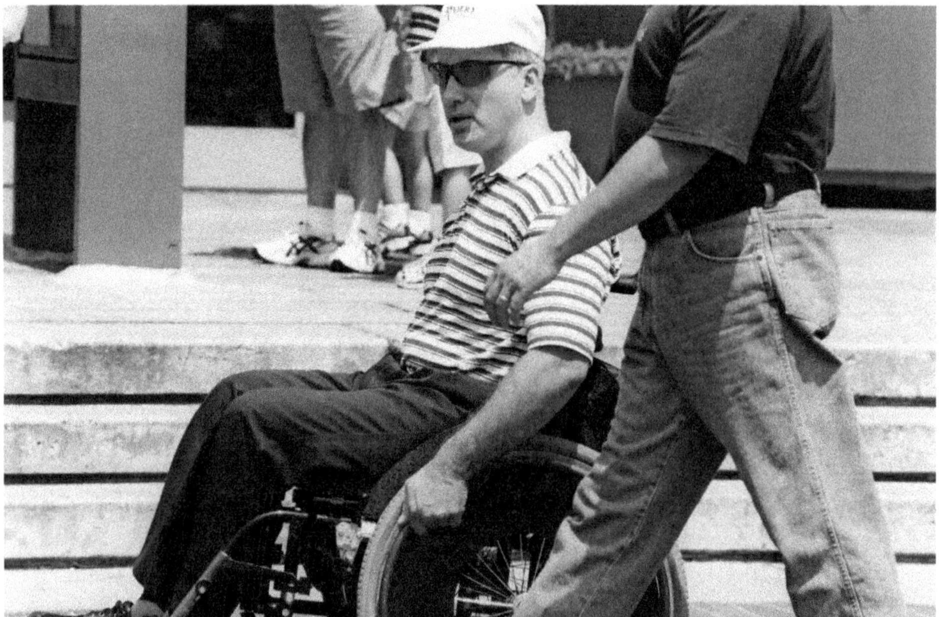

The Americans with Disabilities Act ensures that people with disabilities enjoy the same opportunities to work, shop, travel, and visit public places as enabled people. (U.S. Census Bureau)

they are requested by the employee. The business does not have to change their standard of operation to make such accommodations. The employer reserves the right to meet with the employee if their disability is resulting in poor performance or disciplinary issue. At this time, the employer can inquire how to assist in correcting the negative issues and if the accommodation is ultimately required. If there are multiple accommodations requested, then it is up to the employer to determine the most cost effective or least imposing adjustment to their organization.

The ADA also prohibits the employer's ability to ask medical related questions such as "the existence, nature, or severity of a disability" (Equal Employment Opportunity Commission, 2017). Medical questions can only be asked if it was required during the application process or others with similar position are required to disclose such information. Employers must protect an employee's records especially those relating to health conditions. They are forbidden to provide an employee's direct supervisor any information relating to diagnosis or course of treatment. Finally, employers may not terminate or discriminate against those who have requested, filed a complaint, or actively engaged in litigation under the ADA.

Although employers are bound by the strict regulations of the ADA, the employee also has responsibilities and guidelines to follow. Those who are actively participating in the use of illegal drugs as defined by the federal government or alcohol abuse are covered under the ADA. Furthermore, employers who require drug testing are not in violation of the ADA and can hold those employees accountable.

The Americans with Disabilities Act protects and ensures that any employee with a qualified disability is not discriminated against. To ensure that the regulations are being followed, there are four governmental agencies tasked with enforcing the regulations: the Equal Employment Opportunity Commission (EEOC), the Department of Transportation, the Federal Trade Commission (FFC), and the Department of Justice.

Leapolda Figueroa

See also: Disability; Disability Movement; Health; Leading Health Indicators; National Institutes of Health; Obesity; Public Health Law; Social Security Act

Further Reading

Bayer, R. (2003). Workers' liberty, workers' welfare: The Supreme Court speaks on the rights of disabled employees. *American Journal of Public Health*, 93(4), 540.

Department of Justice, Civil Rights Division. (2017). *Introduction to the ADA*. Retrieved from https://www.ada.gov/ada_intro.htm.

Equal Employment Opportunity Commission. (2017). *Facts about the Americans with Disabilities Act.* Retrieved from https://www.eeoc.gov//eeoc/publications/fs-ada.cfm.

Iezzoni, L. I., & O'Day, B. L. (2006). *More than ramps: A guide to improving health care quality and access for people with disabilities.* New York: Oxford University Press. doi:10.1093/acprof:oso/9780195172768.003.0002.

Longmore, P. K. (1987). Uncovering the hidden history of people with disabilities. *Reviews in American History, 15*(3), 355–364.

Shapiro, J. (1994). From charity to independent living. *No pity: People with disabilities forging a new civil rights movement.* New York: Times Books.

ANCIENT WORLD, PUBLIC HEALTH IN THE

The concept of public health, as we know it today, did not exist in the ancient world. Public health measures were implemented primarily for aesthetic and religious reasons, not as a form of disease control. Sewage was removed because it was unsightly and smelled, bathing was primarily a matter of ritual purity, not cleanliness, and medical care had more to do with magic than science. The study of public health in the ancient world is an interdisciplinary effort engaging researchers from a number of fields including archaeology, paleobiology, history, linguistics, and entomology, to name a few. The knowledge that we have about public health in the ancient world comes primarily through the written records that were left behind, and the archeological evidence that has been uncovered. In all cases, the information is subject to interpretation, and these interpretations can change over time as new information comes to light.

It is believed that humans living in hunter-gather societies were beset by many of the same illness that we still encounter today (Rosen, 1993). However, due to the small size of these groups, and their limited contact with other humans and animals, epidemics of disease are thought to have been minimal, if they occurred at all. As humans began to transition to an agrarian, settled existence, their interactions with other people, and domesticated animals, increased, as did the population. These interactions exposed humans to new and more numerous pathogens and parasites than they had encountered in the past (Sherman, 2006). In addition, nutritional deficiencies arose as diets became restricted to a few staple crops. They also faced food insecurity issues due to the danger of crop failures caused by pestilence or natural disasters. Problems with waste disposal and contaminated water resources also occurred.

In dealing with the myriad of diseases and environmental problems that they faced, most people in the ancient world turned toward ritualistic cures. They viewed disease, famine, and other ills as being caused by a god, spirit, or other supernatural being. Consequently, they thought that the main way to cure the disease, or divert a looming disaster, was to appease the offended entity. This was done with methods as benign as prayers or offerings of food, or on the other extreme, by performing human or animal sacrifices. The ancient peoples also thought that another source of illness and misfortune could occur as a direct result of sorcery or the dead, each of which required its own set of rituals to overcome. A part of this theurgical belief was that cleanliness was a religious rite. People would bathe as a form of purification before entering a temple or performing certain rituals. The Inca purification festival of Citua, for example, required the act of ritual bathing and the purification of homes with maize flour. These rituals were carried out as a means to rid the city and its people of impurities, including illness (Staller, 2010). Many of these religious rituals and rules where codified, and they are known to us, in part, from the surviving records.

Health care professionals in the ancient world ranged from medicine men and shamans to physicians and midwives. In most ancient cultures, physicians used their empirical knowledge in conjunction with magical spells or other rituals. Or, as in Mesopotamia, they often worked in conjunction with a magician (Biggs, 2005). In some regions, such as Sumeria, the priests not only served as religious and political leaders, but they were also responsible for carrying out major public works projects, such as the complex irrigation systems that brought water to farms and helped to control flooding.

In addition, community leaders often used their influence to institute public health projects. It is important to note that almost every ancient settlement that has been studied, no matter its size, shows evidence of some sort of sewage system. These systems include what are thought to be the first flush toilets, dating to about 1850 BCE, which were found in Knossos on Crete. As well, excavations at Skara Brae in the Orkney Islands of Scotland have uncovered small recesses in many of the homes. These recesses, dating to around 3500 BCE, have drains in the floor that lead outside and are thought to be primitive indoor toilets. In addition, most of the large cities studied show evidence of detailed urban planning that included not only the layout of the various towns, but also the development of water and drainage systems, granaries, sewers, household plumbing, and systems to divert storm runoff. A key example of the latter is the moats found around ancient Thai villages that were uncovered at excavations in Ban Non Wat, Thailand. These moats are thought to have served multiple purposes, including protection, but also as a reservoir for water during the dry season and as a way to divert water away from the villages during the wet seasons (Lawler, 2009). Examples of other towns that show extensive urban planning include the ancient city of El Mirador, in Guatemala. This Maya pre-Columbian city is thought to have had more than 100,000 residents at its peak, and it appears to have been carefully laid out to coincide with astronomical alignments of religious and agricultural significance (Sprajc, Morales-Aguilar, & Hansen, 2009). The cities of Mohenjo-Daro and Harappa, located in the Indus River Valley, are also thought to have been preplanned cities. They became major urban centers around 2500 BCE. From the archaeological evidence that has been uncovered, both of these cities featured paved streets, covered sewers, and a complex water system that included indoor bathrooms. In addition, numerous ancient cities uncovered throughout the Near East, Egypt, Asia, and Mesoamerica all show evidence of urban planning.

There are many ancient Chinese medical texts that provide insights into the treatment and theories about medicine in China. Two of them are attributed to mythical emperors whose histories may have some basis in fact. The first of these is the Emperor Shennong, who is credited with writing the *Divine Husbandman's Materia Medica* (*Ben cao jing ji zhu*), which lists various pharmaceuticals and how they were made (Hsu & Harris, 2010). The other is the Yellow Emperor Huang Di, who is credited with writing *The Canon of Internal Medicine* (*Huangdi neijing*), which offers both magical and naturalistic explanations for the causes of various diseases, along with therapeutic treatments (Raphals, 2013). Although both emperors are thought to have lived between 3000 and 2600 BCE, the actual books mentioned are not believed to have been written until much later and are thought to be compilations of earlier oral traditions and written texts (Hsu & Harris, 2010). Other texts that provide insights into how residents of the ancient world viewed and treated illnesses included the medical library of the Assyrian king, Ashurbanipal, held at Nineveh. It includes descriptions of diseases, herbal remedies, and how to make and use various pharmaceuticals. The *Atharva Veda*, a Hindu book of hymns from around 1500 to 1000 BCE, includes spells and incantations that were used for medical purposes. Perhaps one of the best-known texts to have survived from the ancient world is the *Pentateuch* (*Five Books of Moses*), which contains a detailed list of prohibited foods, instructions on cleanliness, and related issues that are thought to have had public health implications (Porter, 1998). Information on public health practices in the past have also been garnered from the Mayan glyphs and Sumerian cuneiform writings, as well as Egyptian medical papyri that include information on both the religious aspects of healing as well as empirical-based observations. The Law Code of Hammurabi includes references to malpractice by physicians. There are letters from Kassite physicians discussing treatments, and many more examples, including the Mari letters, from Mesopotamia, which deal with relocating people to try to stop the spread of contagious illnesses (Biggs, 2005). In addition, there are still texts that have not been translated, such as the writings left by the Harappan civilization that once flourished in the Indus Valley region of ancient India. This is indicative of the fact that we still have much to learn about public health in the ancient world, and that our current understanding of the period is likely to change as new information is discovered.

Rochelle Caviness

See also: Greco-Roman Era, Public Health in the; Hippocrates; Infectious Diseases; Locus of Control; Middle Ages, Public Health in the; Modern Era, Public Health in the; Renaissance, Public Health in the; Rosen, George; Spiritual Health

Further Reading

Biggs, R. D. (2005). Medicine, surgery, and public health in ancient Mesopotamia. *Journal of Assyrian Academic Studies*, *19*(1), 28–46.

Hsu, E., & Harris, S. (Eds.). (2010). *Plants, health and healing: On the interface of ethnobotany and medical anthropology*. Volume 6 of *Epistemologies of healing*. New York: Berghahn Books.

Lawler, A. (2009, February). Bodies of evidence in Southeast Asia. *Smithsonian Magazine*, *39*(11). Retrieved from http://www.smithsonianmag.com/history/bodies-of-evidence-in-southeast-asia-44419614/?no-ist.
Porter, D. (1998). *Health, civilization and the state: A history of public health from ancient to modern times*. New York: Routledge.
Raphals, L. (2013). *Divination and prediction in early China and ancient Greece*. New York: Cambridge University Press.
Rosen, G. (1993). *A history of public health: Expanded edition*. Baltimore: Johns Hopkins University Press.
Sherman, I. W. (2006). *The power of plagues*. Washington, DC: Asm Press.
Sprajc, I., Morales-Aguilar, C., & Hansen, R. D. (2009). Early Maya astronomy and urban planning at El Mirador, Peten, Guatemala. *Anthropological Notebooks*, *15*(3), 79–101.
Staller, J. (2010). *Maize cobs and cultures: History of zea mays l*. New York: Springer.

ANDERSON, ELIZABETH MILBANK (1850–1921)

Elizabeth Milbank Anderson was an American philanthropist who used her wealth and status to develop and promote public health. Elizabeth was born in New York City (NYC) to parents Jeremiah and Elizabeth (Lake) Milbank. Jeremiah Milbank was a wholesale grocer, banker, and financier. In 1858, he financed the struggling New York Condensed Milk Company. The investment quickly paid off when the U.S. government ordered 500 pounds of condensed milk for American Civil War soldiers. When the veterans returned home, they continued to use the familiar product. The company eventually became the Borden Condensed Milk Company with Mr. Milbank as a stockholder. Milbank also invested in and became director of the Chicago, Milwaukee, and St. Paul Railroad. Elizabeth's early life was privileged. She was taught by private tutors, attended religious services at Madison Avenue Baptist Church, and traveled extensively. When her father died in 1884, Elizabeth inherited $10 million, equivalent to $249 million today. In terms of economic power, the influence and power to create further wealth, the inheritance would be equivalent to $15.2 billion today.

On June 15, 1876, Elizabeth married Abraham Archibald Anderson (1846–1940). A. A. Anderson was a portrait painter, born in Hackensack, New Jersey. He spent 10 years in Paris studying art with the masters, Léon Bonnat, Alexandre Cabanel, Fernand Cormon, and Raphaël Collin. The couple had two children, Eleanor (1878–1959) and Jeremiah (c. 1879–1886). Jeremiah died of diphtheria at the age of seven. Elizabeth blamed her son's death on unsanitary conditions in New York City. At the time, urban streets were filled with human waste, horse manure, and animal cadavers. The decaying waste contaminated water sources. Crowded living conditions resulted in multiple epidemics of cholera, diphtheria, typhus, and tuberculosis. The loss of a child instilled a sense of determination. Elizabeth's first public health effort was building bathhouses, a place where the poor could bathe and maintain some degree of personal hygiene. Elizabeth's philanthropy was on the cusp of broader social reforms taking place around the nation. In 1889, steel industrialist Andrew Carnegie published *The Gospel of Wealth,* calling on wealthy people to use their fortunes to benefit the poor. The Progressive Era (c. 1890–1920) was a period when the wealthy attempted to bypass government corruption and give directly to colleges, hospitals, religious organizations, and science and community organizations, which would benefit all of society.

Over time, A. A. Anderson and his wife developed separate interests and separate lives. He split his time between Paris, New York, and their ranch in Wyoming, advocating for preservation of national parks. President Theodore Roosevelt named "Colonel" Anderson the first superintendent of the Yellowstone Forest Reserve. In his 1933 autobiography, *Experiences and Impressions: An Autobiography of Colonel A. A. Anderson,* Anderson allocates three chapters to bear hunts and little description of his wife and daughter (Dickason, 2000). Unhindered by marital responsibilities, Elizabeth took on the mission. In her mind, preventable disease and premature death were the main obstacles to human happiness, and the government was primarily responsible for ensuring public health. Her idea was to fill a void until the city was in a position to provide the necessary social services.

In 1892, Elizabeth made her first major donation of $350,000 to Roosevelt Hospital in New York City. Over the next two decades, she funded the Milbank Public Baths for the New York Association for Improving the Condition of the Poor, subsidized the NYC school hot lunch program, donated to the Children's Aid Society, and became trustee and supporter of Barnard College. During World War I, Anderson supported orphans and homeless children of immigrant Europeans. In 1905, with the help of her cousin, Albert G. Milbank, she established the Memorial Fund Association. The mission of the organization was "to improve the physical, mental and moral condition of humanity and generally to advance charitable and benevolent objects." The foundation's name was changed to the Milbank Memorial Fund in 1921 in memory of her parents. The Milbank Memorial Fund originally supported programs in public health and nutrition and established community health centers and dental clinics. In the 1920s, the fund expanded to support best practices in medical and health care delivery systems and health demonstration projects. Overall, Mrs. Anderson endowed $9,315,175 to the Milbank Foundation. The foundation continues today advancing evidence-based practice in population health and studying social determinants of health.

In 1912, Elizabeth legally adopted her granddaughter, Elizabeth Milbank Tanner. Her daughter, Eleanor, had married medical doctor John Stewart Tanner. Tanner had an extramarital affair and Elizabeth did not want her daughter to experience the same, empty marital relationship, which she had endured. Elizabeth raised her granddaughter while Eleanor studied at Boston University Medical School and interned in NYC and Boston. Eleanor followed in her mother's footsteps of social activism, opening the Judson Health Center (1921) to serve the poor immigrant Italian population living near Judson Memorial Church.

Elizabeth Milbank Anderson died of pernicious anemia on February 22, 1921. At the time of her death, she held stock in Borden Company, Texas & Pacific Coal & Oil Company, and Pacific Mutual Life Insurance Company and Liberty Bonds. The major public health benefactors of her estate were the Memorial Fund Association ($1.5 million), National Committee for Mental Hygiene ($100,000), Association for Improving Conditions of the Poor ($200,000), Henry Street Settlement ($50,000), Harlem Legal Aid Society ($50,000), National Child Labor Committee ($25,000), and Tuskegee Institute ($25,000). Of her $7 million estate, she left $50,000 to her husband, explaining that "ample provision had been made for him previously" (*New York Times*, 1921). In the 1935 Annual Conference of Secretaries of the County Medical Societies of Indiana, Albert G. Milbank remembered his cousin's contributions:

> Elizabeth Milbank Anderson was one of those rare souls who combined a brilliant mind, a love of humanity, a generous nature, and a keen sense of humor. She was an unquestioned individualist but with a profound sense of her social obligations. She mistrusted fads and visionary theories as solutions for current problems but the honesty of her mind made it impossible for her to ignore a problem even when its solution called for changes in an established procedure.

Elizabeth believed that too many charities dealt with the symptoms of poverty, ignoring the underlying urban and social problems. Her hope was that one day the government would recognize the need for social services and finance public health programs.

Elizabeth Milbank Anderson was a philanthropist who supported early public health efforts in urban sanitation, women and children's health, and women's education. Her determination and support created public health programs in disease prevention and health promotion, which benefit many people today.

Sally Kuykendall

See also: Baker, Sara Josephine; Children's Health; Maternal Health; Social Determinants of Health; Winslow, Charles-Edward Amory

Further Reading

Dickason, E. (2000). Eleanor Campbell. In E. Dickason & J. G. Dickason (Eds.), *Remembering Judson House* (pp. 93–99). New York: Judson Church. Retrieved from http://classic.judson.org/images/Judson_House_12_Elly_Dickason.pdf.

Milbank, A. G. (1935, January 27). Annual Conference of Secretaries of the County Medical Societies of Indiana in Indianapolis, IN. Yale University. Milbank Memorial Fund papers, Sterling Library, Series II, Box 25. Retrieved from https://www.ncbi.nlm.nih.gov/pmc/articles/PMC2690275/.

Miller, H. S., & Miller, H. S. (1971). Anderson, Elizabeth Milbank (Dec. 20, 1850–Feb. 22, 1921). In E. James, J. James, & P. Boyer (Eds.), *Notable American women: 1607–1950*. Cambridge, MA: Harvard University Press.

New York Times. (1921, June 30). Half of $7,000,000 estate to public.

ANTIBIOTIC RESISTANCE

Antibiotics could be one of the most important public health advances ever. Before the discovery of antibiotics, infectious diseases were the leading cause of death worldwide. The use of antibiotics to prevent and control bacterial infections significantly increased average life expectancy by reducing death and disability due to communicable diseases. The list of antibiotics approved by Federal Drug Administration (FDA) is extensive, but the main challenge in using antibiotics is that bacteria are living organisms that can adapt to changes in their environment.

Antibiotic resistance is the ability of bacteria to change so it is no longer destroyed by an antibiotic. Resistance develops when a person misses critical doses, stops the doses prematurely, or overuses or misuses antibiotics, such as using an antibiotic for a viral infection rather than bacterial infections. Even though a person may take an antibiotic in the correct manner and for the correct duration, the bacteria may still resist its effect. In 2013, the Centers for Disease Control and Prevention (CDC) reported more than 2 million bacterial-resistant illnesses occur each year, resulting in more than 23,000 deaths (U.S. Department of Health and Human Services, Centers for Disease Control and Prevention, 2013).

Antibiotic resistance is problematic to public health because antibiotic resistant infections require stronger and stronger antibiotics. Yet, developing and testing antibiotics takes many years of pharmaceutical research. Thus, antibiotic resistance becomes a race between pharmaceutical companies to develop effective drugs to keep infectious diseases under control and bacteria that are constantly mutating in an effort to survive.

Antibiotics are categorized as bactericidal or bacteriostatic. Bactericidal is when an antibiotic "kills" the bacteria by interfering with its cell wall and substances within the cell. Penicillin, for example, is bactericidal. Bacteriostatic stops bacteria from multiplying but does not kill the infecting bacteria. It works with the host's own immune system to eliminate the bacteria. Bacteria fall into two main categories: gram positive and gram negative. The goal of an antibiotic is to weaken the cell wall of bacterial cells so the bacteria can no longer replicate, or to kill the bacteria directly. Although antibiotics provide quick and effective relief from what were once deadly diseases, antibiotic use presents a secondary issue of antibiotic resistance.

Antibiotic resistance occurs when the cell wall of the bacteria becomes resistant to the antibiotic and, despite being in the presence of the antibiotic, the cell wall continues to remain intact and unaffected. Multidrug-resistant (MDR) bacteria develop when bacteria find ways to deter the effects of several different antibiotics. *Streptococcus pneumoniae* is one bacteria associated with many infections seen in communities including meningitis, pneumonia, sepsis (bacteria in the blood), and ear infections. *Streptococcus pneumoniae* tends to be resistant to multiple antibiotics, and researchers are studying this resistance (Borg et al., 2009). Antibiotic resistance is not limited to humans. Antibiotics are also used to control bacterial infections among animals. Resistance can be transferred from animal to animal, animal to human, and human to human. One common method is when an animal's feces is used to fertilize food crops. When humans consume the food, resistance is transferred. Drug-resistant bacteria can also remain within meat; improper cooking or handling spreads the infection. Human carriers may then transfer the resistance through poor sanitation (i.e., contaminated hands). Antibiotic resistance can spread rapidly within hospitals or health clinics because the patients served may already be immunocompromised due to cancer, cancer treatments, AIDS, or other disease.

The CDC divides antibiotic resistance into three categories based on threat to public health: urgent, serious, and concerning (Centers for Disease Control and Prevention, 2016). Urgent threats are bacteria that are labeled high consequence because the bacteria can bring significant threat to the health of an individual or community. They require aggressive action by our public health system. These microorganisms are listed as urgent threats: Carbapenem-resistant *Enterobacteriaceae*, *Clostridium difficile*, and drug-resistant *Neisseria* gonorrhoeae. *C. difficile* infects 250,000 people per year, causing 14,000 deaths. The cost to treat these cases exceeds $1 billion per year (USDHHS, CDC, 2013). Serious threats are antibiotic-resistant bacteria that do not rise to the level of urgent, yet require constant surveillance and sustained intervention. There is the potential for serious threats to become urgent threats. Current serious threats include multidrug-resistant *Acinetobacter,* Fluconazole-resistant Candida, drug-resistant *Campylobacter,* extended spectrum ant Candida, causing *Enterobacteriaceae,* Vancomycin-resistant *Enterococcus,* drug-resistant Shigella, Methicillin-resistant *Staphylococcus aureus* (MRSA), and drug-resistant tuberculosis. Multidrug-resistant *Acinetobacter* accounts for 7,300 infections per year and results in 500 deaths. *Acinetobacter* is resistant to three different classes of antibiotics, and we no longer have a pharmaceutical agent that can cure this dangerous strain of bacteria. MRSA, once found primarily in hospital settings, is now found in many different communities. The threat category of "concerning" presents a lower level of danger because alternative treatment options are still available. Bacteria in this category are monitored for incidence, rapid outbreaks, further mutation, or locations. Examples include Erythromycin-resistant Group A *Streptococcus,* Vancomycin-resistant *Staphylococcus aureus,* and Clindamycin-resistant Group B *Streptococcus.* Erythromycin-resistant Group A *Streptococcus* is associated with numerous common infections, such as strep throat, toxic shock syndrome, scarlet fever, rheumatic fever, impetigo, and necrotizing fasciitis, commonly known as "flesh-eating" disease. One to two million people each year suffer from strep throat caused by *Streptococcus.* As more and more antibiotics are manufactured, many mimicking others, bacteria also advance in finding ways to resist not one, but many, antibiotics.

Despite the dire consequences of antibiotic-resistant microorganisms, this serious problem can be controlled through good and sometimes easy public health measures. The primary means of reducing antibiotic resistance is by stopping the spread of infections. Following vaccination guidelines, using good hygiene during food preparation, and proper handwashing are the first line of defense. A practice as simple as good handwashing reduces upper respiratory infections 16 to 21 percent

(Aiello, Coulborn, Perez, & Larson, 2008; Rabie & Curtis, 2006) and diarrhea by 31 percent (Aiello, Coulborn, Perez, & Larson, 2008; Ejemot-Nwadiaro, Ehiri, Meremikwu, & Critchley, 2015).

Local and state public health departments track reportable infectious diseases and track cases to determine the severity of the problem. Tracking enables cases to be handled rapidly and effectively to prevent the spread within a community or to other communities. Good antibiotic stewardship refers to the practice of using antibiotics in humans and animals only when necessary and appropriate to the microorganism, and ensuring the proper disposal of antibiotics. The final line of defense is the search for new, effective drugs that can withstand bacterial resistance. One such antibiotic is teixobactin. Teixobactin is termed a "super antibiotic" because the chemical structure works against bacteria through several modes of action. It is yet to be seen whether teixobactin can withstand resistance (Ling et al., 2015). As bacteria become resistant to antibiotics, researchers are hoping newly developed antibiotics can be effective agents in ceasing bacterial growth with minimal side effects to the patient.

Antibiotic resistance is an area of concern nationally and internationally. As we run out of drugs to treat various infections, we become vulnerable to novel strains of microorganisms. The public health principles of immunizations, food safety, hand hygiene, tracking infectious diseases, and good antibiotic stewardship go a long way in preventing and controlling infectious diseases. When these mechanisms fail, it is important to have an arsenal of effective antibiotics against bacteria.

Eileen L. Sullivan and Sally Kuykendall

See also: Agricultural Safety; Centers for Disease Control and Prevention; Community Health; Disease; Food Safety; Handwashing; Infectious Diseases; Patient Safety; Penicillin; Prevention; Vaccines

Further Reading

Aiello, A. E., Coulborn, R. M., Perez, V., & Larson, E. L. (2008). Effect of hand hygiene on infectious disease risk in the community setting: A meta-analysis. *American Journal of Public Health*, *98*(8), 1372–1381.

Borg, M., Tiemersma, E., Scicluna, E., van de Sande-Bruinsma, N., de Kraker, M., Monen, J., & Grundmann, H. (2009). Original article: Prevalence of penicillin and erythromycin resistance among invasive Streptococcus pneumoniae isolates reported by laboratories in the southern and eastern Mediterranean region. *Clinical Microbiology and Infection*, *15*, 232–237.

Centers for Disease Control and Prevention. (2016). *National antimicrobial resistance monitoring system.* Atlanta, GA: U.S. Department of Health and Human Services, CDC. Retrieved from http://wwwn.cdc.gov/narmsnow/.

Ejemot-Nwadiaro, R. I., Ehiri, J. E., Arikpo, D., Meremikwu, M. M., & Critchley, J. A. (2015). Handwashing promotion for preventing diarrhoea. *The Cochrane Database of Systematic Reviews*, 9; CD004265. doi:10.1002/14651858.CD004265.pub3

Ling, L. L., Schneider, T., Peoples, A. J., Spoering, A. L., Engels, I., Conlon, B. P., & Chen, C. (2015). A new antibiotic kills pathogens without detectable resistance. *Nature*, *517*(7535), 455–459.

Rabie, T., & Curtis, V. (2006). Handwashing and risk of respiratory infections: A quantitative systematic review. *Tropical Medicine & International Health*, *11*(3), 258–267.

U.S. Department of Health and Human Services, Centers for Disease Control and Prevention. (2013). *Antibiotic resistance threats in the United States, 2013*. Retrieved from http://www.cdc.gov/drugresistance/threat-report-2013.

World Health Organization. (2015, October). *Antibiotic resistance fact sheet*. Retrieved from http://www.who.int/mediacentre/factsheets/antibiotic-resistance/en/.

ASSOCIATION OF PUBLIC HEALTH LABORATORIES (APHL)

Public health laboratories are responsible for monitoring food safety; responding to public health emergencies created by natural disaster, terrorist attack, hazardous substances, or emerging infectious diseases; monitoring environmental conditions; and screening all newborns for potentially life-threatening genetic and metabolic disorders. Located in strategic positions throughout the United States, public health laboratories are equipped to monitor and detect numerous health threats. Highly trained scientists must be able to analyze a variety of specimens from different sources and accurately report results. The Association of Public Health Laboratories (APHL) is the national organization networking state and local government health laboratories, companies, laboratory professionals, and students interested in the laboratory sciences.

At the local level, APHL works with local health departments and practitioners to support essential diagnostic services and promote best practices in testing to ensure public health, environmental, agricultural, and food safety. At the national level, APHL works with the Centers for Disease Control and Prevention (CDC), the Environmental Protection Agency (EPA), the Food and Drug Administration (FDA), and the Health Resources and Services Administration (HRSA) to provide surveillance and rapid, effective response to public health threats. APHL also works internationally, consulting with developed and developing countries on strategic planning, training, and quality assurance. APHL member benefits include access to scientific protocols, continuing education courses, publications, leadership development, and the annual meeting where members can share the latest research and practices. As the main professional organization for public health laboratories, APHL is active in public policy, advising decision makers on pending legislation.

One of the many, many critical functions performed in public health laboratories is newborn screening. Four million babies are born every year in the United States and 1 out of 1,500 has an inborn error of metabolism. Inborn errors of metabolism are genetic disorders where the body cannot break down specific components of food for conversion to energy or other functions in the body. The resulting by-products build up and can cause a variety of health or developmental problems. Phenylketonuria (PKU) is an inborn error of metabolism resulting from mutation of the phenylalanine hydroxylase (*PAH*) gene. The *PAH* gene provides instructions for the body to make phenylalanine hydroxylase, the enzyme, which converts the amino acid phenylalanine into tyrosine. Tyrosine is another amino acid, important for neurotransmission and skin and hair pigmentation. Without phenylalanine hydroxylase, phenylalanine builds up in the body and causes seizures and permanent brain damage. PKU is easily treated. The person with PKU must avoid food products with phenylalanine, and food products containing phenylalanine carry a warning label to help people with PKU. To avoid the complications of untreated PKU, every state requires PKU screening within the first days of birth. Public health laboratories screen over 97 percent of the 4 million babies born every year! As with any disease detection, laboratory professionals want to be sure that anyone who screens positive is in fact positive and anyone who screens negative is in fact negative. Thus, laboratories use the most precise equipment, careful procedures, double checking of positive screens, and other procedures to ensure that test results are accurate.

APHL ensures that laboratories and laboratory staff are adequately trained and aware of changes in the field to protect us from environmental, food, genetic, infectious disease, and global health hazards and that public policies on mandatory testing are grounded in the best available science.

Sally Kuykendall

See also: Bioterrorism; Core Competencies in Public Health; Emergency Preparedness and Response; Environmental Protection Agency; Infectious Diseases; Waterborne Diseases

Further Reading

Association of Public Health Laboratories. (2017). Retrieved from https://www.aphl.org/Pages/default.aspx.

Centers for Disease Control and Prevention (CDC). (2012). Good laboratory practices for biochemical genetic testing and newborn screening for inherited metabolic disorders. *Morbidity and Mortality Weekly Report, 61*(2). Retrieved from http://www.cdc.gov/mmwr/pdf/rr/rr6102.pdf.

ASSOCIATION OF STATE AND TERRITORIAL HEALTH OFFICIALS (ASTHO)

The Association of State and Territorial Health Officials (ASTHO) is a national nonprofit network of current and past public health officers in the United States, U.S. territories, District of Columbia, Mexico, and Canada. The main functions of ASTHO are to provide technical assistance to members, to disseminate best practices in public health, and to identify, assess, and educate members on laws and policies impacting public health practice. ASTHO's overall vision is to support public health officials in achieving the goal of "Healthy people thriving in a nation free of preventable illness and injury" (ASTHO, 2016).

The idea of a national association of health officials was first proposed in 1879 at a meeting of health officers from the state boards of health along the Mississippi River. As people migrated west, communicable diseases endemic to other areas of the globe were carried along. Multiple outbreaks of cholera, yellow fever, and smallpox occurred along trade routes and spread inland. In 1878, an outbreak of yellow fever in the Caribbean forced thousands of people to seek refuge in New Orleans. In response, New Orleans health officials established a quarantine station south of the city on the Mississippi River. All incoming ships were fumigated, and all passengers and sailors were checked for disease prior to docking. Ships with sick passengers or sailors were placed in quarantine. Efforts to thwart the virus failed, and yellow fever quickly spread through towns and cities on the river and inland throughout Louisiana, Mississippi, Tennessee, Kentucky, Indiana, Illinois, and Ohio. Current medical treatments of bloodletting, carbolic acid, and quinine were also ineffective. Before the epidemic faded out, 120,000 people contracted yellow fever including 20,000 people who died (WHYY, 2006). In 1879, the Sanitary Council of the Mississippi Valley convened delegates from the state boards of health to discuss measures to control future outbreaks. Although some attendees blamed New Orleans health officials for their inability to stop the disease, overall, the group agreed that a coordinated response was needed. Dr. J. M. Woodworth, Marine Hospital Service Surgeon General compared communicable diseases to enemy attack. Just as the nation used well-planned strategies to guard against enemy attacks, the nation needed prevention and intervention strategies to guard against communicable disease attacks. Over the next 50 years, groups of health officials met formally and informally. They primarily focused on quarantine rules and ways to control epidemics. Under the Social Security Act of 1935, health policies and programs expanded, and health officials needed technical assistance to navigate the many complex federal, state, and local laws. On March 23, 1942, the ASTHO became an official organization.

ASTHO's mission, "To transform public health within states and territories to help members dramatically improve health and wellness," is achieved through several pathways. ASTHO supports state and territorial health officials in becoming leaders, strengthens the capacity of public health agencies, provides a collective voice for state and territorial public health, coordinates public health efforts through dissemination of evidence-based programs and practices, and sustains the health and status of the ASTHO as a professional organization (ASTHO, 2016). In example, in 2011, the ASTHO partnered with the Centers for Disease Control and Prevention (CDC) to develop a toolkit for reducing and preventing healthcare–associated infections (HAI). The toolkit describes why controlling HAI is important and presents the most effective state health policies to eliminate HAI. People go to hospitals and health care centers for treatment of numerous injuries and illnesses. They also bring germs. One in 20 patients contracts an infection during health care treatment. Hospital-acquired infections cost an additional $33 billion in medical treatment every year. Prescribing prophylactic antibiotics or antivirals is not an ideal solution because excessive use produces drug resistance, immunocompromised patients are still at risk, and one cannot guess which antibiotics to prescribe without knowing which pathogens are lurking within or on the health center's doorknobs, waiting rooms, or countertops. The problem becomes more complicated because health care organizations are reluctant to report HAI for fear that people will stop using their facilities. The toolkit suggests a multifaceted approach that includes mandatory and accurate HAI reporting that allows health officials to monitor infections; creation of advisory councils; accreditation, training, and licensure to encourage best practices; and financial incentives and oversight. The interventions may be tailored to fit within various state health systems.

ASTHO serves as a clearinghouse of information for state and territorial health officials. Knowing how other systems effectively address health problems empowers members to fulfill their mission of promoting the health and safety of residents. ASTHO activities strengthen public health partnerships by creating a network of knowledgeable professionals who are engaged in continuous quality improvement of public health systems and practices.

Sally Kuykendall

See also: Administration, Health; Antibiotic Resistance; Core Competencies in Public Health; Epidemic; Health Policy; Infectious Diseases; Modern Era, Public Health in the; National Association of County and City Health Officials; Public Health Departments; Public Health Law

Further Reading

Association of State and Territorial Health Officials. (2016). Retrieved from http://www.astho.org/.

Association of State and Territorial Health Officials and Centers for Disease Control and Prevention. (2011). *Eliminating healthcare associated infections: State policy options.* Retrieved from http://www.cdc.gov/hai/pdfs/toolkits/toolkit-hai-policy-final_03-2011.pdf.

Sanitary Council of Mississippi Valley. (1879). *Minutes of the meeting of organization and proceedings of the Sanitary Council of the Mississippi Valley,* Memphis, April 30, May 1; Atlanta, May 5–9. National Library of Medicine. Retrieved from https://archive.org/details/63230070R.nlm.nih.gov.

Smillie, W. G. (1943). The National Board of Health 1879–1883. *American Journal of Public Health and the Nation's Health, 33*(8), 925–930. Retrieved from https://www.ncbi.nlm.nih.gov/pmc/articles/PMC1527526/pdf/amjphnation00698-0009.pdf.

WHYY. (2006). *The great fever.* American Experience. PBS. Retrieved from http://www.pbs.org/wgbh/amex/fever/peopleevents/e_1878.html.

ATTENTION-DEFICIT/HYPERACTIVITY DISORDER (ADHD)

Attention-deficit/hyperactivity disorder (ADHD) is a neurodevelopmental disorder where the nerve cells leading to the frontal lobe of the brain are missing the normal coating of proteins and phospholipids. This fatty coating known as myelin speeds up nerve transmission to create a superhighway for incoming information. Without myelin, messages are transmitted more slowly and the brain takes longer to process information from the outside world. As a result, people with ADHD can appear impulsive, have poor memory, or have difficulty paying attention. This inability to process information quickly creates serious public health challenges. Children and youth with ADHD are at higher risk of traumatic brain injury, car crashes, poisoning, self-injury, and suicide (Silva, Colvin, Hagemann, Stanley, & Bower, 2014). ADHD can lead to lifelong disability and death. People with ADHD are twice as likely to have other mental health disorders, such as oppositional defiant disorder, conduct disorder, learning disorders, anxiety, and depression (Cuffe, Visser, Holbrook, Danielson, Geryk, Wolraich, & McKeown, 2015). In 2011, 11 percent of children in the United States held a diagnosis of ADHD (Visser et al., 2014). Economists estimate that the total cost of treatment and lost workdays to seek care for ADHD amounted to $31.6 billion in 2000 (Birnbaum et al., 2005). Improved diagnosis and treatment may enable safe, productive, and satisfying lives for those with ADHD.

ADHD-like symptoms were first noted and studied in 1798 by Sir Alexander Crichton. In *An Inquiry into the Nature and Origin of Mental Derangement*, Crichton described an attention disorder (Lange et al., 2010, 242). He believed that the abnormality was due to an increased or decreased "sensibility of the nerves." The British pediatrician, Sir George Frederic Still (1868–1941), described cases of children with normal intelligence who appeared overly defiant and inattentive. Reflecting the values of the Victorian era, Still believed the problem was due to defective moral control. Still's cases typically presented with symptoms prior to age seven and displayed difficulty with delayed gratification and trouble concentrating (Lange et al., 2010, 244). Though Still's description does not completely fit the current definition of ADHD, his descriptions do provide some of the earliest records of the disorder. In 1932, a new disorder call *hyperkinetic disease of infancy* was coined by physicians Franz Kramer and Hans Pollnow (Lange et al., 2010, 247). The physicians described children with hyperkinetic disease as those who are always moving and cannot sit still for a second. The children reportedly ran around the room, climbed to worrisome heights, and were resistant when told to control their impulses. The children were unable to complete a set of tasks and were unresponsive when spoken to. Kramer and Pollnow believed that the disease was not restricted to children and may continue into adulthood.

The *Diagnostic and Statistical Manual of Mental Disorders* (*DSM*) is the primary handbook listing psychiatric problems and the associated symptoms. Psychiatrists and medical doctors use the *DSM* to diagnose mental disorders. The listing of *hyperkinetic reaction of childhood (or adolescence)* first appeared in the *Diagnostic and Statistical Manual of Mental Disorders II* of 1968. The American Psychiatric Association described the disorder as, "characterized by over activity, restlessness, distractibility, and short attention span, especially in young children; the behavior usually diminishes by adolescence" (APA, 1968, p. 50). The third edition of the DSM introduced attention deficit disorder with and without hyperactivity, shifting the focus from hyperactivity to inattention and poor impulse control. The fifth edition of the *DSM* divided ADHD into three subtypes: *predominantly hyperactive-impulsive presentation, predominantly inattentive,* and *combined presentation,* and added criteria to include diagnosis among older adolescents and adults (APA, 2013).

Symptoms of ADHD vary by age, gender, and situation. *Predominantly hyperactive-impulsive presentation* is characterized by excessive activity such as fidgeting, squirming, pacing, running, talkativeness, and impatience. People with *predominantly inattentive* type are easily distracted, messy, forgetful, and have trouble concentrating. They often lose important documents or personal items. On the other hand, the predominantly inattentive type can also be highly focused, remaining on tasks long after others would give up. The symptoms of both subtypes—hyperactivity and inattention—occur equally with *combined presentation*. In order for health professionals to make a diagnosis of ADHD, children must show at least six of the symptoms listed in the *DSM*, adults must show at least five of the symptoms, behaviors must occur in multiple settings (school, home, extracurricular activities, work, and community), symptoms must be severe enough to interfere with everyday life, and symptoms must be present for at least six months. The symptoms of ADHD are embarrassing and exhausting. Without treatment, the delayed ability to self-regulate behavior may impact school, employment, and interpersonal relationships (Brassett-Grundy & Butler, 2004). The person may have a history of suspension, expulsion, or run-ins with the criminal justice system. Over time, the individual can become withdrawn, anxious, depressed, suicidal, or self-medicate with alcohol or stimulant drugs.

Because people with ADHD have a high or normal intelligence, they often learn to compensate for the symptoms. However, as they get older and take on more responsibilities, strategies that were once successful begin to fail. It is important to know that there are effective treatments available, and it is better to seek effective treatment than to develop unhealthy behaviors. The Centers for Disease Control and Prevention (CDC) currently recommend cognitive behavioral therapy (CBT) as the first line of treatment. CBT teaches techniques to eliminate the behaviors that create problems, to make the most of the positive characteristics of the disorder and to learn new strategies to harness the power of hyperactivity or hyperfocus. Parent therapy teaches skills to manage children's behavior and develop a coordinated system of care for children with special health care needs. Evidence-based programs recommended by the CDC are Triple P (Positive

Parenting Program), Incredible Years, Parent-Child Interaction Therapy, and New Forest Parenting Programme. Medications may also be prescribed to speed up mental processes and help people with ADHD process information at a faster rate. Medications have been shown to reduce disruptive behavior, improve social interactions, improve goal-directed behavior and concentration, and reduce aggression. There are drawbacks to medication. Side effects include loss of appetite, weight gain, and trouble sleeping, and there is the potential for misuse of prescription stimulants. Since some of these drugs have not been on the market for very long, the long-term side effects of ADHD medications are still being explored (Martin, 2016).

The causes of ADHD are unknown. There appears to be a strong genetic component. ADHD tends to run in families. Other factors that may contribute to developing ADHD are low birth weight, premature birth or birth complications, and maternal tobacco, alcohol, and substance use while pregnant. Future directions for ADHD research include finding a consistent genetic marker. Some studies are also trying to determine if there are differences in genotypes that distinguish one type of ADHD from another. Longitudinal studies are also in process to research the long-term outcomes of individuals with ADHD.

The goal for public health is not to cure ADHD but to enable individuals to survive their impulses in order to maximize their potential in society. People who live with ADHD can adapt to their environments and situations in highly creative, humorous, and novel ways. They are not afraid to take risks, to challenge how we think about and deal with problems, and to try new, ingenious solutions. Children, youth, and adults with ADHD often struggle to overcome the perceptions and frustrations of others. Through these life experiences, they develop a strong sense of justice, compassion, generosity, humility, and resilience. ADHD creates very powerful and interesting personalities. The challenge for public health is to reduce stigma against those with neurodevelopmental disorders, ensure early identification and diagnosis, and secure early referral to evidence-based treatments.

Alison C. Walensky

See also: Behavioral Health; Children's Health; Genetics; Mental Health

Further Reading

American Psychiatric Association. *Diagnostic and Statistical Manual of Mental Disorders* (2nd ed.). (1968). Washington, DC: American Psychiatric Association.

American Psychiatric Association. *Diagnostic and Statistical Manual of Mental Disorders* (5th ed.). (2013). Arlington, VA: American Psychiatric Association.

Birnbaum, H., Kessler, R., Lowe, S., Secnik, K., Greenberg, P., Leong, S., & Swensen, A. (2005). Costs of attention deficit-hyperactivity disorder (ADHD) in the US: Excess costs of persons with ADHD and their family members in 2000. *Current Medical Research and Opinion*, *21*(2), 195–205.

Brassett-Grundy, A., & Butler, N. (2004). *Prevalence and adult outcomes of attention-deficit/hyperactivity disorder: Evidence from a 30-year prospective longitudinal study.* Bedford Group for Lifecourse and Statistical Studies Occasional Paper: No. 2. London: Institute of Education, University of London.

Cuffe, S. P., Visser, S. N., Holbrook, J. R., Danielson, M. L., Geryk, L. L., Wolraich, M. L., & McKeown, R. E. (2015). ADHD and psychiatric comorbidity: Functional outcomes in a school-based sample of children. *Journal of Attention Disorders.* Retrieved from http://journals.sagepub.com/doi/abs/10.1177/1087054715613437#articleCitationDownloadContainer.

Lange, K. W., Reichl, S., Lange, K. M., Tucha, L., & Tucha, O. (2010). The history of attention deficit hyperactivity disorder. *Attention Deficit and Hyperactivity Disorders*, 2(4), 241–255.

Martin, B. (2016). Future directions in ADHD. *Psych Central.* Retrieved September 13, 2015, from http://psychcentral.com/lib/future-directions-in-adhd/.

Silva, D., Colvin, L., Hagemann, E., Stanley, F., & Bower, C. (2014). Children diagnosed with attention deficit disorder and their hospitalisations: Population data linkage study. *European Child & Adolescent Psychiatry*, 23(11), 1043–1050.

Visser, S. N., Danielson, M. L., Bitsko, R. H., Holbrook, J. R., Kogan, M. D., Ghandour, R. M., & Blumberg, S. J. (2014). New research: Trends in the parent-report of health care provider-diagnosed and medicated attention-deficit/hyperactivity disorder: United States, 2003–2011. *Journal of the American Academy of Child & Adolescent Psychiatry*, 53, 34–46, e2.

B

BAKER, SARA JOSEPHINE (1873–1945)

Sara Josephine Baker revolutionized public health practices to create systems of care for children and infants. Many of the techniques Dr. Baker established are still used today. "Jo" Baker was born to an affluent family in Poughkeepsie, New York. Her father, Daniel Mosher Baker, was a lawyer. Her mother, Jenny Harwood Brown, was alumna of the first degree-granting institution for women in the United States—Vassar College. Jo was expected to follow her mother's example until her father died suddenly. To help support the family, Jo forfeited her scholarship at Vassar and spent a year teaching herself biology so that she could attend the Women's Medical College of the New York Infirmary founded by sisters Elizabeth and Emily Blackwell. Elizabeth was the first female to earn a medical degree in the United States, and Emily graduated from Case Western University School of Medicine after being rejected by 12 other medical schools because she was female. The Blackwells created the medical school to support other females interested in medicine. Although Baker was a good student, she failed one course on "The Normal Child." Retaking the course proved both a frustration and a revelation. Her interest in children was furthered through an internship at the New England Hospital for Women and Children in Boston. In Boston, Jo was exposed to the horrors of poverty, addictions, epidemics, and poor health.

In 1899, Dr. Baker opened a private practice in New York City. Living conditions in New York City were particularly awful for her patients. Thousands of immigrants crowded into squalid tenement houses or lived on the streets. Young orphaned and abandoned children begged, stole, or worked to survive. Children drank beer because it was more freely available and was safer than milk. Since her clients were unable to pay for medical services, Baker took a part-time job as a New York City medical inspector to subsidize her practice. Baker's autobiography, *Fighting for Life*, describes her first experiences in Hell's Kitchen, New York:

> I climbed stair after stair, knocked on door after door, met drunk after drunk, filthy mother after filthy mother and met dying baby after dying baby. . . . There was no dodging the hopelessness of it all. It was an appalling summer, too, with an average of fifteen hundred babies dying each week in the city; lean, miserable, wailing little souls carried off wholesale by dysentery. (1939)

New immigrants accustomed to living on farms with fresh air and nutritious foods were ill-equipped to deal with crowded, urban living and fatal epidemics. In addition to alcoholism and dysentery, health officials battled smallpox, cholera, typhoid,

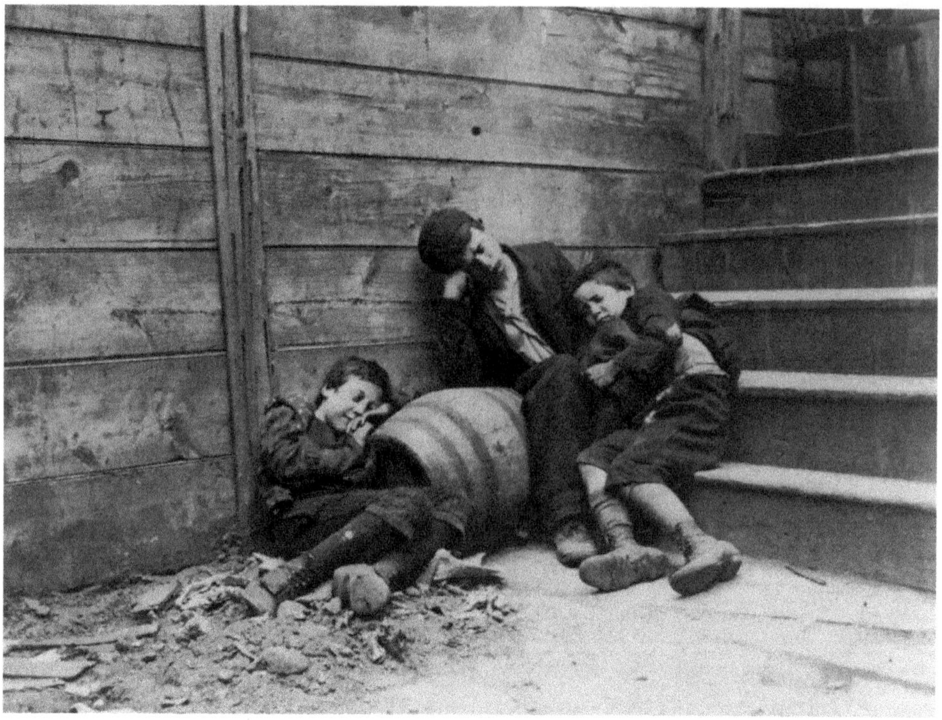

Street children in a tenement neighborhood of New York City, photo by Jacob Riis, ca. 1888. Abandoned children begged, stole, or worked long hours to survive the streets of New York City in the late 1800s. Homeless children drank beer because it was cheap and less contaminated than milk. (Library of Congress)

diphtheria, measles, and political corruption. Some health officials simply resigned themselves to the hopeless situation, neglected patients, and fabricated notes. By 1907, Baker was appointed the assistant commissioner for health. She worked on several projects of smallpox vaccinations and typhoid control. She was also involved in the identification and capture of Mary Mallon, referred to as Typhoid Mary. Within a year, Baker was appointed director of the New York City Bureau of Child Hygiene—the first public health department in the nation to focus exclusively on children's health and welfare.

Through the Bureau of Child Hygiene, Baker revolutionized public health. Previously, health officials tracked down specific incidents of disease and provided individualized treatment or control. Baker created a system of preventive care drawing on ideas from social medicine. The bureau introduced initiatives in midwifery training, visiting nurses, school nurses, health education, disease prevention, well baby care, stations providing safe milk and care for babies, and sibling care programs. Visiting nurses checked on every new mother within a day of delivery providing basic health education. The nurses encouraged mothers to breastfeed rather than giving their infants beer (Epstein, 2013). They taught mothers about germs and how to keep babies safe. The Little Mothers Leagues was a program for girls, aged 12 and over, who were responsible for caring for younger siblings while the mother worked. The bureau's programs were realistic, embracing the reality of life for poor immigrants in New York City while maximizing limited resources. Baker also created a system for administering silver nitrate. Silver nitrate is dropped into the eyes of infants to prevent blindness due to congenital syphilis. The delivery system featured ampules with the correct dose of medication.

In the early 1900s, birth control was nonexistent and abortions were dangerous. Hundreds of newborns were abandoned on the streets every year. Catholic charities refused to accept the orphans under the assumption that the children were born out of wedlock. The Bureau of Child Hygiene opened a special hospital where trained nurses cared for these abandoned infants. Despite qualified care and good nutrition, mortality rates were still high. Approximately 50 percent of abandoned infants died. At the same time, Baker noticed that while the hygiene measures improved life for infants born to poor mothers, infants born to wealthy mothers did not fare as well. Baker hypothesized that in addition to nutrition and hygiene, infants needed love and attention. As an experiment, the bureau paid some of the poor mothers who had worked with the visiting nurses to care for the sickest of the abandoned infants. The experiment was a success. Infant mortality rates among this very vulnerable population were cut in half. Baker proved that a safe, stable, loving home environment is just as critical to healthy childhood development as nutrition and hygiene. By the time Baker retired, infant mortality rate in New York City had decreased from 115 deaths per 1,000 live births to 69 deaths per 1,000 live births (Statistical Analysis and Reporting and Quality Improvements Units of the Bureau of Vital Statistics, 2011). Baker's vision of infant and child care was replicated in other cities and states, although not without controversy. Some politicians and physicians, including representatives of the American Medical Association, objected to Baker's social medicine. Opponents believed that the high infant mortality rate of poor communities was eugenics, a way to eliminate undesirable genetic traits. After retirement Baker continued to advocate for children and disadvantaged populations. She represented the United States at the League of Nations, was active in professional organizations, and wrote numerous books and articles on children's health.

What is particularly remarkable about Baker's achievements is that she envisioned and implemented major changes within a system dominated by male politicians, health administrators, and physicians. Baker, like many other women of her era, was all too familiar with gender discrimination. To blend into the system, she kept her hair short and parted in the middle and wore men's suits with collared shirts and ties. The strategy worked because Baker joked that some of her male colleagues forgot that she was female. In 1915, the dean of New York University and Bellevue Medical College asked Baker to teach the child hygiene course as part of the doctorate in public health program. Although the school only accepted males, Baker negotiated a condition that she be allowed to take courses in the program. Through the program, she earned her doctorate in public health and continued to teach for another 15 years.

Although Baker was a fearless role model for female physicians, Hansen (2002) notes that Baker was a missed opportunity to serve as a role model for LGBTQ youth interested in the sciences. Despite dedicating her life to children, Baker never had children of her own and never married. After retiring, Baker and her long-term partner, novelist Ida Wylie, moved to New Jersey to live with Louise Pearce, another female physician. Baker and Wylie were members of a group where many of the members were openly lesbian. Hansen speculates that although Baker kept her sexuality private, there is a need to acknowledge and honor the achievements of LGBTQ individuals within public health. Recognizing the achievements of individuals from minority sexual groups encourages others to achieve incredible feats.

Sara Josephine Baker's achievements in social medicine made her a leading figure in public health. Many of her programs in child welfare are still used today. Visiting nurses is now recognized as a leading evidence-based program in child development with lifelong benefits of reducing substance abuse, health care costs, and poverty. The concepts that Baker used, strategically using limited resources to empower people within the community to prevent disease, are highly applicable to current public health challenges.

Sally Kuykendall

See also: Anderson, Elizabeth Milbank; Blackwell, Elizabeth; Children's Health; Infant Mortality; Mallon, Mary; Maternal Health; Public Health in the United States, History of

Further Reading

Baker, S. J. (1939). *Fighting for life*. New York: Macmillan.

Epstein, H. (2013). The doctor who made a revolution. *The New York Review of Books*. Retrieved from http://www.nybooks.com/articles/2013/09/26/doctor-who-made-revolution/.

Hansen, B. (2002). Public careers and private sexuality: Some gay and lesbian lives in the history of medicine and public health. *American Journal of Public Health, 92*(1): 36–44. Retrieved from https://www.ncbi.nlm.nih.gov/pmc/articles/PMC1447383/.

National Library of Medicine. (n.d.). Dr. S. Josephine Baker. Retrieved from https://www.nlm.nih.gov/changingthefaceofmedicine/physicians/biography_19.html.

Statistical Analysis and Reporting and Quality Improvements Units of the Bureau of Vital Statistics. (2011). *Summary of vital statistics 2010, the City of New York: Population and mortality.* Retrieved from http://www.nyc.gov/html/records/pdf/govpub/6551as_2010_final_population_&_mortality.pdf.

BEERS, CLIFFORD WHITTINGHAM (1876–1943)

During the middle of the 19th century, pioneering mental health reformer Dorothea Lynde Dix created state mental hospitals to remove mentally ill people from prisons and jailhouses. Over time, these new mental institutions struggled with intractable chronic illness, lack of funding, and bad publicity. Society slipped back into old beliefs that people with mental illness had done something wrong to deserve such a horrific fate and state mental hospitals fell into disrepair and disrepute. Suffering from bipolar disorder, paranoia, and delusions, Clifford Whittingham Beers spent three years in such institutions. His chronicles of thoughts, experiences, and treatment revealed the world of a confused mind, greedy, negligent doctors, and unqualified, abusive attendants. Beers's autobiography challenged society to examine current attitudes and care of the mentally ill. His efforts reignited the field of mental health, leading to the creation of the National Institute of Mental Health.

Clifford was born on March 30, 1876, in New Haven, Connecticut, to Ida Cook and Robert Beers. Ida was the oldest daughter and primary caregiver of her birth family. When she moved from her parent's home in Marietta, Georgia, to live with her husband in New Haven, her four unmarried sisters and one brother followed. Ida's siblings did not work. Despite being of modest means, Mr. Beers dutifully provided for the household's needs. There was no history of mental illness on the father's side. Mr. Beers was 27 years older than his wife, quiet, and conflict avoidant and otherwise healthy. Members of the Cook family suffered from depression and were known for exhibiting eccentric or erratic behavior. In those days, doctors avoided assigning a diagnosis of mental illness for fear of stigmatizing the client and the family. Of Ida and Robert's six children, one died during infancy, one died of a brain tumor, and three died in mental institutions. Two of the sons committed suicide. Clifford experienced emotional ups and downs as a child and adolescent. The mood swings did not affect him academically or socially. In school, he was an average student who excelled when pushed. He did fear that his father might commit suicide because of financial pressures. Otherwise, his childhood was atraumatic and unremarkable.

In June 1894, as Clifford was preparing for college entrance exams, his older brother Samuel had a grand mal seizure. Since Clifford was a student and available during the day, he became his brother's main caregiver. As Clifford nursed his brother through publicly embarrassing tonic-clonic seizures and loss of consciousness, he became increasingly obsessed with the idea that he may also develop epilepsy, a disease once believed to be a form of mental illness. While attending classes at Yale's Sheffield Scientific School, Clifford experienced paralyzing anxiety attacks. He stopped attending lessons and only returned after sympathetic professors promised not to call on him. Despite struggles and hypochondriacal fears, Clifford was socially active. He held prestigious positions and wrote for the school newspaper. After graduating, Clifford moved to New York City. On June 15, 1900, while working as a clerk at Bankers Life Insurance Company, he experienced a severe anxiety attack. His voice was paralyzed, and his handwriting wobbly. Convinced that something was horribly wrong, he requested two weeks' vacation, went back to his residence, destroyed personal papers, and journeyed back to New Haven.

In the family home, Sam was dying of a brain tumor. Clifford spent the week in bed, depressed and contemplating suicide. On June 23, he climbed out of his third-story bedroom window, hung off the window ledge, and dropped to the ground.

His arms scraped against the house as he fell, breaking his fall. Missing the sidewalk by inches, he landed on his feet on soft ground. His point of impact was in front of the dining room window where the family was eating lunch. Clifford recalled that his hypochondriacal obsessions were immediately replaced by paranoid delusions. He believed that he had committed some unknown crime and everyone around him was a detective or spy attempting to gather evidence for his upcoming trial. He refused to speak and was diagnosed with manic depression, now known as bipolar disorder.

The Beers family arranged for Clifford's physical and emotional recovery in a sanatorium. Sanatoriums were private, for-profit institutions managed by doctors. Families paid a basic per capita fee with additional charges for incidentals or private duty care. Since little was known about mental illness, the physician-administrators were less interested in treatment and primarily concerned with making money. Patients were crowded into rooms with a few untrained, supervising attendants. In 1901, the Beers family took Clifford out of the sanatorium and paid one of the attendants to care for Clifford in his home in Wallingford. The Beers family visited frequently. The attendant and his family were kind. However, Clifford's paranoia, delusions, and hallucinations continued. He believed that everyone in the village knew of his imagined crime and that the people who came to see him were not really his family but impersonators trying to trick him.

Seeing that he was not recovering in Wallingford, the Beers family committed Clifford again, this time to a private, nonprofit mental institution. His brother, George Merwin Beers, assumed power of attorney. Clifford was comforted by a regular routine. However, his mind continued to deceive him. He believed that the staff and other patients were detectives conspiring against him and that the George who visited him was an imposter. Clifford refused to speak to the visitor George and devised an elaborate scheme to get a message to the real George. He convinced a patient with outside privileges to get George's address from the New Haven directory. He wrote a letter to his brother and asked another patient to address the envelope so that his imagined spies would not intercept it. In the letter, Clifford explained his delusions and instructed his brother to bring the letter as proof that he was George. On August 30, 1902, George appeared for the planned visit and produced the letter. Clifford described a moment of epiphany:

> Untruth became Truth. A large part of what was once my old world was again mine. To me, at least, my mind seemed to have found itself, for the gigantic web of false beliefs in which it had been all but hopelessly enmeshed I now immediately recognized as a snare of delusions. That the Gordian knot of mental torture should be cut and swept away by the mere glance of a willing eye is like a miracle. (Beers, 1907, p. 85)

As the depression dissipated, Clifford progressed into mania. While attending church, he heard the scripture and got the idea that God was sending him on a crusade to reform the mental health system. Clifford became extremely hyperactive, slept only two to three hours a day, wrote long letters to relatives and friends, and started fighting the attendants who abused patients. Doctors placed him in a straight jacket and moved him to a ward for violent patients.

On November 8, 1902, George arranged for Clifford's transfer to a state-funded mental hospital. This third institution was the worst. The guards were unqualified, petty, and spiteful. They yelled at, choked, beat, and unnecessarily restrained patients. It was not long before Clifford was placed on the violent ward again. For four months, he lived in a small, barred cell with no bed. Personal hygiene was restricted. At times, he was not able to shower for up to three weeks. When he finally transferred out of the locked ward, he was granted outside privileges. With freedom to walk into town under attendant supervision, Clifford purchased writing paper. He wrote a 32-page letter to the governor of Connecticut describing the conditions of the state hospital. On his next visit to the city, he slipped the letter into an unsold copy of the *Saturday Evening Post* with instructions to mail the letter. He also included a warning that since he had attached a two cent stamp to the envelope, not mailing the letter would be a federal crime because one was interfering with the U.S. Postal Service. The shop clerk found and mailed the letter. In the letter, Clifford introduced himself:

> I take pleasure in informing you that I am in the Crazy Business and am holding my job down with ease and a fair degree of grace. Being in the Crazy Business, I understand certain phrases of the business about which you know nothing. (Beers, 1907, p. 196)

The letter described staff abuses against patients, including fatal assaults. He called for reform of the state mental hospital system and threatened to contact the press if the state failed to investigate. The governor contacted the superintendent of the asylum and conditions improved temporarily. Clifford realized that in order to bring about real reform, he needed to get well. He wrote graphic descriptions about his experiences and relationships, and on September 10, 1903, he was discharged. His enlightened employer at Bankers Life Insurance Company offered him his job back. The man believed that illness is illness and it did not matter whether an employee was physically ill or mentally ill. He encouraged Clifford to take care of himself and to rest as needed.

At the time, mental illness was considered a sign of moral impairment, and many people even believed that mental illness was caused by masturbation. Thus, few people were willing to disclose personal struggles or history. Beers consulted with colleagues at Yale and preeminent psychiatrists of the day. The director of the Psychiatric Institute of the New York State Hospital system, Adolf Meyer, and William James, professor of philosophy and psychology at Harvard University, encouraged Beers to publish his experiences. In 1908, Beers published *A Mind That Found Itself*. The autobiography described Beers's delusions, paranoid responses, and treatment. He intentionally did not name the institutions because he wanted readers to focus on the abuse of power and human rights atrocities rather than blaming one specific institution. Although Clifford did not condone the abuse, he understood it. Without proper training, guards developed harsh treatments as a way to manage the large, crowded inpatient wards. Motivating through fear seemed quicker and more effective than reasoning with a confused mind. Furthermore, power corrupts. As the guards realized their uncontested power over other human beings, ethical boundaries blurred and egos inflated. Beers's calm, simple, and direct style of writing aroused public sympathy and protest.

In 1908, Beers founded the Connecticut Society for Mental Hygiene, the organization that eventually became the National Institute of Mental Health (1946). Its mission was to improve public attitudes, improve services, prevent mental illness, and promote mental health. The first task was counting the number of mentally ill patients in the country and medical professionals who could treat them. Subsequent surveys and reports on the conditions of state mental hospitals prompted changes such as hiring more social workers. In 1913, Beers founded the Clifford Beers Clinic, the first outpatient mental health clinic in the United States. And in 1930, he organized the International Congress on Mental Health. Over time, Beers's paranoia returned. His beloved brother George committed suicide after going to a psychiatrist and being told that his complaints did not rise to hospitalization. Clifford was severely affected. The disease he had worked to prevent had claimed the life of another loved one. Clifford was hospitalized once again and eventually died of bronchopneumonia.

Clifford Whittingham Beers led a crusade against mental illness, advocating for humanity and compassion for those suffering from mental illness. His willingness to reveal his own vulnerability created a movement that recognized the rights of those with mental illness and ways to prevent the downward spiral.

Sally Kuykendall

See also: Behavioral Health; Disability; Dix, Dorothea Lynde; Mental Health; Mental Illness; Substance Abuse and Mental Health Services Administration; *Controversies in Public Health:* Controversy 2

Further Reading

Beers, C. W. (1907). *A mind that found itself*. New York: Longmans, Green.

Beers, C. W. (2010). A mind that found itself: An autobiography. *American Journal of Public Health, 100*(12), 2354–2356.

Capps, D. (2009). Mental illness, religion, and the rational mind: The case of Clifford W. Beers. *Mental Health, Religion & Culture, 12*(2), 157–174. doi:10.1080/13674670802398543

Dain, N. (1980). *Clifford W. Beers, advocate for the insane*. Pittsburgh: University of Pittsburg Press.

BEHAVIORAL HEALTH

Behavioral health is the medical science and art that relates personal behaviors to health and well-being. This interdisciplinary field combines aspects of psychology, sociology, health, and medicine to identify and apply effective ways to promote health-enhancing behavior. There is a wide range in severity and outcomes of behavioral health problems. An estimated one out of seven children (ages two to eight) is diagnosed with a mental, behavioral, or developmental disorder (Bitsko, Holbrook, Robinson, Kaminski, Ghandour, Smith, & Peacock, 2016). In transition to adulthood, the individual may mask socially unacceptable behaviors through substance abuse, overeating, physical inactivity, smoking, or self-harm. Long-term behavioral problems interfere with social relationships, education, and employment and increase risk of early mortality. Two-thirds of nursing home residents exhibit emotional and behavioral problems (U.S. Department of Health and Human Services, Administration on Aging, 2001). There is an increasing need for behavioral health specialists who work with elderly clients to manage behaviors related to dementia, incontinence, depression, and anxiety as well as life transitions, death of loved ones, chronic illnesses, or family discord. Regardless of age, early diagnosis and intervention are important to deconstruct negative behaviors and learn new, health-enhancing behaviors. Often used interchangeably with mental health, behavioral health goes beyond the psychiatric diagnosis to include psychosocial care. The goal of therapy is to help the individual attain normal developmental milestones, enjoy healthy social interactions, and practice positive coping strategies. Criticisms of behavioral health are that practices focus on symptoms rather than underlying causes. Putting the responsibility for change on the individual, rather than society, dismisses the impact of discrimination, poverty, or abuse on mental and behavioral health. Public health addresses primary behavioral issues of attention-deficit/hyperactivity disorder (ADHD), conduct disorder, and oppositional defiant disorder (ODD), as well as secondary problems of smoking, drinking, or overeating.

Behavioral health encompasses a range of neurological conditions and behaviors. Among children and adolescents, ADHD, conduct disorder, ODD, and self-harm are some of the classic behavioral health problems. ADHD is a neurodevelopmental disorder where the nerve cells of the brain lack the fatty coating needed to expedite nerve transmission. The ADHD brain takes longer to take in and process information. As a result, people with ADHD appear impulsive or inattentive. Conduct disorder is an emotional disorder characterized by aggressiveness, destructiveness, deceit, and persistent violation of normal social boundaries. ODD is excessive and persistent rejection of authority with overly argumentative or vindictive behavior. Self-harm is a behavioral condition where the individual purposely injures himself or herself through cutting or burning. Behavioral health treatments vary based on diagnosis and severity. Psychotherapy focuses on helping the client to find positive ways to express and control negative emotions. Treatment focuses on changing problem behaviors, building skills to help the individuals manage their behaviors, and helping parents to manage children's behavior.

Although psychotherapy focuses on the individual client, public health uses a population-based approach to prevent behavioral health problems and their sequelae. Pediatric health clinics are a great opportunity to screen for mental, behavioral, and developmental disorders (MBDDs) and to refer the patient for treatment. Population-based approaches are visiting nurses, parent training classes, and early childhood education programs. A large-scale study of more than 35,000 children found that inadequate health care coverage, fair or poor parental mental health, living in a family struggling to pay bills, difficulty in attaining child care, lack of neighborhood social support, and lack of access to recreational amenities were risk factors for MBDDs (Bitsko, Holbrook, Robinson, Kaminski, Ghandour, Smith, & Peacock, 2016). Results suggest that improving access to health care, supporting families, and community improvement may promote healthy child development and reduce the need for some behavioral health services.

Many chronic and acute health problems are related to personal lifestyle choices and behavior. Smoking causes chronic obstructive pulmonary disease and lung cancer. Alcohol abuse causes pancreatitis, hepatitis, cirrhosis, and cancers of the mouth, esophagus, breast, and liver. Physical inactivity and overeating cause cardiovascular disease, diabetes, and hypertension. Public health uses aspects of behavioral health to change behaviors. There are numerous ways to change behaviors—scientific research, food or health warning labels, financial incentives, cigarette or alcohol taxes, even "nudges" (Galizzi, 2014). Simple nudges, such as putting fruits and vegetables near the cafeteria checkout line rather than candy and cookies; using 100-calorie packs to limit caloric intake; or using smaller plates or dark-colored plates are subtle, noncoercive ways to encourage good nutrition. The media, particularly public service announcements on television, can effectively create behavioral change (Das, 2016). The transtheoretical model is one of many models used to create population-based behavioral change. By deconstructing misconceptions, educating and empowering, people can stop smoking or adopt healthy behaviors. Future directions are to investigate the most effective ways to achieve population-based changes.

Lifestyle and cognition affect physical and mental health. Behavioral health is a field of medicine and public health that addresses the unique conduct of individuals and the impact on health. The symptoms and consequences of behavioral health problems can be seen from early childhood to late adulthood. Public health works to prevent behavioral health disorders by supporting populations with special needs and ensuring access to effective treatment programs.

Sally Kuykendall

See also: Adverse Childhood Experiences; Attention-Deficit/Hyperactivity Disorder; Child Maltreatment; Children's Health; Community Health Centers; Mental Health; Mental Illness; National Institutes of Health; State, Local, and Territorial Health

Departments; Substance Abuse and Mental Health Services Administration; Social Determinants of Health; Transtheoretical Model; *Controversies in Public Health:* Controversy 2

Further Reading

American Psychological Association. (n.d.). *Mental and behavioral health and older Americans.* Retrieved from http://www.apa.org/about/gr/issues/aging/mental-health.aspx.

Bitsko, R. H., Holbrook, J. R., Robinson, L. R., Kaminski, J. W., Ghandour, R., Smith, C., & Peacock, G. (2016). Health care, family, and community factors associated with mental, behavioral, and developmental disorders in early childhood—United States, 2011–2012. *Morbidity and Mortality Weekly Report*, 65(9), 221–226. doi:10.15585/mmwr.mm6509a1

Das, S. (2016). Television is more effective in bringing behavioral change: Evidence from heat-wave awareness campaign in India. *World Development*, *88*, 107–121. Retrieved from http://dx.doi.org.ezproxy.sju.edu/10.1016/j.worlddev.2016.07.009.

Galizzi, M. M. (2014). What is really behavioral in behavioral health policy? And does it work? *Applied Economic Perspectives and Policy*, *36*(1), 25–60.

Oyama, O. N., & Burg, M. A. (2016). *The behavioral health specialist in primary care: Skills for integrated practice.* New York: Springer.

U.S. Department of Health and Human Services, Administration on Aging. (2001). *Older adults and mental health: Issues and opportunities.*

BELMONT REPORT, THE

The principles within *The Belmont Report* represent the most important ethical guidelines for conducting biomedical and behavioral human research in the modern United States. The purpose of *The Belmont Report* was to summarize the ethical principles and guidelines essential to protecting the safety and well-being of patients and human participants in research. This was particularly important in the post-Tuskegee syphilis experiment era of the United States. The scientific community was struggling with the ethical horrors of the Tuskegee Syphilis Study, Willowbrook Hepatitis Studies, and the cancer studies at New York City's Jewish Chronic Disease Hospital. In Tuskegee, Alabama, doctors did not use readily available cures for patients with syphilis so that they could study the effects of untreated syphilis on an African American community. *The Belmont Report* was commissioned to help prevent such unethical research from ever occurring again. *The Belmont Report* guidelines are still used by researchers and research institutions in the United States.

In 1974, the National Commission for the Protection of Biomedical and Behavioral Research was created by the National Research Act in 1974. One of the major responsibilities of the commission was to identify the basic ethical principles that should underlie how biomedical and behavioral research with human participants is conducted (Office for Human Research Protections, 2016). Issued in 1978, *The Belmont Report* outlined three core ethical principles: respect for persons, beneficence, and justice. These core ethical principles are essential to contemporary research, particularly because they ensure that human participants are protected from the harms and dangers of unethical research. These recommendations and guidelines still form the foundation of how research is conducted and regulated by the Department of Health, Education, and Welfare. Additionally, institutional review boards throughout the country rely on *The Belmont Report* to guide their decision making for allowing or rejecting research studies.

The first of these core principles, respect for persons, involves the protection of individual autonomy and the need for research scientists to treat human participants with dignity and honor participants' right to make their own decision regarding study participation. Respect for persons means that the researcher will provide the participant with easily understandable information on the nature and purpose of the study, what to expect during the study, potential risks or discomforts, anticipated benefits, and alternatives to participating in the study and that participants have the right to ask questions, to not take part in the study or withdraw from a study at any time, and be free of pressure to participate. As a result of *The Belmont Report*, research scientists must provide informed consent to all human study participants whenever there are risks—even minor ones—to well-being as a result of study participation. Informed consent is an ongoing process. As the study evolves, researchers are obligated to keep participants advised of risks and changes to the study.

The second core ethical principle, beneficence, involves the responsibility of the researcher to not harm human participants. This is done by minimizing risks, maximizing benefits, and not carrying out research that is inappropriately harmful or detrimental to human health. This ethical principle was likened within *The Belmont Report* to the Greek maxim of "do no harm" and prohibits research that would seriously harm participants. Under the principle of beneficence, research like that done in the Tuskegee syphilis experiment would not have been carried out due to the patient harm that occurred from prolonged syphilis infection. A modern-day example of beneficence in contemporary biomedical research is during clinical trials with new medications; as soon as one medication in the trial shows greater efficacy than the others, all patients must be switched to that medication to maximize their well-being, and likewise, if one medication shows worse outcomes than the others, then the patients are asked to cease taking that medication. According to the concept of justice in *The Belmont Report*, it would be unethical to withhold human participants from a beneficial medication and likewise, it would be unethical to ask human participants to continue taking a known harmful medication. In this way, beneficence ensures that the well-being and protection of individual human research participants is protected at all phases of the research endeavor.

The third principle outlined by *The Belmont Report* is that of justice. The concept of justice concerns which populations receive the benefits of research and which populations bear the burden of research. Justice means that research does not exploit vulnerable populations and that all populations in society deserve to benefit from the findings of biomedical and behavioral research. One example of the importance of justice is how research scientists recruit human participants for their research. It would be unjust for patients from one population to bear all of the burdens of research so that a different population will benefit. Therefore, research scientists attempt to ensure that the burdens of research are evenly and appropriately spread throughout the population, and that the findings of research are distributed equitably. Justice does not only include interracial justice, but intergender, intersocioeconomic, and other social differences.

The Belmont Report and its underlying ethical principles and guidelines have been tremendously influential in shaping how modern research is ethically regulated and protected from ethical misconduct. In this way, *The Belmont Report* represents one of the most important ethical documents in the domain of human research in the world.

Shayan Waseh

See also: Code of Ethics; Ethics in Public Health and Population Health; Greco-Roman Era, Public Health in the; Hippocrates; Research; Tuskegee Syphilis Study

Further Reading

National Institute of Health. (2016). *Protecting human research participants.* Retrieved from https://phrp.nihtraining.com/codes/02_codes.php.

Office for Human Research Protections. (2016). *The Belmont Report.* Retrieved from https://www.hhs.gov/ohrp/regulations-and-policy/belmont-report/index.html.

Sims, J. M. (2010). A brief review of the Belmont Report. *Dimensions of Critical Care Nursing, 29*(4), 173–174.

BIOSTATISTICS

Biostatistics is a specialty field, a branch of applied mathematics that focuses on converting complex biomedical data into usable information. For example, many people fear dying by plane crash, lightning, or assault with a firearm. Using biostatistics to calculate the probability of fatal injuries, the odds of dying by plane crash (1 in 96,566), lightning strike (1 in 164,968), or assault with a firearm (1 in 358) are much less than motor vehicle crash (1 in 112) (National Safety Council, 2016). Knowing the potential for death by motor vehicle crashes emphasizes safe driving techniques, such as wearing a seat belt, respecting speed limits, not driving under the influence, and not using a cell phone while driving. Public health practitioners use biostatistics to understand the extent of a health problem and to identify effective treatment or prevention programs. Because biostatistics deals with critical health issues, biostatisticians follow ethical guidelines in research.

Biostatistics is a portmanteau, created by blending the words "biology" and "statistics." In practice, biostatistics encompasses other disciplines beyond biology. Biostatistical techniques are used in medicine, sociology, psychology, pharmacology, health policy, program planning, and health education. These statistical analyses study real-world problems as opposed to mathematical theory or abstract mathematical concepts. Biostatisticians partner with program planners, community organizations, nonprofit groups, clinical staff, and public health practitioners to plan, gather, and analyze data.

To create data for analysis, raw data are collected using the scientific method. To review, the scientific method is the systematic process used by scientists to investigate, explore, describe, or explain concepts. The scientific method commences with an in depth review of the current literature in the field of interest, reading and studying scholarly articles and books. The literature review spotlights what is known and what needs to be known next to alleviate the problem. Scientists take ideas of what needs to be studied and create the research hypothesis or research question. The research hypothesis is used to design the research study and methods of collecting the data. Once results are collected, statisticians use mathematical formulas to convert the raw numbers into a form that tests the hypothesis. In public health, common statistical calculations are means, medians, modes, standard deviations, probabilities, confidence intervals, t-tests, analysis of variances (ANOVA), relative risk, odds ratios, incidence, and prevalence rates. Once the study results are analyzed, researchers can draw logical inferences. Scientists can determine whether two or more variables are correlated, existing together at the same point or within the same group of people; whether a health problem is caused by a specific factor; or whether one program or treatment is more effective than other treatments. Biostatistics allows scientists to resolve questions of whether the results are significant enough to qualify as a true difference. Imagine that the National Safety Council develops a media campaign to reduce driving while intoxicated, speeding, and distracted. After one year, deaths from motor vehicle crashes decrease from 1.3 per 100 million miles traveled to 1.2 per million miles traveled. Biostatistics can determine whether the program made a significant impact on deaths due to motor vehicle crashes.

In order to perform the correct mathematical calculation, the statistician must know how data are constructed, collected, analyzed, and interpreted. For example, it is impossible to calculate the average age of study participants from a survey that asks study participants to check their age group from the following options: 18 to 29 years, 30 to 39 years, 40 to 49 years, or 50 years and above. Statisticians and researchers know what one can legitimately do with specific types of data. Failure to correctly analyze data could lead to misinformation and faulty decision making. In public health, doctors could order medications that do not work, health policies could be created that aggravate the health problem, or effective programs may be displaced by ineffective programs. Therefore, in addition to understanding data and mathematical calculations, biostatisticians follow a code of ethics to ensure accurate and honest reporting of data.

Biostatistics is a specialized field of study within public health that takes raw health data and converts the data into a form that is more easily understood. As new health issues and ways to measure health emerge, biostatisticians are challenged to develop new methods to analyze data and promote public health.

Sally Kuykendall

See also: Administration, Health; Certified in Public Health; Code of Ethics; Core Competencies in Public Health; Degrees in Public Health; Epidemiology; Infant Mortality; Research; Wegman, Myron Ezra

Further Reading

American College of Epidemiology. (2017). Retrieved from https://www.acepidemiology.org/.
American Statistical Association. (2017). Retrieved from http://www.amstat.org/.
Department of Biostatistics, Vanderbilt University. (n.d.). *What is biostatistics?* Retrieved from https://medschool.vanderbilt.edu/biostatistics/content/what-biostatistics.
International Society of Clinical Biostatistics. (2017). Retrieved from http://www.iscb.info/.
National Center for Health Statistics. (2017). Retrieved from http://www.cdc.gov/nchs/.
National Safety Council. (2016). *Odds of dying*. Retrieved from http://www.nsc.org/act/events/Pages/Odds-of-Dying-2015.aspx.

BIOTERRORISM

Bioterrorism is the intentional transmission of bacteria, viruses, or other pathogenic organisms in order to incapacitate or kill a person or group of people. Advancements in genetic technology created the potential for manipulation of naturally occurring organisms. Enhancing toxicity, modes of transmission, or treatment resistance can create a weaponized organism, which is difficult to detect and easily transmitted through air, water, or food. The victims may not realize they have been attacked until symptoms occur hours or days later, or they may never realize that they were intentionally sickened. Although any organism may be engineered, commonly weaponized organisms are *Bacillus anthracis* (anthrax), *Clostridium botulinum* toxin (botulism), *Ricinus communis* (ricin toxin), *salmonella*, smallpox, and *Yersinia pestis* (plague). The concept of intentionally developing and harvesting pathogenic organisms is completely contrary to public health, which works to control and eliminate infectious diseases. In order to address the issue of bioterrorism and ensure public safety, the specialized field of *public health preparedness and response* plans, prepares, and practices for public health emergencies, including bioterrorism attacks. The Division of Strategic National Stockpile maintains a stockpile of more than $7 billion worth of drugs and medical supplies to respond to infectious diseases, radiation/nuclear emergencies, chemical attacks, and natural disasters.

From a military perspective, bioterrorism is ideal for covert attacks. Military historians believe that feuding tribes used human cadavers or dead animals to contaminate the water sources of enemies. The first documented bioterrorism occurred in 600 BCE when the Assyrians poisoned wells with rye ergot fungus. In 1346, Muslim soldiers chased Christian Italian merchants to Kaffa, a Crimean city on the

Black Sea. The citizens of Kaffa closed the city gates to protect the Italians. The army was suffering from the plague. Soldiers catapulted corpses over the walls in hopes of spreading disease and weakening the city. The city eventually succumbed to the plague. The Italians fled to Constantinople and Asia Minor on merchant ships and so commenced the Black Death. During the French and Indian War (1754–1763), British field marshal Jeffrey Amherst contrived to distribute smallpox-infected blankets to indigenous people. The Delaware and Shawnee tribes were decimated because they had no natural immunity. Amherst was later chastised by military leaders for using such cowardly strategies.

World War II brought renewed interest in bioterrorism. In 1930, the Japanese Unit 731 developed and tested biological agents in Northeast China. Scientists tested weaponized agents on criminals, allied prisoners of war, political prisoners, and local Chinese, Russian, and Korean citizens gathered by the military police. In 1942, British military scientists at Porton Down tested anthrax on sheep placed on Gruinard Island, Scotland. All 80 sheep died. The island remained contaminated until mass decontamination efforts in 1986 and final safety testing in 1990. In 1943,

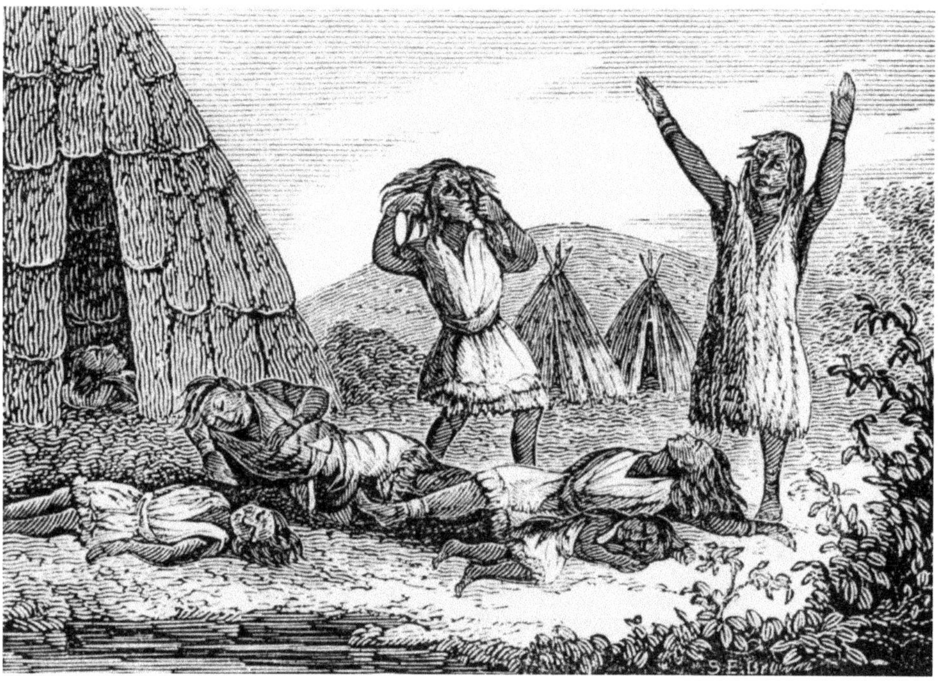

The Wampanoag people of Massachusetts are stricken by smallpox. Millions of indigenous people died as European explorers brought deadly germs to the New World. British field marshal Jeffrey Amherst exploited disease susceptibility by distributing smallpox-contaminated blankets to Native Americans during the French and Indian War. (North Wind Picture Archives)

the United States started their own biological weapons program engineering seven lethal agents. Nazi Germany also pursued the development and use of biological weapons.

On November 25, 1969, President Nixon renounced the use of biological weapons. Within two years, U.S. bioterrorism facilities closed and weaponized agents were destroyed. In 1975, the international treaty banning biological weapons, the Convention on the Prohibition of the Development, Production and Stockpiling of Bacteriological (Biological) and Toxin Weapons and on Their Destruction (now known as the Biological Weapons Convention) went into effect. In April 2, 1979, anthrax leaked from a military facility in Sverdlovsk, Russia, resulting in 100 deaths. The event demonstrated that some countries were continuing to produce weapons of mass destruction despite international agreements. Under Saddam Hussein, the Al Hakum facility in Iraq began mass production of weaponized anthrax in 1989 and is estimated to have produced half a million liters of weaponized organisms. In 1992, Dr. Kanatjian Alibekov (later known as Ken Alibek) defected to the United States. Alibekov was the former deputy chief of Biopreparat, the Soviet program studying, developing, and stockpiling biological warfare. After immigrating to the United States, Alibek worked with the U.S. government to develop biodefense strategies. In 1995, the cult group Aum Shinrikyo released sarin gas in the Tokyo subway. In September 2001, letters containing anthrax were sent to news offices and U.S. senators. In total 22 people were infected including 5 people who died. The FBI traced attacks to Bruce Edwards Ivins, a scientist working at Fort Detrick in Frederick, Maryland. Ivins committed suicide in 2008. Although nations have voluntarily agreed not to develop, test, or stockpile biological weapons, the possibility for attacks by rogue individuals or groups continues.

The public health system detects and responds to bioterrorism through surveillance of communicable diseases, investigation of outbreaks, and mobilization of the national stockpile. Bioterrorism agents are classified into three categories. Category A agents are highly lethal, easily transmitted, and likely to result in panic and disruption of society. Anthrax, botulism, plague, smallpox, tularemia, and the viral hemorrhagic fevers—Ebola, Marburg, and dengue—are Category A agents (Baylor College of Medicine, n.d.). Category B agents are moderate priority, easy to transmit, and carry lower mortality. Norovirus, *E. coli*, hepatitis A, ricin toxin, *salmonella,* and West Nile Virus are Category B agents. Category C agents are pathogens that are easily produced and engineered for high lethality. Influenza, rabies, multidrug resistant tuberculosis, yellow fever, severe acute respiratory syndrome (SARS), and Middle East respiratory syndrome (MERS) are examples of Category C agents.

The Health Alert Network (HAN) is a communication network. HAN disseminates trustworthy information during public health emergencies. Messages are classified as health alerts (high priority), health advisories (warnings), health updates, and general information. Health alerts on weaponized organisms are tailored to the specific agent, providing background information, at-risk groups or regions, and recommendations for treatment and prevention. The information is sent to federal, state, territorial, and local health officers and public health practitioners. The Crisis & Emergency Risk Communication (CERC) uses evidence-based practices to communicate with the public. The disastrous events of Hurricane Katrina (2005) helped government agencies, emergency responders, and public health professionals to see that they needed to do a better job in issuing warnings. During a natural or man-made disaster, the public needs clear, concise, and accurate information. CERC provides training, resources, and materials in how to communicate with the public and to empower people to make wise, life-saving decisions. The Department of Homeland Security, CERC, the Office of Public Health Preparedness and Response, and the Centers for Disease Control and Prevention work with state, local, and other federal agencies to coordinate responses to public health emergencies. Because of lessons learned from Hurricane Katrina, the response to Hurricane Sandy (2012) was very different. Days before Hurricane Sandy was predicted to make landfall, residents were instructed to evacuate, police went door to door, news agencies listed shelters that allowed pets, and utility trucks immediately outside of the path of the hurricane were standing by to repair damaged power and communication lines.

Public health works to eliminate deadly pathogens. In 1796, Edward Jenner tested his immunological theory by using cowpox serum to inoculate eight-year-old James Phipps against the deadly smallpox virus. In 1950, the Pan American Health Organization developed the goal of eradicating smallpox on the American continent and by 1979, the World Health Organization officially declared global smallpox eradication. In the heat of conflict, weaponized organisms may be seen as a highly effective and covert means of disarming and destabilizing the enemy. Fortunately, nations around the globe realized that bioterrorism crosses the line between humanity and inhumanity and developed the Biological Weapons Convention. Today, bioterrorism is a health event that we hope will never happen. Unfortunately, it is necessary for public health systems to plan for and prepare for such possibility. The lessons learned and systems developed to respond to incidents of bioterrorism are also valuable for natural disasters or other man-made disasters.

Sally Kuykendall

See also: Centers for Disease Control and Prevention; Emergency Preparedness and Response; Environmental Health; Global Health; Infectious Diseases; Smallpox; State, Local, and Territorial Health Departments; World Health Organization; Zombie Preparedness; *Controversies in Public Health:* Controversy 3; Controversy 4

Further Reading

Baylor College of Medicine. (n.d.). *Potential bioterrorism agents.* Retrieved from https://www.bcm.edu/departments/molecular-virology-and-microbiology/emerging-infections-and-biodefense/potential-bioterrorism-agents.

Centers for Disease Control and Prevention. (2007). *Emergency preparedness and response: Bioterrorism overview.* Retrieved from https://emergency.cdc.gov/bioterrorism/overview.asp.

International Physicians for the Prevention of Nuclear War. Retrieved from http://www.ippnw.org/.

Lillibridge, S. (2000). A public health response to bioterrorism. *Medicine & Global Survival,* 6(2), 82–85. Retrieved from http://www.ippnw.org/pdf/mgs/6-2-lillibridge.pdf.

U.S. Department of Health and Human Services, Centers for Disease Control and Prevention. (2001). *The public health response to biological and chemical terrorism: Interim planning guidance for state public health officials.* Retrieved from https://emergency.cdc.gov/Documents/Planning/PlanningGuidance.PDF.

U.S. Department of Homeland Security. Retrieved from https://www.ready.gov/.

BIRTH DEFECTS

Birth defects, also known as congenital disorders, are health problems that develop before a baby is born. These can include a variety of conditions such as congenital heart defects, developmental disorders, neural tube defects, and more. Although different birth defects vary in their incidence rates, birth defects are overall relatively common and occur in approximately 1 out of every 33 children (Centers for Disease Control and Prevention [CDC], 2008). Globally, at least 8 million children are born each year with a birth defect, and more than 3 million of these children die each year before the age of five (Weinhold, 2009). There is a wide range in the severity of different birth defects, with some causing mild or superficial effects and others causing life-threatening or life-ending conditions.

Birth defects can be the result of any one of many different factors. There are a diverse variety of genetic conditions that can be passed from parents to their children, and there is also a wide array of environmental factors that can greatly influence the child's development in the womb. Birth defects due to genetic conditions are often caused when two parents are heterozygous for a recessive mutation. Although each parent's dominant alleles may protect them from the genetic condition during their lifetime, their child may inherit both parents' recessive allele and therefore exhibit the signs of the birth defect. Additionally, there are a variety of environmental factors that impact the development of the embryo or fetus. Toxic substances and exposure to pollutants can play a large role in causing birth defects by harming developmental processes during gestation. Even lifestyle decisions such as smoking, alcohol intake, exercise levels, and weight can all play a role in increasing the risk of having a child with a birth defect.

Throughout modern history, several environmental health cases related to birth defects have brought great societal attention to the field of public health. The birth defect crisis from the use of the antinausea medication Thalidomide was one such event. In the late 1950s to the early 1960s, thousands of children throughout the world were born with congenital deformities such as limb malformation. It was only later discovered that Thalidomide acted as a teratogenic in pregnant mothers. Teratogens are compounds that cause birth defects through toxic actions on the developing embryo or fetus. Since Thalidomide was marketed as an antinausea medication, particularly for pregnant mothers suffering from morning sickness, many children were negatively affected and developed moderate to severe birth defects. In the United States, the refusal of the Food and Drug Administration to approve Thalidomide for distribution was key in preventing the birth defect effects from affecting large numbers of children. The case of Thalidomide in the United States serves to highlight the role that public health and other regulatory agencies can play in protecting populations from health problems such as birth defects.

Nonetheless, contemporary birth defect rates in the United States and internationally are still relatively high and carry an immense associated cost. Therefore, they are a matter of great interest to public health professionals and society as a whole. Birth defects affect approximately 120,000 babies each year in the United States alone and the cost of health care for a child born in the United States with spina bifida, a birth defect of the backbone, can be more than $20,000 (Radcliff et al., 2012). The medical costs for a child born with Down syndrome can be approximately 10 to 12 times higher than for children without Down syndrome (Kageleiry, Samuelson, Duh, Lefebvre, Campbell, & Skotko, 2017). Additionally, since many of these congenital disorders can be prevented through well-timed and effective interventions, the role that public health can play in alleviating birth defects is vital.

Many public health campaigns have therefore been initiated to reduce key behaviors that place mothers at a higher risk of giving birth to a child with a congenital disorder. For example, some public health interventions have sought to reduce the number of women who drink alcoholic beverages during pregnancy. This is because the children of mothers who drink alcohol during pregnancy are much more likely to suffer from a wide range of congenital health problems, including fetal alcohol syndrome. Additionally, primary care physicians and other health care providers encourage mothers to take nutritional supplements to prevent nutritional deficiencies from causing birth defects. Maternal folate deficiency, for example, is implicated in a variety of congenital neural tube defect disorders such as spina bifida. To prevent folate-deficiency-related congenital disorders, pregnant mothers are often placed on a regimen of folic acid supplementation throughout their pregnancy. Many public health educational interventions and medical association guidelines have therefore been established to promote the prescribing of folic acid supplementation regimens for pregnant mothers. Some health centers and clinics even offer free screenings and health services to mothers in order to encourage them to follow proper folate supplementation protocols.

Since the child's body is undergoing extensive development during the mother's pregnancy, it is in a susceptible state to influences such as environmental threats and maternal behaviors. Although many causes of birth defects can be mitigated through genetic screenings, positive lifestyle decisions, and other beneficial actions, chance mutations and unknown environmental exposures can still cause many different types of congenital disorders. Even errors in the cell division of the gametes proceeding the conception of a child can cause congenital disorders. Down syndrome is a classic example of this type of birth defect.

Since birth defects are a relatively common phenomenon throughout the world, greater attention is being given to effective interventions and policies in order to mitigate the opportunities for congenital disorders to develop. More work is needed to accomplish greater reductions in preventable congenital disorders going forward. The collaboration of government, health care, and families is essential to combating the avoidable causes of birth defects. By instituting policies that limit environmental toxins, promote proper screening and nutrition, and encourage healthy lifestyle choices, the current birth defect rates can be reduced and more children can enjoy fully healthy lives.

Shayan Waseh

See also: Air Pollution; Alcohol; Children's Health; Disability; Environmental Protection Agency; Epidemiology; Family Planning; Genetics; Infant Mortality; Leading Health Indicators; Maternal Health; Nutrition; Roosevelt, Franklin Delano

Further Reading

Centers for Disease Control and Prevention. (2008). Update on overall prevalence of major birth defects. *Morbidity and Mortality Weekly Report,* 57(1), 1–5.

Centers for Disease Control and Prevention. (2016). *Birth defects.*Retrieved from https://www.cdc.gov/ncbddd/birthdefects/index.html.

Kageleiry, A., Samuelson, D., Duh, M. S., Lefebvre, P., Campbell, J., & Skotko, B. G. (2017). Out-of-pocket medical costs and third-party healthcare costs for children with Down syndrome. *American Journal of Medical Genetics, Part A, 173*(3), 627. doi:10.1002/ajmg.a.38050

National Center on Birth Defects and Developmental Disabilities.Retrieved from https://www.cdc.gov/ncbddd/index.html

Pitkin, R. M. (2007). Folate and neural tube defects. *American Journal of Clinical Nutrition, 85*(1), 285S–288S.

Radcliff, E., Cassell, C. H., Tanner, J. P., Kirby, R. S., Watkins, S., Correia, J., et al. (2012). Hospital use, associated costs, and payer status for infants born with spina bifida. *Birth Defects Research Part A: Clinical and Molecular Teratology, 94,* 1044–1053.

Weinhold, B. (2009). Environmental factors in birth defects: What we need to know. *Environmental Health Perspectives, 117*(10), A440–A447.

BLACKWELL, ELIZABETH (1821–1910)

Dr. Elizabeth Blackwell was the first female to earn a medical degree in the United States. Her persistence and hard work improved care of women and children and created opportunities for other female leaders in medicine. Elizabeth was born on February 3, 1821, the third of nine children of Hannah Lane and Samuel Blackwell. The Blackwell family lived in Bristol, England, a city that thrived on the African slave trade. Samuel Blackwell was partner in a series of sugar refinery businesses. Sugar refineries imported sugar cane from slave plantations in the West Indies and refined the product for use in food and drink, including tea.

Despite a series of unsuccessful business ventures, the family was modestly affluent. Elizabeth and her siblings were homeschooled by private teachers. In 1832, the family immigrated to the United States so that Samuel Blackwell could work toward the abolishment of slavery. With the help of old and new business partners, Blackwell opened the Congress Steam Sugar Refinery in New York City. He was unable to pay loans on the business. His business partner bought him out, and the Blackwell family moved to Cincinnati. Samuel died of malaria in 1838, leaving the family without any means of support. Hannah and Elizabeth's two older sisters took jobs teaching and later opened a school. These early experiences of fortune, hardship, risk-taking, and interest in social reform left a lasting impression. As adults, all of the Blackwell siblings were involved in the abolitionist movement or women's rights.

Elizabeth was not initially attracted to the field of medicine. She found the study of the human body vulgar and preferred history and metaphysics. From 1845 to 1847, she worked as a teacher in Kentucky, North Carolina, and South Carolina. The idea of attending medical school came as a friend was dying from a gynecological disorder. Elizabeth's friend believed that a female physician may have been more empathetic to her complaints and alleviated some of her suffering. Elizabeth did not want to get married and believed that she could avoid matrimony by going to medical school. She consulted with six prominent physicians on next steps. All of them discouraged her noting, "That it was utter impossibility for a woman to obtain a medical education; that the idea though good in itself, was eccentric and utopian, utterly impracticable!" (Blackwell & Blackwell, 1863, pp. 4–5). Friends and colleagues recommended that she either disguise herself as a male or move to Paris where there were opportunities for female physicians. Believing that the Quaker community might be supportive, Elizabeth moved to Philadelphia. She borrowed medical books from friends and obtained a tutor in anatomy and physiology. When it came time to apply to medical school, Elizabeth applied to all of the medical schools in New York City and Philadelphia as well as 12 other schools in the Northeastern region. She was rejected by 29 schools. Geneva Medical College (now Hobart and William Smith Colleges) in upstate New York was the only school that did not reject her outright. The admissions committee was unable to agree on her application and decided to put the question to the all-male student body for a vote. If just one of the 150 students voted against her, the application would be denied. The students thought it was a joke. They voted unanimously to approve her admission, and in 1847 Elizabeth started medical school. Her struggles did not end there. Ms. Blackwell was scorned by people in town who labeled her as "a bad woman whose designs would gradually become evident, or that, being insane, an outbreak of insanity would soon be apparent" (Blackwell, 1895, pp. 70–73). Although other students at the college harassed her, the medical students came to respect her. Professors noted that the medical students who were normally loud and crude became quiet and studious when Elizabeth was present. She found it difficult to gain clinical experience. Professors banned her from anatomy and physiology labs, and patients refused to allow her to examine them. To get experience, Elizabeth worked summers at Blockley Almshouse in Philadelphia. Located in a dangerous section of the city, Blockley treated Philadelphia's poor, disabled, elderly, and mentally ill populations. Her doctoral thesis examined typhus fever, a disease contracted on coffin ships used by Irish immigrants fleeing the Great Famine of Ireland (1845–1852). On January 23, 1849, Elizabeth graduated first in her class from Geneva Medical College. The graduation ceremony was a curiosity. Townspeople and academics watched with anticipation as the humble and slightly embarrassed Dr. Blackwell accepted her diploma. Over the next three years 20 other women graduated from American medical schools, including Emily Blackwell (1826–1910), Elizabeth's younger sister.

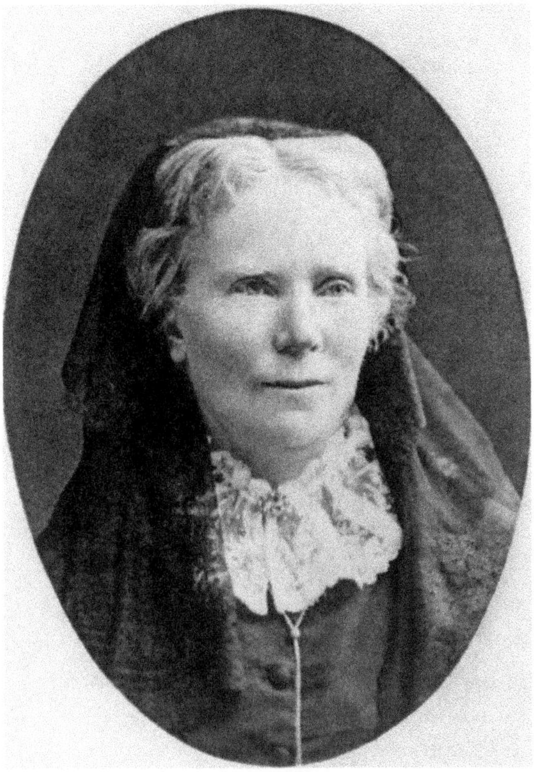

Refusing to yield to gender discrimination and oppression, Elizabeth Blackwell became the first woman to earn a medical degree in the United States. Her persistence improved the care of women and children, and created opportunities for other females in medicine. (Library of Congress)

After graduation, Elizabeth moved to Paris to gain medical experience and eventually specialize in surgery. While assisting with a delivery at La Maternité, gonorrhea-infected vaginal fluids splashed into her face. Elizabeth suffered a purulent eye infection that resulted in permanent blindness in one eye. The loss of depth perception meant that she could no longer safely perform surgery. Unyielding, Elizabeth turned to hygiene and sanitation as a specialty. The prevention of communicable diseases was a natural extension of her work in the almshouse, her interest in social reform, her doctoral thesis, and her own disabling experience at La Maternité. In 1850, Elizabeth returned to London to work at St. Bartholomew's Hospital with the famous surgeon Dr. James Paget (1814–1899). She was allowed to work in all wards except the gynecology and pediatrics wards. In England, she was befriended by many progressive women of the time, including Florence Nightingale (1820–1910). Nightingale and Blackwell shared an interest in hospital sanitation and hygiene and professionalism of women in health and medicine. Nightingale wanted Elizabeth to use her knowledge and skills to train nurses. Elizabeth was intent on training female medical doctors.

In 1851, Elizabeth moved to New York City to start her own private medical practice. She soon found that she was blacklisted as an abortionist, medical colleagues excluded her from educational opportunities, and patients were reluctant to seek the services of a female physician. She applied for a position at the city's women's clinic and was rejected. Undeterred, she worked as a freelance writer, publishing a series of works entitled *The Laws of Life, with Special Reference to the Physical Education of Girls.* In 1853, Quaker friends helped Elizabeth to start a health clinic treating indigent patients three afternoons each week. Within four years, the clinic grew from a small rented room near Tompkins Square in Manhattan to the New York Infirmary for Women and Children. The infirmary attracted other female physicians including Drs. Emily Blackwell and Marie Zakrzewska (1829–1902). Emily eventually took over day-to-day management of the hospital leaving Elizabeth free to pursue her passion of women's medical education.

In 1860, Elizabeth published *Medicine as a Profession for Women.* The essay argued that the stereotypical female roles of housekeeper and teacher were also relevant to the field of medicine. Reflecting the social values of the time, the article explained that women who knew how to keep a house clean would also know how to prevent communicable disease transmission. The American Civil War (1861–1865) helped to advance women in medicine. Infection was one of the leading causes of death. The overcrowded, unsanitary conditions of civil war hospitals resulted in high postoperative infection and mortality rates. Modeling Nightingale's experiences and methods of controlling infection during the Crimean War (1853–1856), the American government established the U.S. Sanitary Commission to care for wounded soldiers. Elizabeth helped to organize the sanitary commission and the Woman's Central Relief Association. The general public started to envision female nurses as the primary caregivers of diseased and injured men. The idea of women in medicine, albeit in subservient roles, was no longer a utopian dream. Emily and Elizabeth's *Address on the Medical Education of Women* (1864) argued for a medical school designed exclusively for female physicians. The sisters presented the widely accepted view that there was a need for nurse training programs and explained that female physicians were an ideal group to advance nurse training. In

1867, the infirmary opened a medical college and offered both medical training and clinical experience for women. Elizabeth ensured high standards in admission and clinical training. In 1869, Elizabeth returned to London to establish a private medical practice and to work toward women's medical education in Great Britain. In collaboration with Dr. Sophia Jex-Blake, a student of the New York Infirmary, she established the London School of Medicine for Women (1874). The following year, she was appointed professor of gynecology at the London School of Medicine for children. She was the first woman to have her name listed on the British Medical Register.

Reflecting on her life, Elizabeth noted an overwhelming loneliness. She was often the target of harassment and institutional discrimination. Few colleagues understood or recognized the obstacles she faced in society, in medicine and as a woman. Where many people would have given up, she kept going. The persistent humiliation and disparagement created a very fierce and relentless character. She was often at odds with people, including her own sister, Emily. In 1856, while establishing the New York Infirmary, Elizabeth adopted Katherine "Kitty" Barry, an Irish orphan. Elizabeth cared for Kitty, but she also used Kitty as a domestic servant and never allowed Kitty to flourish on her own. The two women remained together until Blackwell's death on May 31, 1910. When Kitty died in 1930, she called Elizabeth her "true love."

Elizabeth Blackwell was an Anglo-American woman who broke gender barriers by becoming the first woman to graduate from a recognized medical school in the United States. As a doctor, she worked to ensure sanitary conditions in hospitals, to prevent communicable diseases, and to advance women's health care. By developing training opportunities for women in medicine, she advanced the fields of nursing and medicine.

Sally Kuykendall

See also: Baker, Sara Josephine; Children's Health; Handwashing; Infant Mortality; Infectious Diseases; Maternal Health; Patient Safety

Further Reading

Blackwell, E. (1895). *Pioneer work in opening the medical profession to women: Autobiographical sketches by Dr. Elizabeth Blackwell* (pp. 70–73). London: Longmans, Green.

Blackwell, E., & Blackwell, E. (1863, December 19). *Address on the medical education of women.* New York: Baptist & Taylor, Book and Job Printers. Retrieved from https://iiif.lib.harvard.edu/manifests/view/drs:2582644$1i.

Hobart and William-Smith Colleges. (2016). *Elizabeth Blackwell.* Retrieved from http://www.hws.edu/about/blackwell/.

U.S. National Library of Medicine. (2015). Dr. Elizabeth Blackwell. *Changing the face of medicine.* Retrieved from https://cfmedicine.nlm.nih.gov/physicians/biography_35.html.

BODY MASS INDEX (BMI)

The body mass index (BMI)—also known as the Quetelet index—is a convenient and inexpensive way to estimate body composition calculated from an individual's weight and height. BMI ranks the person's body size relative to other people. Although BMI is not a diagnostic test, health practitioners can use BMI to screen and monitor health status. High BMI suggests high body fat or adipose tissue and is associated with higher risk of chronic diseases, such as Type 2 diabetes, heart disease, osteoarthritis, stroke, gallstones, hypertension, breathing problems, sleep apnea, and breast and colon cancer. Diseases associated with high BMI are some of the most common in the United States and very costly to health care systems. When a patient registers a high BMI, the health care provider will initially assess the patient's diet, physical activity, and family history to determine factors that may be related to high BMI. If initial screening suggests high body fat, more extensive laboratory testing is done to decide the extent of any problems and levels of risk for obesity-related diseases. In addition to monitoring disease state, BMI can also be used to monitor progress of people who are adapting healthier lifestyles.

The formula to calculate BMI was developed by Lambert Adolphe Jacques Quetelet (1796–1874). Quetelet was a Belgian mathematician, statistician, and astronomer with an interest in social phenomena, art, and the human body. Quetelet used his training as a mathematician and astronomer to study similarities in people, an approach that was fairly novel at the time. While managing several large-scale studies of human development, Quetelet observed recurring body shapes and frames that matched what he had seen as a painter and sculptor. In analyzing the data sets of height and weight, Quetelet recognized a mathematical pattern. With the exception of childhood and puberty, when growth spurts occur, body weight increases relative to the square of height. The Quentelet index was published in 1832. The calculation was not fully appreciated until more than a century later when scientists discovered connections between body weight and heart disease. Hoping to reduce one of the leading causes of death in the United States, experts sought ways to define healthy weight ranges. The Quetelet index was recognized as an accurate way to assess body fat with the major advantage that it does not require expensive equipment. In 1972, Ancel Keys, a prominent nutrition scientist, renamed the Quentelet index the body mass index.

BMI calculators are available online, but the formula for an adult is the following:

$$\text{BMI} = \text{weight (kg)} / [\text{height (m)}]^2$$

or

$$\text{BMI} = \text{weight (lb)} / [\text{height (in)}]^2 \times 703$$

Although BMI calculation is universal, the cutoff values indicating risk vary by country. In the United States, an adult BMI of less than 18.5 is underweight, suggesting possible malnutrition. BMIs between 18.5 and 24.9 are considered average, healthy values. BMIs between 25 and 29.9 are classified as overweight and at risk for obesity-related health problems. BMIs between 30 and 34.9 are classified as moderately obese (also referred to as Class I obesity). BMIs between 35 and 39.9 are severely obese or Class II obesity, and BMI above 40 is very severely obese or Class III obesity. Adult BMI values cannot be applied to youth because the characteristic patterns of childhood and adolescent growth might give falsely high or low results. Children and adolescents grow in periodic spurts, rather than as a constant consistent process. With adequate nourishment, the body gains weight immediately before a height spurt. Thus, the same child could be classified as overweight before a height spurt and underweight after the height spurt. To account for normal childhood growth patterns, medical professionals use BMI-for-age where BMI is converted to a percentile and standardized to age and gender. BMI-for-age percentile of 4 percent or less suggests the child is underweight. Healthy weight range is 5 to 84.9 percent. A BMI-for-age percentile of 85 to 94.9 percent is classified as overweight. A BMI-for-age of 95 percent or greater is considered obese. As in adults, high BMI-for-age in children is not a perfect diagnostic tool. High BMI warns the health care provider to explore diet, exercise, and further diagnostic testing.

Although BMI is an easy and accurate form of measuring body fat, there are some instances where the measure may be misleading. BMI calculation uses a person's weight, and it does not differentiate weight of adipose tissue from weight of muscle or bone tissue. Muscle tissue is heavier by volume than adipose tissue. This means that a very muscular person may register BMI in the overweight range. (It is unlikely a muscular person would have a BMI in the obese range.) Therefore, highly muscular people such as athletes may need to use other methods of measuring body composition. Furthermore, a person with a large skeletal frame has more skeletal muscle, and this may falsely elevate BMI into the overweight range; whereas someone with a small frame and excess adipose tissue may rank as normal weight. Body fat also varies by gender and age. Women tend to have a higher percentage of body fat than men. In the female body, the hormone estrogen directs fat to the breasts, hips, waist, and buttocks. In males, fat is directed to the chest, abdomen, and buttocks. Percentage of adipose tissue also varies with age. With nutritious diet and adequate exercise, muscle tissue increases until the mid-twenties. After the age of 50, the body loses muscle mass, a process known as age-related sarcopenia. Thus, there are limitations to using BMI to interpret individual health. Alternative ways to measure body composition include skinfold thickness, waist circumference, densitometry, isotope dilution (hydrometry), dual energy X-ray absorptiometry, bioelectrical impedance analysis, and magnetic resonance imaging. Each method has advantages and disadvantages with respect to accuracy, accessibility, expense, and ease of use.

Beyond assessing individual health risk, public health professionals use BMI to study the general health of various populations. The Centers for Disease Control and Prevention and National Center for Health Statistics currently collect BMI data and develop maps, which allows epidemiologists to identify trends in obesity and distribution by geography or other factors. Through such large-scale BMI studies, program planners can develop programs for high-risk communities, public health officials can develop policies, and local governments can plan neighborhoods that promote healthy weight.

Sally Kuykendall

See also: Diabetes Mellitus; Disease; Eating Disorders; Food Insecurity; Heart Disease; Heart Truth® (Red Dress) Campaign, The; Hypertension; Obesity; Physical Activity

Further Reading

Eknoyen, G. (2008). Adolphe Quetelet (1796–1874): The average man and indices of obesity. *Nephrology Dialysis Transplantation*, *23*(1), 47–51.

U.S. Department of Health and Human Services, Centers for Disease Control and Prevention, Division of Nutrition, Physical Activity and Obesity. (2015). *Body mass index (BMI)*. Retrieved from http://www.cdc.gov/healthyweight/assessing/bmi/.

U.S. Department of Health and Human Services, Centers for Disease Control and Prevention, Division of Nutrition, Physical Activity and Obesity. (2015). *Data, trends and maps*. Retrieved from http://www.cdc.gov/obesity/data/prevalence-maps.html.

BOUSFIELD, MIDIAN OTHELLO (1885–1948)

Midian Othello Bousfield was a physician, insurance executive, and foundation officer who promoted public health, medical, and nursing training among African Americans and advocated for the health needs of people of color. Midian was born in Tipton, Missouri, to Cornelia Catherine Gilbert and Willard Hayman Bousfield. The older Bousfield was a barber and businessman. In 1907, Midian earned a bachelor's degree from the University of Kansas followed by a medical degree from Northwestern University. He completed his internship and residency at Freedmen's Hospital in Washington, DC. Freedmen's Hospital was affiliated with Howard University School of Medicine, serving the medical needs of African Americans, many of whom were former slaves or children of former slaves. After medical residency, Dr. Bousfield moved to Kansas City where he worked in the city hospital. In 1911, he traveled to Brazil to establish a medical practice for African Brazilians. During the slave trade, Brazil imported more Africans than any other country. Slaves were used to work on sugar plantations, in gold and diamond mining, and ranching. From a business perspective, there should have been a great need for health services. However, Bousfield's efforts to open a private practice were unsuccessful. He even tried panning for gold without success. After a year, Bousfield returned to Kansas City.

In 1914, Bousfield met Maudelle Tanner Brown, a public school teacher. They married and moved to Chicago where Bousfield started private practice, worked as a health officer for the Chicago Public School District, and was on staff at Provident

Hospital. From 1915 to 1920, Bousfeld served as secretary of the Railway Men's International Benevolent Industrial Association. Railroads were the main mode of transportation, and Chicago was a major gateway between the East and the West. Many Chicago residents worked for the railway—jobs that demanded long dangerous hours and provided little job security. Starting in the mid-1800s the white railway workers started unionizing and striking for better working conditions (Thale, 2005). The union of master mechanics was followed by unionization of engineers, freight handlers, track workers, and switchmen. One of the last groups to unionize was the African American porters. The porters' income came solely from tips. The railway companies expected the porters to set up or clean up the restaurant and sleeping cars without any additional reimbursement. The railway companies also charged the porters for food, sleeping quarters, and uniforms, a sum that amounted to approximately half of their income. And porters were responsible for reimbursing the company if a passenger stole towels or kitchenware. When the porters attempted to unionize, the Pullman Company hired spies to squelch the labor movement. However, the Railway Men's International Benevolent Industrial Association met secretly, organized, and hired outside organizers, beyond the reach of Pullman. The Railway Men's International Benevolent Industrial Association later became the Brotherhood of Sleeping Car Porters (BSCP), one of the first African American labor unions chartered by the American Federation of Labor. The BSCP founders also became leaders in the black civil rights movement.

In 1919, Bousfield founded Liberty Life Insurance. The company was designed to serve the needs of African Americans. At the time, life insurance for African Americans would not have been a lucrative business. By 1939 (the first year that data on income by race was recorded), the average annual income of African Americans was $537, half the annual income of whites, $1,234.41 (Maloney, 2002). Life span was also much shorter. Whites born in 1900 had a life expectancy of 47.6 years (46.6 years for males and 48.7 years for females), while African Americans had a life expectancy of 33.0 years (32.5 years for males and 33.5 years for females) (U.S. Census Bureau, 1999). The Liberty Life Insurance later merged with other companies to become Supreme Life Insurance Company. Dr. Bousfield served as medical director and vice president of Supreme and chairman of the public health committee of the National Negro Insurance Association. In 1934, Bousfield became the first African American to address the American Public Health Association (APHA) annual meeting. This historic speech called attention to the living and working conditions of African Americans. Bousfield described overcrowding, lack of fresh air and recreational spaces, racial health disparities, segregated hospitals, refusal to treat black patients, and limited health services. Bousfield encouraged public health professionals to partner with black communities to provide treatment and preventive health services. Bousfield's ideas were inspired by W. E. B. Du Bois, a sociologist who advocated for solidarity among African Americans, education, and activism. Bousfield envisioned education as a way to promote health and wellness and to reduce health disparities. There is no doubt that Bousfield was also inspired by his wife.

Maudelle Bousfield made her own mark in history by becoming the first African American high school principal in Chicago. In 1940, white males had an average of nine years of education while African American males had an average of six years of education (Maloney, 2002).

In 1935, Bousfield became director of the Negro Health Division of the Julius Rosenwald Fund. In this role, he was able to work toward his vision. He focused grant funds on supporting African American health services and hospitals and expanded training opportunities in public health, nursing, and medicine and postgraduate education for African American health professionals. Bousfield was also instrumental in developing the Infantile Paralysis Units at Tuskegee Institute and Provident Hospital. From 1933 to 1934, he served as president of the National Medical Association (NMA), the national organization of African American physicians. He was elected president of the Chicago Urban League in 1936 and appointed as the first African American to serve on the Chicago School Board in 1939. In 1942, he joined World War II efforts as the first African American colonel in the Army Medical Corps. He commanded Station Hospital in Fort Huachuca, Arizona. Station Hospital was a segregated hospital that served the medical and health needs of 14,000 African American military personnel. His time in the military was difficult. Bousfield was criticized for contributing to segregated hospitals. He retired in 1945, and died on February 16, 1948, of acute coronary disease.

Dr. Midian Othello Bousfield was a key figure in calling attention to the plight of African Americans post-slavery. As a physician and life insurance executive, Bousfield provided insights into social injustice and racial health disparities. Within his lifetime, Bousfield was able to achieve some progress. By 1945, the gap in life expectancy had started to narrow. The average life expectancy of African Americans increased to 58 years while life expectancy of whites increased to 67 years (U.S. Census Bureau, 1999). However, socioeconomic differences persisted where African Americans continued to earn half that of whites. Today, Bousfield's message is acknowledged and embraced. Reducing health disparities is a primary goal of public health professionals.

Sally Kuykendall

See also: Epidemic; Epidemiology; Health Disparities; Smith, James McCune; Social Determinants of Health; Tubman, Harriet

Further Reading

Bousfield, M. O. (1934). Reaching the Negro community. *American Journal of Public Health, 24*, 209–215. Retrieved from https://www.ncbi.nlm.nih.gov/pmc/articles/PMC1558597/pdf/amjphnation00913-0031.pdf.

Ewbank, D. C. (1987). History of black mortality and health before 1940. *The Milbank Quarterly, 65*, 100.

Gamble, V. N., & Brown, T. M. (2009). Midian Othello Bousfield: Advocate for the medical and public health concerns of Black Americans. *American Journal of Public Health, 99*(7),

1186. Retrieved from http://ajph.aphapublications.org/doi/abs/10.2105/AJPH.2009.163709?journalCode=ajph.

Maloney, T. (2002). African Americans in the twentieth century. R. Whaples (Ed.), *EH.Net Encyclopedia*. Retrieved from https://eh.net/encyclopedia/african-americans-in-the-twentieth-century/.

Thale, C. (2005). Railroad workers. *Encyclopedia of Chicago*. Chicago Historical Society. Retrieved from http://www.encyclopedia.chicagohistory.org/pages/1038.html.

U.S. Census Bureau. (1999). *Statistical abstract of the United States, annual and national vital statistics reports*. Retrieved from https://www.census.gov/library/publications/1999/compendia/statab/119ed.html.

BOWDITCH, HENRY INGERSOLL (1808–1892)

Dr. Henry Ingersoll Bowditch was a Boston physician who established the first state board of health in the United States. He encouraged colleagues to use scientific reasoning in medical practices and authored numerous books and brochures on topics ranging from use of the stethoscope, physical examination techniques, supporting the medical education of women, and advocating for emergency medical teams to expedite treatment of wounded soldiers. Bowditch's expertise in pulmonary diseases greatly advanced the diagnosis and treatment of tuberculosis, bronchitis, pneumonia, and pneumothorax. Although his accomplishments in medicine are historic and noteworthy, his most important contributions to society and public health were in the area of social reform. Bowditch was a leader in the anti-slavery movement. Working alongside notable abolitionists, Bowditch founded a secretive paramilitary force to foil slave hunters and drafted the Massachusetts state law protecting fugitive slaves from recapture.

Henry was born on August 9, 1808, in Salem, Massachusetts, to Mary (Polly) Ingersoll and Nathaniel Bowditch. The Bowditch family history is relevant to understanding Henry's interests, talents, and values. Henry's grandfather, Habakkuk Bowditch, was the captain of a merchant ship. He was not very successful and the Bowditch family often relied on aid from the Salem Marine Society to pay their bills. On the nights that Habakkuk was at sea, Nathaniel sat in the window with his mother, watching the moon and the stars. When Nathaniel was 10, his mother died and Nathaniel had to leave school to work in his father's new business venture, making wooden barrels. This business was also unsuccessful and after two years, Habakkuk indentured Nathaniel to a ship chandler for a period of nine years. Nathaniel had an amazing ability to calculate numbers in his head. During times when the shipping business was slow, Nathaniel taught himself algebra, calculus, Latin, and French. He quickly advanced from bookkeeper to supercargo, the title given to the ship owner's representative. At sea, Nathaniel continued his self-study, translating major literary works into English. However, he did not simply translate the works, he also corrected errors, thereby improving and sometimes rewriting the books. After completing his covenant, Nathaniel continued to work on ships, managing the books, reading, and studying the stars and ocean. His enthusiasm for learning was contagious. Onboard one ship, he taught the entire crew, including the cook, to navigate by the stars. Nathaniel wrote *The New American Practical Navigator*, an encyclopedia of navigation, which is still used today. He is also credited with introducing America to the field of astronomy. Harvard University acknowledged Mr. Bowditch's accomplishments with an honorary master's degree. When Nathaniel married Polly Ingersoll, he settled into the prestigious position as head of the Massachusetts Hospital Life Insurance Company. By the time his children were born, Nathaniel had worked his way from an impoverished family and nine years of indentured servitude to become one of the most prestigious and influential members of Boston society.

Henry attended the Public Latin School and Harvard University where he completed his bachelor's degree (1828) and medical degree (1832). Part of his medical training involved studying in London and France with the preeminent physicians Gabriel Andral, Auguste Francois Chomel, and Pierre Charles Alexandre Louis. In Paris, Henry and fellow classmate Oliver Wendell Holmes developed a lifelong professional connection with Dr. Louis. Louis taught his students how use a stethoscope, different sounds to listen for when auscultating the heart and lungs, and the benefits of postmortem examinations. Louis spoke out against the popular therapy of bloodletting, believing that the doctor's role was to support natural recovery. His theories and practices using the *numerical method* in medicine were the start of the field of epidemiology. Bowditch was instrumental in sharing Louis's ideas and philosophies with physicians in the United States. In 1846, Bowditch wrote *The Young Stethoscopist or the Student's Guide to Auscultation* and later translated Louis's groundbreaking book, *Anatomical, Pathological and Therapeutic Researches upon the Disease Known under the Name of Gasto-Enterite.*

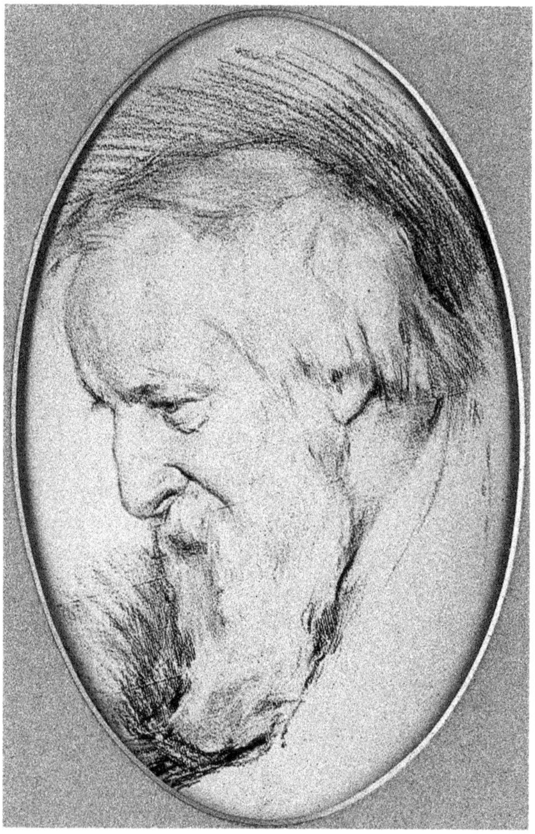

Massachusetts General Hospital threatened to revoke Dr. Henry Ingersoll Bowditch's staff privileges when he admitted the first African American patient to the hospital. Bowditch designed the first state board of health in the United States. (Wellcome Collection)

While Bowditch was in Europe, the British Parliament enacted the Slavery Abolition Act 1833, a law that abolished slavery in the British Empire and compensated slave owners for business losses because of losing slaves. The movement was led by member of Parliament William Wilberforce. Wilberforce was a deeply religious man who believed that the use and abuse of slaves in the West Indies and the depraved lifestyle of slave owners were an embarrassment to Great Britain and an affront to Christianity. People admired Wilberforce's ability to act on his faith. When Wilberforce died, Bowditch attended his funeral and was deeply moved toward the abolition of slavery.

On return to Boston, Bowditch resumed his position within Boston society. He married Olivia Yardley, whom he had met in London, started a medical practice with staff privileges at Massachusetts General Hospital, and participated in charities supporting the poor and less fortunate. Against hospital rules, Bowditch attempted to admit an African American patient with pulmonary problems. Massachusetts General Hospital refused the admission and the hospital board passed a policy revoking staff privileges of any doctor who admitted African American patients. Bowditch resigned in protest, forcing the board to withdraw the policy.

Bowditch joined the anti-slavery cause in 1835 after witnessing the attack and attempted hanging of journalist William Lloyd Garrison. Garrison was scheduled to speak to the Female Anti-Slavery Society of Boston when an angry pro-slavery mob interrupted the meeting and dragged Garrison through the streets. Bowditch saw the angry mob attacking Garrison. Their violent and abusive behavior would have been repulsive to anyone who worked to help and heal people. Authorities intervened and warned Garrison to leave Boston. The event was a turning point for many Bostonians creating a foundation for the anti-slavery movement. In 1842, fugitive slave George Latimer and his pregnant wife, Rebecca, fled to Boston. They were recognized and reported to slaveholder James B. Gray. Gray traveled from Virginia to reclaim Latimer and was met by serious resistance from the Boston abolitionists. Latimer sat in jail through a series of legal maneuvers intended to stop Gray from reclaiming Latimer. Bowditch served on the Latimer Committee, a group established to secure Latimer's freedom. Frustrated, Gray eventually agreed to sell Latimer for $400. The work of the Latimer Committee continued, drafting the first law protecting fugitive slaves. The 1843 Personal Liberty Act banned Massachusetts state officials from arresting or holding suspected slaves. The Personal Liberty Act was overruled when Congress passed the Fugitive Slave Act of 1850. The Fugitive Slave Act required free states to cooperate with the capture and return of slaves. In 1854, Anthony Burns was captured under the Fugitive Slave Act. Burns was a Baptist minister and fugitive slave living and working in Boston. When officials arrested Burns, Bostonians protested with riots, demonstrations, and attacks on the federal courthouse. Efforts to keep Burns in Boston were unsuccessful, and the city was placed under martial law while Burns was escorted to a ship returning him to the South. After Burns left Boston, abolitionists continued attempts to purchase and free Burns. However, the slaveholder refused. Eventually, Burns's freedom was secured through a series of purchases. In response to Burns's case, Bowditch, Samuel Gridley Howe, Bronson Alcott, and other prominent Bostonians established the Anti-Man-Hunting League. The league was a secret society of more than 100 people who devised plans to surround, overcome, and capture slave hunters while the fugitive slave was moved to safety (Massachusetts Historical Society, n.d.).

During the Civil War, Bowditch served as medical examiner, screening soldiers for the Massachusetts regiment. His beloved son, Nathaniel, joined the cavalry and was severely injured during a charge at Kelly's Ford, Virginia. Two surgeons saw Lieutenant Bowditch fall but had no means to carry him off the battlefield. Another soldier eventually draped Nat over the neck of his horse and carried him to a wagon waiting to transport wounded soldiers. Nat died in the wagon without receiving medical care. Bowditch was convinced that Nat may have survived if he had received proper medical attention. In his sorrow, Bowditch wrote *A Brief Plea for an Ambulance System for the Army of the United States.* The government responded by establishing an ambulance corps, which greatly reduced morbidity and mortality of both Confederate and Union army soldiers.

After the war, Bowditch turned his attention to mending the division between Northern and Southern physicians. He served as vice president and president of the American Medical Association (AMA) where he proposed a medical code of ethics and advocated for medical schools to accept women and former slaves. He taught at Harvard Medical School and published numerous medical reports on tuberculosis, inoculations, and public health. In 1869, Bowditch founded the Massachusetts State Board of Health. He served as chairman of the board for 10 years until he was appointed to the National Board of Health. He resigned from the National Board of Health when President Chester A. Arthur cut funding. Bowditch died in 1892. As he lay on his deathbed, the widow of Lewis Hayden, a former slave and patient of Bowditch's, insisted on sitting by his side. Mrs. Hayden was determined that Dr. Bowditch should not die alone.

Dr. Henry Ingersoll Bowditch was a physician, social reformer, and father who worked tirelessly to raise up those who society viewed as lesser than or not deserving of the same rights and privileges. Despite ostracism by friends, colleagues and patients, Bowditch held firmly to his beliefs that all men and women should have equal rights to health, education, and life's liberties. His knowledge and efforts advanced medical practice, founded state boards of health, and led to critical social changes.

Sally Kuykendall

See also: American Medical Association; Shattuck, Lemuel; State, Local, and Territorial Health Departments; Tubman, Harriet

Further Reading

The Boston Medical and Surgical Journal (January 21, 1892). Obituary: Henry Ingersoll Bowditch, M.D., *126*(3), 67–70.

Bowditch, H. I. (1846). *The young stethoscopist or the student's guide to auscultation.* New York: J. & H. G. Langley. Retrieved from https://archive.org/details/63630550R.nlm.nih.go.

Bowditch, H. I. (1863). *A brief plea for an ambulance system for the army of the United States, as drawn from the extra sufferings of the late Lieut. Bowditch and a wounded comrade.* Boston: Ticknor and Fields. Retrieved from https://archive.org/details/briefpleaforambu00bowd.

Bowditch, H. I. (1881). The medical education of women. *Boston Medical and Surgical Journal, 105*(5), 109–110. Retrieved from http://www.nejm.org/doi/full/10.1056/NEJM188109291051301.

Cumbler, J. T. (2008). A family goes to war: Sacrifice and honor for an abolitionist family. *Massachusetts Historical Review, 10,* 57–84.

Felts, J. H. (2002). Henry Ingersoll Bowditch and Oliver Wendell Holmes: Stethoscopists and reformers. *Perspectives in Biology and Medicine*, *45*(4), 539–548.

Massachusetts Historical Society. (n.d.). *Collections online: Diagram to show the drill the Anti-Man-Hunting League had for running off of a slave or man-hunter.* Retrieved from https://masshist.org/database/1668.

Rodriguez, J. P. (2007). Bowditch, Henry Ingersoll. In J. Rodriguez, *Encyclopedia of emancipation and abolition in the transatlantic world.* London: Routledge.

C

CANCER

Cancer is characterized by the abnormal growth of cells in the body. Typically, the cells of the human body are well regulated and their growth is tightly controlled by a series of molecular signals and processes. However, when these guidance systems and protective mechanisms are disrupted, the cells of the human body can proliferate inappropriately. This abnormal proliferation of cells is then labeled as cancer. Neoplasm is another term used to describe abnormal growths or cancers.

Cancers or neoplasms can be benign or malignant. Benign neoplasms still involve the abnormal growth of cells, but these inappropriately proliferating cells remain localized to one area, do not invade the surrounding tissue, and are generally not harmful unless they restrict blood vessels, nerves, or other important body structures. Malignant neoplasms, however, are aggressively proliferative and invade the surrounding tissue. They are often able to metastasize through the bloodstream and grow to damage important body structures such as the lungs or brain. Typically, it is malignant neoplasms that are thought of as the stereotypical example of deadly cancer.

The causes of cancer are diverse and can include genetic, behavioral, and environmental factors. The genetic code of cells is essential for the regulation of cell growth and behavior. Mutations in genes responsible for cellular growth and regulation are implicated in causing a variety of cancers. These mutations can be inherited from parents or developed throughout a person's lifetime. Additionally, a variety of behaviors and lifestyle decisions can contribute to the frequency and nature of genetic mutations. Tobacco use, for example, often results in lung damage and the ingestion of mutation-causing chemicals. With repeated tobacco usage, genetic mutations can build up in the smoker's cells and eventually result in cancer. In fact, nearly a quarter of all cancer deaths are related to the use of tobacco (World Health Organization, 2017). Finally, environmental factors such as air pollution, toxic chemicals, and even unprotected sun exposure can increase the incidence of cancer through a variety of mechanisms that result in genetic damage and subsequently lead to the development of cancer.

Cancer, which has become the second leading cause of death in the contemporary world, has afflicted populations and been studied by physicians for thousands of years. The term "cancer" itself derives from the Greek word *karkinos*, which was used by Hippocrates to describe tumors. Even ancient Egyptian case records as far back as 1500 BCE include mentions of breast cancer (Sudhakar, 2009). Throughout different periods of time, new explanations and theories related to how cancer occurs were developed. In Hippocrates's time through the Middle Ages, the prevalent belief was that human health was governed by the balance between four different types of bodily fluids and that the disruption of this balance could cause cancer. In the 17th century, lymph theory was developed that proposed that cancer formation was through the body's lymph fluid. Johannes Peter Muller and Rudolf Virchow however, in the 1800s, demonstrated that cancer is made up of cells and not of lymph. They determined that cancer cells were derived from other cells, and Virchow proposed that chronic irritation was the principle cause of cancer. In the following century, scientists proposed a series of different potential causes of cancer. It was believed to be caused by trauma to the body. Then, it was believed to be caused by infectious parasites. Finally, in the middle of the 20th century, as scientists began to discover and understand DNA and genetics, it became more well understood that DNA damage could lead to unrestricted cellular growth and result in cancer. The modern theory of cancer has now evolved to be more complex, but it is still centered around the idea that the role of DNA and the genetic code is to effectively regulate and control the growth of cells in the body. This scientific paradigm stresses the importance of public health approaches that mitigate the causes of cellular and genetic damage that are at the root of cancer.

The public health impact of cancer is keenly felt throughout the modern world. Over one and a half million new cases of cancer are diagnosed each year in the United States alone, and national expenditures for cancer care in the United States are expected to reach over $150 billion a year by 2020 (Quintiles IMS Institute, 2017). More than a third of all men and women are estimated to be diagnosed with cancer at some point in their lifetimes (National Cancer Institute, 2017). Cancer, with its associated social, emotional, and financial challenges, is therefore a large interest of public health interventions and professionals seeking to reduce its incidence.

The prognosis, or course of disease, of patients diagnosed with cancer is often largely impacted by the stage of their cancer. The later that patients are diagnosed, the worse their prognosis tends to be. Therefore, many public health interventions seek to improve the rate of cancer screenings so that patients are diagnosed in the earliest stages of disease when treatments such as chemotherapy are the most effective. These interventions have targeted screening rates through a variety of strategies, including launching awareness campaigns about the importance of screening, promoting the development of guidelines encouraging health care professionals to recommend screening, and carrying out lobbying for the inclusion of screening costs into health insurance plans to promote affordable access. The success of these efforts has shown such approaches to be effective. The British health care system, for example, launched a Breast Screening Programme in 1988 to invite all women between the ages of 50 and 70 to be screened for breast cancer. Evaluation of the program has shown that an estimated 1,400 lives are saved because of the program each year (Advisory Committee on Breast Cancer Screening, 2006).

Although cancer is one of the biggest causes of death in the world, there are tens of billions of dollars spent each year on cancer research with the hope of discovering and developing new and improved cancer therapies. The discoveries of these research scientists, coupled with the implementation and work of public health professionals, will serve to alleviate a portion of the contemporary health burden of cancer.

Shayan Waseh

See also: Addictions; Adverse Childhood Experiences; Air Pollution; Alcohol; Behavioral Health; Birth Defects; Chronic Illness; Environmental Health; Environmental Protection Agency; Epidemiology; Genetics; Health Disparities; Healthy Places; Hepatitis; Human Immunodeficiency Virus and Acquired Immune Deficiency Syndrome; Leading Health Indicators; Men's Health; Modern Era, Public Health in the; National Cancer Institute; Nutrition; Prevention; Skin Cancer; Surgeon General; Women's Health; Wynder, Ernst Ludwig; *Controversies in Public Health:* Controversy 2

Further Reading

Advisory Committee on Breast Cancer Screening. (2006). Screening for breast cancer in England: Past and future. *Journal of Medical Screening, 13,* 59–61.

National Cancer Institute. (2017, March). *Cancer statistics.* Retrieved from https://www.cancer.gov/about-cancer/understanding/statistics.

Quintiles IMS Institute. (2017). *Global oncology trends 2017: Advances, complexity and cost.* Retrieved from http://www.imshealth.com/en/thought-leadership/quintilesims-institute/reports/global_oncology_trends_2017.

Ryerson, A. B., Eheman, C. R., Altekruse, S. F., Ward, J. W., Jemal, A., Sherman, R. L., . . . Anderson, R. N. (2016). Annual report to the nation on the status of cancer, 1975–2012, featuring the increasing incidence of liver cancer. *Cancer, 122*(9), 1312–1337.

Siegel, R. L., Miller, K. D., & Jemal, A. (2016). Cancer statistics, 2016. *CA: A Cancer Journal for Clinicians, 66*(1), 7–30.

Sudhakar, A. (2009). History of cancer: Ancient and modern treatment methods. *Journal of Cancer Science Therapy, 1*(2), 1–4.

World Health Organization. (2017, February). *Cancer fact sheet.* Retrieved from http://www.who.int/mediacentre/factsheets/fs297/en.

CARE, ACCESS TO

Access to care is a concept in public health policy that describes the means of entry, ease of use, and receipt of basic health care services and provisions by an individual or population. Access to care is defined as "the extent a population can reach and utilize health services." The concept is particularly important in public health because it reflects the quality of life, disease detection, treatment, and disease and disability prevention efforts of society. Experts divide access to care into four main categories: affordability, availability, acceptability, and physical accessibility. Failure to adequately address these factors can present barriers that impact public health (Jacobs, Ir, Bigdeli, Annear, & Van Damme, 2012). Barriers to care can be alleviated through national policies related to health financing and socioeconomic status. In the United States, health programs and policies, such as the Patient Protection and Affordable Care Act (PPACA) and Medicare regulate the level of access to care, utilization, and coverage of health care costs.

Affordability is the minimal cost a patient or client can afford to pay for needed medical care without suffering financial hardship. One out of 20 Americans do not get needed medical treatment due to cost (Ward, Clarke, Nugent, & Schiller, 2016). Affordability is determined by income, insurance, health care funding agreements, and minimal cost payments. The United States uses a multi-payer mode with health care financing by public and private payers dependent on market competition. Working adults may be covered by employer-sponsored health insurance programs. However, not all employer-sponsored programs are affordable (Levesque, Harris, & Russell, 2013). Out-of-pocket payments may be prohibitive for low-income workers or those with high monthly expenses. Taking time off work to travel to medical appointments or receive treatment can also impact earning potential and affordability. Government policies, resources, and funding allocation can improve affordability. The PPACA removed some barriers in access to care by providing subsidies for eligible beneficiaries and eliminating restrictions on preexisting conditions. Programs offering free maternal and child health care, HIV/AIDS treatment, or other community-based treatment or prevention programs can also assist those who are struggling to earn a living wage. In comparison to the U.S. system, other developed countries use a single-payer health model dependent on community-based financing. Taxes are used to create a national system of care for protection during disease or disability.

Availability of services refers to the geographic location of providers in relation to the patient population, hours of operation, service wait times, accessible technology, qualified staff, and treatment interventions. The hours of operations and service wait times are a reflection of system efficiency. Efficiency or capacity can be improved through medical technology, telemedicine, human resources management, and strategic planning. The Electronic Health Record (EHR) improves efficiency by reducing the time needed for interdisciplinary collaboration and communication. Having well qualified medical professionals with adequate equipment and technology creates quality care. Yet, health professionals are in high demand, and human resources must work to find effective and creative ways to attract and retain qualified staff. Utilization review programs are used to assess the length of hospital stays, preadmission certifications, disease management programs, and second opinions for surgery or authorized referrals. This information is used to determine the best ways to proactively manage population needs.

Acceptability of services refers to the ethical, social, and cultural values that influence a person's decisions in accessing and accepting health services. Religious, social, and cultural values associated with healing and treatment, language, communication, diversity, gender, sexual preference, and ethnicity play a crucial role in patient care and treatment. For example, some followers of conservative Islamic or Jewish faiths will only permit female medical professionals to treat and provide care to female patients. Understanding cultural values can reduce reluctance to seek care and facilitate prevention and early diagnosis. Schools and programs in public health integrate cultural competence and gender sensitivity into health professional training in order to promote acceptability of services.

Physical accessibility is the ability to reach and utilize health services throughout all stages of care and treatment and to access health information in a timely manner. Physical accessibility relates to how the environment or geographic location affects the timely delivery of health services. A good transportation network, personal means of transportation or mobility, and duration of travel are important factors in measuring physical accessibility. To assess accessibility, location of available health facilities or providers are compared to the targeted population density, population distributions and settlements, transport network, and duration of time in seeking care. Such assessments help determine resource allocation, distribution, and the extent of access to care.

Access to care is a complex concept with many moderating factors. Health policy, funding arrangements, education, employment, income, physical environment, and housing are all important in evaluating access to care. Societal and cultural values also play a role. Cultural values such as beliefs, languages, and traditions are imperative in determining the effectiveness of treatments and communication that enhances health service delivery among patients and providers. Developing a public health workforce that reflects the cultural diversity of the community they serve is critical in promoting access to care.

Godyson Orji

See also: Affordable Care Act; Children's Health; Community Health Centers; Health Care Disparities; Health Disparities; Health Policy; Immigrant Health; Medicare; Rural Health; Social Determinants of Health; World Health Organization; *Controversies in Public Health:* Controversy 1; Controversy 5

Further Reading

Centers for Disease Control and Prevention. (2016). *Access to health care.* Retrieved from http://www.cdc.gov/vitalsigns/healthcareaccess.

Healthy People 2020. (2016). *Access to health services.* Retrieved from https://www.healthypeople.gov/2020/topics-objectives/topic/Access-to-Health-Services.

Jacobs, B., Ir, P., Bigdeli, M., Annear, P. L., & Van Damme, W. (2012). Addressing access barriers to health services: An analytical framework for selecting appropriate interventions in low-income Asian countries. *Health Policy and Planning,* 27(4), 288–300. doi:10.1093/heapol/czr038

Levesque, J. F., Harris, M. F., & Russell, G. (2013). Patient-centred access to health care: Conceptualizing access at the interface of health systems and populations. *International Journal for Equity in Health, 12*(1), 1. doi:10.1186/1475-9276-12-18

Ward, B. W., Clarke, T. C., Nugent, C. N., & Schiller, J. S. (2016). *Early release of selected estimates based on data from the 2015 National Health Interview Survey.* National Center for Health Statistics. Retrieved from http://www.cdc.gov/nchs/nhis.htm.

CAUSALITY

Causality looks at the relationship between one factor (the cause) and a subsequent phenomenon (the effect). In public health, cause-effect relationships arouse particular interest because cause-effect defines risk factors for disease, identifies at-risk groups, and enables prevention efforts. However, public health researchers struggle when investigating and reporting etiology, causes of disease. Scientists want to be certain that Risk Factor A causes Disease A before they encourage people to stop using a product or to make lifestyle changes. Premature assumptions about cause and effect create confusion and distrust. Therefore, in order to say that a factor causes a specific health problem, the relationship must meet certain conditions of time sequence (cause must precede effect), scientific credibility, consistency with other research, covariation between the two factors, and other plausible causes are ruled out (Hennekens, Buring, & Mayrent, 1987). Only when the causal factor meets most of these conditions will public health practitioners take steps to ameliorate the causal factor.

Early studies of the safety of the artificial sweetener saccharin demonstrate the importance of honoring the conditions of causality. Saccharin was discovered in 1879 by Dr. Constantin Fahlberg. Fahlberg was working late in the Johns Hopkins University laboratory when he suddenly realized that he was about to miss his dinner. He rushed home, forgetting to wash his hands. During the meal, he noticed that the bread tasted sweet. Wiping his mouth with his napkin and drinking a gulp of water, he realized that his napkin was also sweet, even sweeter than sugar. He realized that the sweetness came from chemicals he had spilled on his fingers during the day. He returned to the lab, tasting each specimen until he found the source. (Fahlberg was apparently not a good model for occupational safety.) Thankfully, none of the chemicals were corrosive, and saccharin became a major breakthrough in food chemistry. Artificial sweeteners are used to sweeten bitter medicine, in food preservation, to disguise inferior products in commercial goods, and improve food taste for people who are diabetic or on special diets. Because saccharin was discovered unintentionally, safety testing came later. Many scientists and members of the public speculated that this artificial (unnatural) chemical was unsafe. In 1977, a group of researchers published the Canadian Saccharin Study (Arnold, Moodie, Stavric, Stoltz, Grice, & Munro, 1977). Study results indicated that saccharin caused bladder cancer in laboratory rats. The study was highly publicized, and other scientists, including those from the National Cancer Institute, endorsed the generalization that saccharin would also cause bladder cancer in humans. In an effort to protect the millions of people who used saccharin as a sweetener, the federal government immediately listed saccharin as a carcinogen. All products containing saccharin were required to have a warning label, and people were advised to avoid ingestion. When other researchers attempted to repeat the study, they found that rats have a unique mechanism of breaking down and excreting saccharin. Humans do not have the same biological mechanism. Thus, saccharin causes bladder cancer in rats, not humans. When the later study results were released, nonscientists were confused and questions lingered. Was saccharin safe? It took almost two decades for the federal government to delist saccharin as a carcinogen and remove the warning. The saccharin studies show the impact of publicizing study results before the conditions of causality are met. Researchers, eager to make a name for themselves, are tempted to release results. True science is careful, patient, and thoughtful.

The first condition of causality, *time sequence*, means that the causal factor will always occur before the outcome. For Factor A to cause Disease A, Factor A must occur *before* Disease A. Using the example that tobacco smoking causes lung cancer, smoking (the cause) occurs before the lung cancer (the effect). Time sequence can be difficult to detect when there is a long time period between the cause and the effect. For example, the period between exposure to human immunodeficiency virus (HIV) and seroconversion, when antibodies are first detected, is normally three weeks to six months. In some cases, seroconversion may not occur for up to 12 months. The long and varying time sequence made it difficult for early AIDS researchers to identify the cause of AIDS. The second condition, *scientific credibility*, means that science supports a logical connection between the cause and effect. The idea that red wine lowers risk of heart disease seems contrary to what we know about alcohol and health. Alcohol impairs fat metabolism and increases risk of heart disease. On further investigation, red wine contains antioxidants that remove harmful molecules known to cause heart disease. In moderation, the antioxidants of red wine lower the risk of heart disease. In higher doses, the damaging effects of alcohol override positive antioxidant effects. Scientific credibility is limited by what we know about the human body. In some instances, credibility cannot be established until knowledge catches up with research findings. The third condition of causality, *consistency with other research*, refers to the idea that different studies of the same problem conclude similar results. The later safety studies of saccharin failed to support earlier conclusions. The fourth condition of causality, *covariation between the two factors*, means that as dose or exposure to the causal factor increases, the effect also increases. With cigarette smoking and lung cancer, the more a person smokes, the greater the risk of lung cancer and other chronic lung diseases. Covariation is also referred to as a dose-response relationship, where the higher the dose, the greater the response. The final condition of causality is *other plausible causes are ruled out*, which means the outcome cannot be explained by another factor. Social researchers struggle with this criterion. There are so many factors and interactions between factors that influence health, making it very difficult to rule out other possible causes. A problem such as childhood obesity is caused by anything that increases calorie intake beyond energy expenditure. Fast food companies can easily argue childhood obesity is not caused by fast food but by the lack of safe places to play and increased screen time. It is difficult for scientists to separate out exposures in order to draw a direct line between cause and effect.

Knowing what causes a particular disease empowers health practitioners to take efforts to stop, prevent, or reduce the risk or causal factor. Knowing that binge drinking is associated with motor vehicle crashes, sexual assault, sexually transmitted diseases (STDs), drownings, suicide, homicide, and meningitis allows health educators to target binge drinking to reduce multiple health issues. However, proving causality is a long and tedious process, and, even when scientists do collect enough evidence, they are cautious in how to present the results. Before public dissemination, results should by reviewed and confirmed by other scientists, a process known as peer review. Only after multiple researchers have studied the problem and come to similar conclusions can health professionals claim causal relationships and advocate for health policy and practices.

Sally Kuykendall

See also: Epidemiology; Koch, Heinrich Hermann Robert; Population Health; Research; Social Determinants of Health; Wynder, Ernst Ludwig; *Controversies in Public Health:* Controversy 4

Further Reading

Arnold, D. L., Moodie, C. A., Stavric, B., Stoltz, D. R., Grice, H. C., & Munro, I. C. (1977). Canadian Saccharin Study. *Science*, *197*(4301), 320.

Hennekins, C. H., Buring, J. E., & Mayrent S. L. (Eds.). (1987). *Epidemiology in medicine.* Boston: Little, Brown and Company.

Reuber, M. D. (1978). Carcinogenicity of saccharin. *Environmental Health Perspectives*, *25*, 173–200.

CENTERS FOR DISEASE CONTROL AND PREVENTION (CDC)

The Centers for Disease Control and Prevention (CDC) is a unit of the U.S. Department of Health and Human Services (DHHS) responsible for disease surveillance, treatment, and prevention and response to man-made and natural disasters. Because diseases and pathogens do not conform to man-made boundaries, the CDC is also active in global disease prevention. The CDC offers accurate and up-to-date information to the general public and health professionals. The CDC website and publications feature evidence-based programs and resources on emerging, remerging, and potential health hazards. The agency is widely recognized as one of the preeminent institutions promoting health and well-being, nationally and internationally.

The idea that the nation needed a central organization to monitor and manage health challenges arose from an outbreak of amebic dysentery in 1933 (Andrews, 1946). Approximately 8.5 million people attended the Chicago World's Fair. Cases of fever, chills, severe abdominal pain, and bloody diarrhea were first reported in

August and followed by other cases spread widely across the nation. Without a formal network of communicating unusual outbreaks of disease, local doctors did not suspect a rare parasitic organism. Doctors suspected more common illnesses, such as appendicitis or colitis. Patients were referred for surgery, which spread the pathogen into the abdominal cavity, causing sepsis and death. By November, health officials connected the cases and tracked the source to two hotels in Chicago. Inspectors found old, rusty pipes. One sewer pipe passed over the drinking water tanks of both hotels, contaminating the drinking water. Officials estimated 160,000 hotel and restaurant guests were exposed to the tainted water, 1,704 people were infected, and 98 people died. It was clear that the nation needed a centralized system of reporting and tracking disease.

The organizational and physical structure of the CDC developed from the Malaria Control in War Areas (MCWA) program. After the attack on Pearl Harbor, military and support personnel were mobilized to training bases in the southern states. Personnel from the North did not have resistance to malaria that was endemic within the southern states. Malarial infection could cause illness or death. The MCWA, U.S. Public Health Service (USPHS), and state health departments joined together to clear the areas surrounding military bases of mosquito vectors. The project immediately hit an obstacle. Many qualified personnel were already involved with other parts of the war effort. The MCWA had to train personnel. Workers were taught

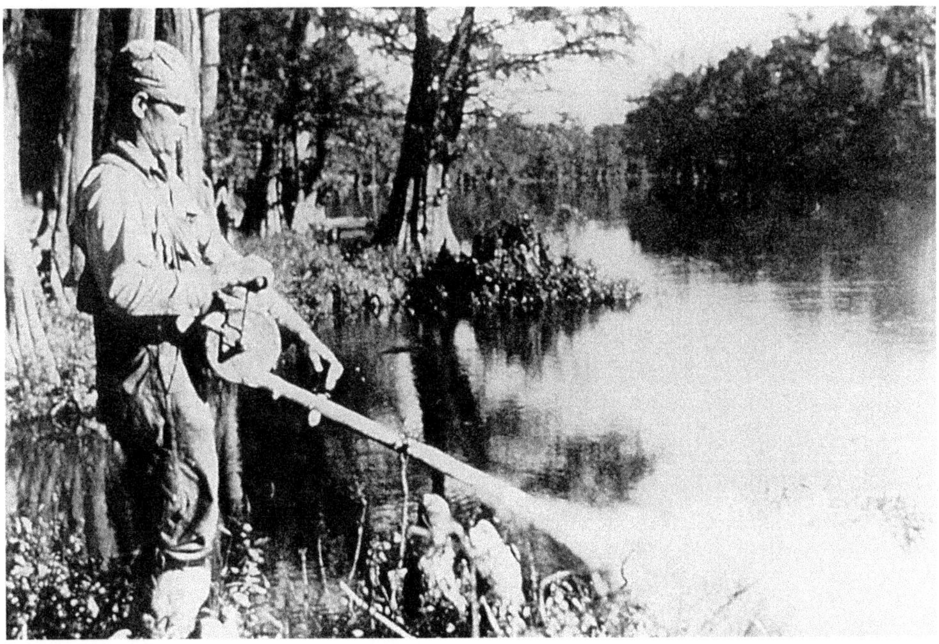

A worker sprays pesticide around a pool of standing water as part of the National Malaria Eradication Program of 1958. The first mission of the new Centers for Disease Control and Prevention (CDC) was to eradicate mosquito breeding grounds near military bases. (Courtesy CDC/Smith Collection/Gado/Getty Images)

safe and effective application of DDT, identification and elimination of mosquito breeding grounds, and working with members of the public to eliminate standing water, places where mosquitos breed. The MCWA project was highly successful. However, a second malaria threat arose when military personnel, including prisoners of war, returned from tropical battlegrounds. With the potential for malaria spreading to new areas, Dr. Joseph Mountin, chief of the USPHS's Division of Domestic Quarantine, advocated expanding MCWA efforts throughout the susceptible southern states.

The Communicable Disease Center (CDC) officially opened on July 1, 1946, with 369 staff of primarily entomologists and engineers. The initial budget of $10 million was used to purchase DDT, shovels, sprayers, and trucks. Workers received specialized training in epidemiology and disease surveillance. For logistical reasons, the CDC was located in Atlanta while other federal organizations were located in or near Washington, DC. The chairman of the board of Atlanta-based Coca-Cola, Robert W. Woodruff, took a special interest in the organization. His favorite hunting land was infested with mosquitos. Here was an opportunity to resolve his problem. Woodruff convinced Emory University to sell 15 acres of land to the CDC for a token payment of $10. CDC employees collected the money themselves. By 1949, workers had sprayed 4.6 million homes with DDT, drained numerous mosquito breeding areas, and the nation was declared malaria free (Centers for Disease Control and Prevention, 2012). The center's responsibilities quickly expanded to other infectious diseases: rabies, tuberculosis, typhus, dysentery, poliomyelitis, plague, and histoplasmosis. Internal support and networks developed. Laboratory staff researched ways to control and combat pathogens. Dr. Alexander Langmuir, the director of the epidemiology division, started a national surveillance program. Local doctors became the front line staff, reporting cases of unusual diseases to the CDC.

The CDC programs and focus adapted to meet the nation's health needs. In 1947, the CDC moved into disaster response when a cargo ship carrying ammonium nitrate exploded in Texas City, Texas. The initial blast ignited a chain reaction spreading to other ships, the oil terminal, freight trains, local businesses, and homes. Over 5,000 people were injured and 581 people died. The Texas City Disaster is considered one of the worst industrial incidents in U.S. history and forced the CDC into the role of official government agency for disaster response.

The strategies that the CDC uses to respond to health issues, epidemiology (investigating outbreaks), the use of science to guide responses and developing multilevel, planned responses are effective against numerous seemingly diverse health issues. In 1950, CDC staff traveled to Southeast Asia to provide technical assistance in malaria control. In 1955, the CDC led the investigation into the Cutter Incident, an outbreak of polio caused by contaminated polio vaccine. Other highlights include the First Surgeon General's Report on *Smoking and Health* (1964), famine relief during the Biafran War (1968), development of national health objectives (1978), global eradication of smallpox (1980), investigation of early AIDS cases (1982), elimination of polio in the Americas (1994), response to World Trade Center and anthrax attacks (2001), response to the earthquake in Haiti (2010), response to the Ebola outbreak in West Africa (2015), and response to lead contamination in the Flint, Michigan, water supply (2016). As advancements in sanitation, vaccines, and antibiotics reduced deaths due to infectious diseases, the CDC expanded efforts into chronic disease prevention, maternal and child health, nutrition, and occupational safety and health. The name of the institution changed to reflect changes in responsibilities. In 1967, the Communicable Disease Center was renamed the National Communicable Disease Center (NCDC). In 1970, the NCDC became the Center for Disease Control and in 1992, the Centers for Disease Control and Prevention emerged. Throughout the name changes, the center has maintained the universally recognized initials, CDC.

Today, the Centers for Disease Control and Prevention works with local government partners to monitor disease outbreaks (surveillance), and to intervene and prevent health threats using evidence-based practices and programs. The CDC publishes numerous journals, resources, and toolboxes. *The Morbidity Mortality Weekly Report* (*MMWR*) communicates timely, accurate, and objective health information to more than 250,000 public health and medical professionals, academics, and researchers. *MMWR* consistently ranks as one of the most influential publications in the field of public, environmental, and occupational health. The CDC website provides a wealth of resources on acute and chronic diseases and other health issues. Information is listed in an easy to navigate A to Z index or by topic category.

Throughout the past 70 years, the CDC has crafted a unique niche as a national and international leader in public health, disease prevention, health promotion, and disaster preparedness. Although the organization is part of the federal government and susceptible to changes in political opinions and climate, efforts are evidence-based. This means that the CDC attempts to remain apolitical, using science and action to address health problems.

Sally Kuykendall

See also: Bioterrorism; Cutter Incident, The; Emergency Preparedness and Response; Maternal Health; National Institutes of Health; Public Health in the United States, History of; State, Local, and Territorial Health Departments; Surgeon General; Tuskegee Syphilis Study; U.S. Department of Health and Human Services; U.S. Public Health Service; Zombie Preparedness; *Controversies in Public Health:* Controversy 4

Further Reading

Andrews, J. M. (1946). *Development of the Communicable Disease Center.* Atlanta: CDC Bulletin. Retrieved from http://www.globalhealthchronicles.com/archive/files/d3dc844d0235d315f0766d4c9521cb3b.pdf.

Centers for Disease Control and Prevention. (2012). *Elimination of malaria in the United States (1947–1951).* Retrieved from https://www.cdc.gov/malaria/about/history/elimination_us.html.

CENTERS FOR MEDICARE AND MEDICAID SERVICES (CMS)

The Centers for Medicare and Medicaid Services (CMS) is a division of the U.S. Department of Health and Human Services (DHHS) responsible for managing programs that finance health services for the elderly, people with special health needs, those with limited income, or those who are not covered by employer-sponsored health plans. Federally sponsored health care programs were first signed into law in 1965 as an amendment to the Social Security Act. The Health Insurance for the Aged (Medicare) Act and Medicaid provided hospital, extended care, and home health care to all Americans aged 65 and over. In 1977, the Health Care Financing Administration (HCFA) was established to manage the Medicare and Medicaid programs. In 2001, HCFA was renamed the Centers for Medicare and Medicaid Services (CMS). Over time, federally sponsored health care has changed as needs change and medical advances provide new and better opportunities for care. CMS currently manages Medicare, Medicaid, the Children's Health Insurance Program (CHIP), and the Health Insurance Marketplace programs. One out of three Americans is currently enrolled in a CMS program. The agency works to promote optimal medical and health care, reduce health disparities, and prevent fraud.

Sally Kuykendall

See also: Affordable Care Act; Children's Health; Emergency Medical Treatment and Labor Act (EMTALA); Family Planning; Health Disparities; Health Literacy; Medicaid; Medicare; Public Health Law; Roosevelt, Eleanor; Roosevelt, Franklin Delano; Stark Law; Social Security Act; U.S. Department of Health and Human Services

Further Reading

Centers for Medicare and Medicaid Services.Retrieved from https://www.cms.gov.

Shalala, D. (2000). Remarks by the Hon. Donna E. Shalala, Former U.S. Secretary of Health and Human Services at the 35th Anniversary Event, Hubert H. Humphrey Building, U.S. Department of Health and Human Services, Washington, DC, pages 2–7. Retrieved from https://www.cms.gov/About-CMS/Agency-Information/History/Downloads/CMS 35thAnniversary.pdf.

Tapia Granados, J. A., & Diez Roux, A. V. (2009). Life and death during the Great Depression. *Proceedings of the National Academy of Sciences of the United States of America*, *106*(41), 17290–17295. Retrieved from http://doi.org/10.1073/pnas.0904491106.

CERTIFIED IN PUBLIC HEALTH (CPH)

Professional certification in public health is achieved by successfully passing the Certified in Public Health (CPH) exam. The exam contains 200 questions on basic principles in public health. The principles reflect foundational skills that every public health professional should possess in order to function efficiently within the system. Core areas are biostatistics, environmental health sciences, epidemiology, health policy and management, and social and behavioral health sciences. Cross-cutting areas are communication and informatics, diversity and culture, leadership, public health biology, professionalism, program planning, and systems thinking. The exam is offered by the National Board of Public Health Examiners (NBPHE). Experienced public health professionals and graduates of the Council on Education for Public Health (CEPH) accredited public health programs are eligible to take the CPH. Professional credentialing demonstrates mastery of the basic concepts of public health and a personal commitment to public health practice. The credential is maintained by completing 50 CPH-approved continuing education credits every two years. Continuing education credits are earned by attending public health professional events or workshops; reading articles on public health research and practice; completing college level courses in public health or approved massive open online courses (MOOCs); writing grants, articles, or books; completing a dissertation, fellowship, or residency; or completing unpaid service related to public health. To ensure that the CPH accurately measures the knowledge and skills necessary for public health practitioners, in 2014, the NBPHE completed a job analysis study. Researchers surveyed 4,850 public health practitioners representing diverse fields of public health. Respondents provided feedback on the content of the exam. Suggestions for improvement were to consider the roles of entry level practitioners in sanitation, hygiene, and program planning as well as integrating more clinical biomedical research and scientific methods into the core competencies. As the field of public health continues to evolve, the examination will also need to evolve.

Sally Kuykendall

See also: Administration, Health; American Public Health Association; Core Competencies in Public Health; Council on Education for Public Health

Further Reading

Council on Linkages between Academia and Public Health Practice. (2014). *Core competencies for public health professionals.* Retrieved from http://www.phf.org/resourcestools/pages/core_public_health_competencies.aspx.

National Board of Public Health Examiners. (2016). *Certified in public health.* Retrieved from https://www.nbphe.org/.

CHADWICK, EDWIN (1800–1890)

Sir Edwin Chadwick was a lawyer, civil servant, and crusader who wrote some of the most important and influential documents in public health. In 1760, rapid expansion of the textile industry, invention of the steam engine, factories, railroads, and a new economic system of capitalism fueled the start of England's Industrial Revolution. In pursuit of factory jobs, working men crowded into the inner cities bringing their families with them. Available housing failed to keep up with demand.

Between 1837 and 1841, Manchester's population grew 47 percent while housing increased 15 percent (Bloy, 2016). Bradford's population grew 78 percent while housing grew 12 percent (Bloy, 2016). In Liverpool, 39,000 people lived in 7,800 cellars (an average of five people per cellar), and 86,000 people lived in 2,400 courtyards or alleyways (an average of 36 people per courtyard) (Bloy, 2016). Aging water and waste systems could not handle the increasing demand. People shared sleeping quarters with chickens, pigs, and sheep; refuse piled up in the streets; sewage spewed from gutters; cholera, typhoid, and other communicable disease epidemics were rampant. In his role of public servant, Chadwick laboriously investigated, analyzed, and documented the health of England's poor working families. Using detailed statistics and graphic descriptions, he provided a clear and unquestionable image of what life was like for the typical working-class individual. Yet, Chadwick did not stop at investigating the problem. He suggested long-term sustainable and affordable solutions. He advocated for public water systems, sewers, flush toilets, street cleaning, and city disposal of trash and refuse. Without any training in medicine or civil engineering, Chadwick created systems of sanitation that saved numerous lives and are still used today.

Edwin Chadwick was born on January 24, 1800, in Longsight, Manchester. His mother died when he was young. His father, James Chadwick, was a newspaper editor and the son of Andrew Chadwick, a close friend of the founder of methodism, John Wesley. Edwin attended public and boarding school until his family moved to London in 1810. In London, he was taught by private tutors, self-study, and his father. Because both his father and grandfather held radical, reformist political views, Edwin was enculturated with a strong sense of courage and public duty, empathy for the disadvantaged, and contempt for power and wealth. As a young man, Edwin apprenticed in a law office. He supplemented his meager earnings with income moonlighting as a journalist. In 1823, Chadwick joined the Honourable Society of the Inner Temple. By this time, his publications on life assurance, sanitation, and prevention drew the attention of well-known radicals, John Stuart Mill, Nassau Senior, and Jeremy Bentham. Chadwick became a protégé of Bentham's, moving into his house and working with the social reformer until Bentham's death in 1832. The founder of utilitarianism, Bentham believed that society should maximize utility where utility is defined as the sum of all pleasure created by an action minus the sum of all suffering created by an action. Chadwick progressed beyond Bentham's philosophical viewpoint to actually *achieve* the greatest good for the greatest number of people.

In 1832, Chadwick was appointed to the Poor Law commission with Nassau Senior. The commission was responsible for administrating the New Poor Law. In 1834, Chadwick and Senior wrote the *Report on the Poor Law,* which recommended reforms in how the poor who were unable to work were cared for. When administrators changed, Chadwick frequently found himself disagreeing with the philosophy of his superiors. The job of the Poor Law administrators was to keep the poor working so that they could support production and national progress. The assumption was that poor people were lazy and immoral and the role of the administrators was to get the poor working and to keep them working. One way to achieve this was by making the alternative to not working, living in a workhouse, very unpleasant. Chadwick believed that preventing poverty and suffering was preferable to housing and feeding people who were already in poverty. To examine poverty and develop solutions, Chadwick proposed a detailed and impartial inquiry into poverty, disease, and crime. His superiors, who had already labeled him as unsafe and impractical, isolated him from the resources and functions of the office.

Unstoppable, Chadwick joined efforts with Dr. Thomas Southwood Smith. He used his own funds, resources, and energy to investigate sanitary conditions. In 1838, Chadwick commissioned James Kay and Neil Arnott to investigate the causes of fever and prevention measures. London had suffered a series of severe cholera outbreaks. Although Chadwick believed in miasma, he also believed that sanitation measures could prevent further outbreaks. In 1840, Chadwick published the *Report on the Result of a Special Inquiry into the Practice of Interment in Towns* followed by *The Report on the Sanitary Conditions of the Labouring Population of Great Britain* (1842), commonly known as *Chadwick's Report*. Despite the fact that *Chadwick's Report* was not an official document, the report had enormous impact. Thoughtful data and detailed descriptions of the deplorable living and working conditions of laboring class presented a convincing argument of the need for reform. The report outlined the high mortality of working men, whose average life span was 29 years lower than wealthy men. The researchers calculated that occupational hazards and poor living conditions created 43,000 new widows and 112,000 new orphans per year. *Chadwick's Report* proposed government investment in sewer improvements, trash removal from houses and roads, clean drinking water, and a medical officer in each town. He argued that since a lot of poor relief went to families of working men who died of infectious diseases, society could reduce spending through sanitary measures. The report formed the basis of Britain's public health system, a system that was later replicated in other countries.

Through utilitarian logic, Chadwick countered commonly accepted policies, practices, and beliefs over and over again. In one study, Chadwick investigated the practice of sending prisoners to the Australian penal colonies to alleviate overcrowding in prisons. Merchant ships were paid a flat rate per prisoner. The ship owners packed as many men as possible onto a ship. Since the owners were paid in advance, there was no incentive to keep the prisoners alive. Approximately half of the men died along the journey. Chadwick recommended a payment based on the number of convicts who arrived safely, and the ship owners quickly developed safety measures and strategies to keep the prisoners alive and safe. In one case, the ship owner hired a doctor to accompany voyages. Deaths were reduced. In 1846, Chadwick studied worker fatalities during railroad construction. He found that companies hired the least skilled and educated workers because labor was cheaper. The lack of knowledge and experience resulted in high rates of injury. Disabled workers and widows and children of workers who died were supported by society. Chadwick advocated shifting financial responsibility onto the construction company, and companies voluntarily implemented training and safety programs. In a study of water usage, Chadwick showed that unsanitary conditions among the poor were not a matter of choice but a matter of economic necessity. Poor people would pay for drinking water delivery but would not pay for water for sanitation. Chadwick proposed piping water directly into homes, allowing the price of water delivery for drinking to offset the price of waste water for sewage disposal. Using policy and economics, Chadwick repeatedly sought the greatest good for the greatest number of people.

After another cholera epidemic, the Public Health Act was passed in 1848. The act established a Central Board of Health and local boards of health in districts where the death rate was above 23 per 1,000 (Parliament, UK, n.d.). Chadwick became chief member of the General Board of Health. However, his time on the board was brief and tenuous. He had created many enemies, businessmen and politicians with vested interests, supervisors who held tight to stereotypes against the poor, and civil engineers who questioned aspects of the sewer pipeline. Chadwick's dogmatic approach and unrelenting push for centralized services made him an easy target for vilification. In 1854, he was deposed from the General Board of Health. He continued his work investigating and reporting on numerous health issues. Through recognition by Prince Albert of Saxe-Coburg and Gotha, Chadwick was awarded a knighthood in 1889.

Sir Edwin Chadwick was a public health crusader with enormous energy and conviction. In his role as a civil servant, Chadwick's primary aim was to increase efficiency and minimize waste. Philosophically, Chadwick focused on achieving the greatest good for the greatest number of people. Without any training in medicine or civil engineering, he carefully collected and used public health statistics to advocate for policies improving safety and sanitation. His ability to identify social problems and see solutions led to massive transformations in urban structure, buildings, and functions that we still enjoy today.

Sally Kuykendall

See also: Cholera; Health Policy; Infectious Diseases; Modern Era, Public Health in the; Nightingale, Florence; Snow, John; Social Determinants of Health

Further Reading

Bloy, M. (2016). *The Sanitary Report, 1842.* A web of English history. Retrieved from http://www.historyhome.co.uk/peel/p-health/sanrep.htm.

Finer, S. E. (1952). *The life and times of Sir Edwin Chadwick.* London: Methuen.

Hamlin, C. (1992). Edwin Chadwick and the engineers, 1842–1854: Systems and antisystems in the pipe-and-brick sewers war. *Technology and Culture*, *33*(4), 680.

Lewis, R. A. (1950). Edwin Chadwick and the railway labourers. *The Economic History Review*, *3*(1). 107.

Parliament, UK (n.d.). *The 1848 Public Health Act.* Retrieved from http://www.parliament.uk/about/living-heritage/transformingsociety/towncountry/towns/tyne-and-wear-case-study/about-the-group/public-administration/the-1848-public-health-act.

CHILD MALTREATMENT

Child maltreatment is an umbrella term for the abuse and neglect of children. The definition of child maltreatment varies between different organizations, professionals, and advocates. Child maltreatment is defined by the Federal Child Abuse Prevention and Treatment Act (CAPTA) as "any recent act or failure to act on the part of a parent or caretaker that results in death, serious physical or emotional harm, sexual abuse or exploitation; or an act or failure to act, which presents an imminent risk of serious harm" (Child Welfare Information Gateway, 2014). According to the Centers for Disease Control and Prevention (CDC), child maltreatment includes abuse and neglect of a child less than 18 years of age by a parent, caregiver, or another person in a custodial role. The World Health Organization (WHO) estimates that approximately 40 million children are victims of maltreatment worldwide annually. According to the *Child Maltreatment Report 2014,* compiled by the Children's Bureau of the U.S. Department of Health and Human Services, there were more than 3 million reports of suspected child maltreatment made to Child Protective Services (CPS) with 702,000 confirmed victims.

Public policies against child maltreatment trace back to the Middle Ages in Europe with laws forbidding infanticide. Child mistreatment and exploitation were common. Children were sold to provide money for families that struggled with poverty and famine. The first documented cases of child abuse charges against parents and the removal of children from unfit homes were in the 1670s. In 1869, the Illinois Supreme Court ruled that a parent treating a child inhumanely was punishable by law after a father in Illinois was charged for locking his blind son in a cold basement. During the Industrial Revolution, children were forced to work long hours in awful and often hazardous conditions. By 1900, every state in the United States passed legislation that addressed the issues of child labor, but it was not until 1941 when the U.S. Supreme Court passed the Fair Labor Standards Act that limited child labor (McCoy & Keen, 2009).

In 1912, the Children's Bureau was founded to explore all issues regarding child welfare. In 1944, the Supreme Court ruled in *Prince v. the Commonwealth of Massachusetts* that states have the right to interfere in family relationships to protect children. In 1974, the United States passed its first federal law on child abuse, the Child Abuse Prevention Treatment Act (CAPTA), which provided funding for the investigation and prevention of child abuse as long as states had mandated reporting laws. CAPTA also established the National Clearinghouse on Child Abuse and Neglect (NCCAN) that serves as a national resource for professionals regarding child maltreatment (McCoy & Keen, 2009).

According to the Children's Bureau, there are four main types of child maltreatment: *physical abuse, sexual abuse, emotional abuse*, and *neglect. Physical abuse* is the use of intentional physical force against a child that can potentially result in physical injury. Physical abuse includes hitting, kicking, shaking, burning, or other use of force. Symptoms of physical abuse include unexplained injuries, injuries inconsistent with the history provided by the parent or caregiver, or the child seems frightened of the caregiver. *Sexual abuse* is defined as engaging a child in sexual acts or attempting sexual contact, including fondling, rape, and exposing a child to other sexual activities. *Emotional abuse* is defined as behaviors that harm a child's self-worth or emotional well-being. Examples include name-calling, degrading, rejecting, threatening, belittling, and isolating the child. *Neglect*, the most common form of child maltreatment, is the failure to meet a child's basic needs or the failure to protect a child from harm or potential harm. There are many forms of neglect. Physical neglect includes the failure to provide adequate nutrition, clothing, hygiene, or a safe living environment. Psychological or emotional neglect is the lack of emotional support or bonding from the parent or caregiver. Medical neglect is the failure to seek health care or the delay of medical care by the parent or caregiver. Educational neglect is when the parent or caregiver fails to enroll a child in an educational institution or allows frequent school absences. Abandonment is when a child is left alone for an extended period of time given the child's age and capacities, including leaving a child in a locked vehicle or incapacitation of the parent or caregiver due to alcohol or substance use. Neglect also encompasses the lack of guidance, defined as exposing a child to criminal activity, illicit drug use, or other risk-taking behaviors by the parent or caregiver. Exposure to intimate partner violence is also considered a form of child maltreatment by many public health professionals.

Knowing at-risk groups empowers health professionals to prevent abuse or to be vigilant for potential cases. Children under the age of four years are at greatest risk for severe injury and death from abuse. The group with the highest rate of child victimization is infants in their first year of life. Approximately 27 percent of victims of child maltreatment and 70 percent of deaths due to child abuse occurred in children under the age of three years (CDC, 2014). Traits that may increase the likelihood of child maltreatment include persistent crying or having special needs, such as a physical disability, an intellectual disability, or a chronic illness. Risk factors that increase the likelihood of a parent or caregiver to abuse or neglect a child include stress in the home due to violence, drug or alcohol abuse, mental illness, poverty, and chronic health problems. Parents who are young, single parents, have a history of maltreatment as children, experience financial difficulties, and/or are of low educational status have higher risk for perpetration. Community risk factors involve neighborhood violence and crime, weak social connections among neighbors, high unemployment rates, and high density of alcohol or illicit drug use. Protective factors, factors that guard against child maltreatment, include supportive and stable family and community environments, parental employment, and adequate housing and access to health care.

Child maltreatment has long-term detrimental effects on child victims and their families. Many studies have shown that child maltreatment can impact brain development. Child victims demonstrate behavioral, physical, and mental health problems such as increased aggression, anxiety, depression, post-traumatic stress disorder, cognitive delays, problems in school and with peers, and disruption in nervous system and immune system development. As adults, child victims are predisposed to mental illnesses, smoking, alcohol and drug use, high-risk sexual behaviors, sexually transmitted diseases, unintended pregnancy, obesity, and heart disease (CDC, 2016). Experiences as a maltreated child influence relationships in adulthood. Victims are at risk for either perpetrating violence or being a victim of violence as an adult. Socially, child maltreatment has a significant economic impact, including costs of hospitalizations, child welfare and criminal justice systems involvement, and long-term health care and mental health treatment. The CDC estimates the total lifetime financial costs associated with one year of confirmed cases of child maltreatment is approximately $124 billion (Fang et al., 2012).

All states in the United States have laws regarding mandatory reporting of suspected child maltreatment. Individuals that are considered mandated reporters may include physicians, nurses, health care workers, teachers, social workers, counselors, therapists, child care providers, and law enforcement officers. In approximately 18 states and Puerto Rico, any person who suspects child maltreatment is mandated to report. However, any concerned individual can report suspicions of child abuse or neglect, and an investigation into the situation will determine if intervention is necessary. Information about how each state addresses reporting suspected child abuse can be found on the Child Welfare Information Gateway website (www.childwelfare.gov). The Childhelp National Child Abuse Hotline is also available 24 hours a day, seven days a week with trained counselors who have access to numerous emergency, social service, and support resources.

Child maltreatment prevention entails a multifaceted approach. The CDC and the World Health Organization (WHO) identify several strategies to prevent child maltreatment. These strategies aim to strengthen economic supports to families, change social norms to support positive parenting, provide quality care and education early in life, enhance parenting skills, and intervene to prevent future harm. Visits by nurses to parents and children in their homes, parent education, and teaching children the difference between safe and unsafe are also some effective methods that can be implemented in programs in health care, schools, and social work.

Kim L. Nguyen and Maria DiGiorgio McColgan

See also: Adverse Childhood Experiences; Children's Health; Hamilton, Alice; Injuries; Intimate Partner Violence; Violence

Further Reading

Centers for Disease Control and Prevention (CDC). (2014). *Child maltreatment: Facts at a glance.* Retrieved from https://www.cdc.gov/violenceprevention/pdf/childmaltreatment-facts-at-a-glance.pdf.

Centers for Disease Control and Prevention (CDC). (2016). *Child maltreatment.* Retrieved from http://www.cdc.gov/violenceprevention/childmaltreatment/index.html.

Child Welfare Information Gateway. (2014). *Definitions of child abuse and neglect.* Washington, DC: U.S. Department of Health and Human Services, Children's Bureau. Retrieved from https://www.childwelfare.gov/pubPDFs/define.pdf.

Fang, X., Brown, D. S., Florence, C. S., & Mercy, J. A. (2012). The economic burden of child maltreatment in the United States and implications for prevention. *Child Abuse & Neglect*, *36*(2), 156–165.

McCoy, M. L., & Keen, S. M. (2009). *Child abuse and neglect*. New York: Psychology Press.

U.S. Department of Health & Human Services, Administration for Children and Families, Administration on Children, Youth and Families, Children's Bureau. (2016). *Child maltreatment 2014*. Retrieved from http://www.acf.hhs.gov/programs/cb/research-data-technology/statistics-research/child-maltreatment.

World Health Organization. (2016). *Child maltreatment*. Retrieved from http://www.who.int/mediacentre/factsheets/fs150/en/.

CHILDREN'S HEALTH

The health of children is always an important issue for any country, since children are the future. There have been a number of important reviews of children's health in the United States and commissions to discuss issues linked to the health of children. One of the most important is the work of the National Research Council and Institute of Medicine (2004). In that work, which began with a review of the available literature as well as a consideration of important issues, the committee agreed on some important guiding principles, repeated below:

- children are vital assets of society;
- critical differences between children and adults warrant special attention to children's health;
- children's health has effects that reach far into adulthood;
- the manifestations of health vary for different communities and different cultures; and
- data on children's health and its influences are needed to maximize the health of children and the health of the adults they will become. (National Research Council and Institute of Medicine, 2004)

It is helpful to understand more about why it is in the national interest to have healthy children. If children are healthy, they are more likely to be ready and able to learn and, as adults, to be healthy and able to contribute to the workforce and the overall vitality of society. In earlier eras, disease and death in children were due largely to infections. Childhood deaths were common. In the 20th century, both childhood mortality and infectious disease rates in the United States have been drastically lowered; it is now uncommon for a child to die in childhood whereas in the late 1800s, many families experienced the death of at least one child.

There are some interim health problems that have seen improvement in the United States more recently, especially since 1970. One of the most important of these is the reduction in negative health effects from lead as well as efforts in reduction of infant mortality and morbidity and accidental causes of injury. There have also been improvements in increasing access to health care for children and reducing other environmental contaminants.

In the area of improvement in ill effects from lead, major improvements have been made in understanding how environmental contaminants such as lead impact children and lead to adverse impacts on children's developments and reductions in the ambient lead amounts and reduced childhood blood lead levels. Average concentrations of lead in the blood of children younger than five dropped 78 percent between 1976 and 1980, and between 1992 and 1994, and there was a decrease of 93 percent by 2011–2012, as compared with 1976–1980 (U.S. EPA, 2015).

Infant mortality, that is, deaths in the first year of life, are understood to be both an important indicator of overall health in a country and an important indicator of child health. In the United States, following a plateau from 2000 through 2005, the U.S. infant mortality rate declined 12 percent from 2005 through 2011. Infant mortality declined for four of the five leading causes of death during the 2005–2011 period (MacDorman, Hoyert, & Mathews, 2016).

Other areas of improved child health are in the areas of access to care, absences from school due to ill health, and teenage pregnancy. About 85 percent of school-aged children 5 to 11 years of age are now reported as in excellent or very good health. Slightly over 3 percent (3.2) of school-aged children 5 to 11 years of age missed 11 or more days of school in the past 12 months because of illness or injury. Partially due to greater coverage of children from aspects of the Affordable Care Act (also sometimes referred to as Obamacare) and the related expansions of Medicaid and the Children's Health Insurance Program since 2009, only 5.1 percent of children under 18 years of age were without health insurance, and only 4.0 percent of children under 18 years of age were without a usual source of health care (National Center for Health Statistics, 2017).

Another area of improvement is that fewer adolescents are having babies—in 1999, the teenage pregnancy rate reached the lowest recorded rate since 1976. Rates continued to improve, with 24.2 births for every 1,000 adolescent females aged 15 to 19 in 2014, or 249,078 babies born to females in this age group. Nearly 89 percent of these births occurred outside of marriage. The 2014 teen birth rate indicates a decline of 9 percent from 2013 when the birth rate was 26.5 per 1,000. The teen birth rate has declined almost continuously since 2000. Teen birth rates differ substantially by racial and ethnic group. Birth rates are higher among Hispanic and black adolescents than among their white counterparts. In 2014, Hispanic adolescent females aged 15 to 19 had the highest birth rate (38 births per 1,000 adolescent females), followed by black adolescent females (34.9 births per 1,000 adolescent females), and white adolescent females (17.3 births per 1,000 adolescent females). Although Hispanics currently have the highest teen birth rates, they have had a dramatic recent decline in rates. Since 2007, the teen birth rate has declined by 50 percent for Hispanics, compared with declines of 44 percent for blacks and 36 percent for whites (Office of Adolescent Health, 2016).

The picture on usage of tobacco products is more complex, with some improvement but also the introduction of new tobacco-related products and more usage of those. Looking across several decades, daily cigarette use fell by more than 50 percent (from 10 to 5 percent) among 8th-grade students between 1996 and 2002, and by more than two-fifths (from 18 to 10 percent) among 10th-grade students. From 2011 to 2015, current cigarette smoking declined among middle and high school students. By 2015, about 2 of every 100 middle school students (2.3 percent) reported that they smoked cigarettes in the past 30 days—a decrease from 4.3 percent in 2011. By 2015, about 9 of every 100 high school students (9.3 percent) reported that they smoked cigarettes in the past 30 days—a decrease from 15.8 percent in 2011. However, current use of electronic cigarettes increased among middle and high school students from 2011 to 2015. Around 5 percent of middle school students reported in 2015 that they used electronic cigarettes in the past 30 days—an increase from 0.6 percent in 2011. There was even more increase for high school students, with 16 of every 100 high school students reporting in 2015 that they used electronic cigarettes in the past 30 days—an increase from 1.5 percent in 2011. Use of other smoking products such as hookahs also increased from 2011 to 2015 (Centers for Disease Control, 2016).

Although some trends are positive or mixed, others are negative. Replacing the problems of the previous 150 years of infectious diseases in the last 50 years is the increase of some more serious chronic diseases, along with a number of health problems that are a result of the interaction of genetics, behavior, and the environment. Childhood obesity, diabetes, and asthma rates in the United States are among the highest in the world and are increasing rapidly. Intentional and unintentional injuries, mental health disorders, and attention deficit disorder are highly prevalent. A few illustrations of some of these issues are that there are increases in obesity among children with 17.4 percent of children 6 to 11 years of age who are obese by 2013 to 2014. The number of children with asthma is now more than 6.2 million, and the percent of children with asthma is 8.4 percent (National Center for Health Statistics, 2017). Attention-deficit/hyperactivity disorder (ADHD) has also been increasing since 1990. Currently, 10.4 percent of children 5 to 17 years of age have been diagnosed with ADHD in 2013–2015, with more boys (14.2 percent) diagnosed as compared to girls (6.4 percent) (National Center for Health Statistics, 2017).

Diabetes is a serious chronic disease, both for adults and children. Although the majority of children under 21 with diabetes have Type 1 (what at one time was known as juvenile diabetes), the major concern as an indicator of increases in poor health in children are linked to the rise of Type 2 diabetes in children 10 and over, a condition almost unheard of as recently as 20 years ago (Gebel, 2012). Type 2 diabetes in 10- to 19-year-olds increased 21 percent between 2001 and 2009, mostly in Hispanic and non-Hispanic white youth.

Although more than a decade has passed since the National Research Council and Institute of Medicine report, their goals are still important for future efforts. Future systems need to incorporate a better conceptualization of children's health that considers prominent developmental characteristics of children as well as positive aspects of health, along with a greater focus on collection of data on child health problems.

Jennie Jacobs Kronenfeld

See also: Adverse Childhood Experiences; Behavioral Health; Birth Defects; Centers for Medicare and Medicaid Services; Child Maltreatment; Dunham, Ethel Collins; Family Planning; *Healthy People 2020*; Infant Mortality; Maternal Health; School Health; Social Determinants of Health; Truth Campaign, The; Vaccines; Violence; Wald, Lillian; *Controversies in Public Health:* Controversy 2; Controversy 3

Further Reading

Centers for Disease Control. (2016). *Youth and tobacco use.* Retrieved from https://www.cdc.gov/tobacco/data_statistics/fact_sheets/youth_data/tobacco_use/.

Gebel, E.. (2012). More kids than ever have type 2 diabetes. *Diabetes Forecast.* Retrieved from http://www.diabetesforecast.org/2012/nov/more-kids-than-ever-have-type-2-diabetes.html 2012.

MacDorman, M. F., Hoyert, D. L., & Mathews, T. J. (2016). *Recent declines in infant mortality in the United States, 2005–2011.* Centers for Disease Control. Retrieved from https://www.cdc.gov/nchs/data/databriefs/db120.htm#x2013;2011%3C/a%3E.

National Center for Health Statistics. (2017). *Faststats.* Retrieved from http://www.cdc.gov/nchs/fastats/child-health.htm.

National Research Council and Institute of Medicine. (2004). *Children's health, the nation's wealth: Assessing and improving child health.* Washington, DC: National Academies Press. doi:10.17226/10886

Office of Adolescent Health. (2016). *Reproductive health.* Retrieved from http://www.hhs.gov/ash/oah/adolescent-health-topics/reproductive-health/teen-pregnancy/trends.html.

U.S. EPA. (2015). America's Children and the Environment (ACE). *Biomonitoring: Lead.* Indicator B1. Retrieved from https://www.epa.gov/ace/biomonitoring-lead.

CHOLERA

Cholera is an intestinal infection caused by the bacterium *Vibrio cholera.* This bacterium is a type of facultative anaerobic organism that secretes cholera toxin or choleragen in the digestive system. Symptoms of the disease range from mild diarrhea and vomiting to severe dehydration depending on the variety of *Vibrio cholerae* involved. The disease is spread predominantly through drinking water that has been contaminated by sewage. Historically, instances of the disease were related to human waste infiltrating the water supply. Cholera affects millions of individuals each year, usually in developing countries where sanitation and preventative measures are insufficient or nonexistent. In the past, the disease reached epidemic proportions of 50 percent or higher mortality rate (World Health Organization, 2008). Today, mortality may be as low as 1 percent for those who receive early treatment. Although modern bacteriology and public health measures have eliminated or reduced waterborne illnesses in many developed countries, this deadly disease remains a threat throughout the world and serves as a model for prevention and control of similar acute infectious diseases.

Cholera is mainly transmitted through water or food in areas where poor or inadequate sanitation exists. The microorganism moves from the initial human host, also known as a reservoir, to the new susceptible host via the water table or water source. The pathogen leaves the initial carrier through diarrhea. The infected fecal matter contaminates the local water source. People either drink the infested water or certain varieties of seafood—plankton and shellfish—drawn from the water transmit the bacteria. Not everyone who ingests the bacterium will become infected. Susceptibility is related to a number of factors, including acidity of the intestinal tract, age, amount of the bacterium ingested, exposure to other infectious pathogens, and chronic diseases or genetic conditions such as cystic fibrosis. The bacteria attack the carrier by embedding in the lining of the intestine. In order to get into the lining, the bacteria must survive the stomach's first line of defense, the highly acidic gastric juices. The pathogens protect themselves from stomach acids by conserving energy, primarily limiting protein production. Upon arrival in the small intestine, they increase protein output to produce the toxin choleragen. The interplay of chloride and sodium ions renders the interior of the intestine saline, or like salt water. This process creates osmotic pressure. The osmosis pulls gallons of water from the body of the host, resulting in large volumes of diarrhea and subsequent dehydration. If fluid and electrolytes are not replaced, death can occur.

Public health professionals diagnose cholera by the characteristic symptoms and laboratory testing. The telltale symptoms of the disease are profuse diarrhea and vomiting to such an extent that the excretions are nearly clear in appearance. In some places, this excretion is nicknamed "rice water" because of its resemblance to the by-product of boiled rice. In its most severe cases, the disease can cause up to three or four gallons of diarrhea to be passed by the host in a single day. This extreme loss of fluids produces the second grouping of visible symptoms, namely dehydration and its related symptoms. The symptoms of dehydration include wrinkled skin on the extremities, sunken eyes, and skin with a bluish hue. Cholera was traditionally called the "Blue Death" because of this change in skin color. The loss of electrolytes affects all of the body organs and can decrease heart rate, impair the muscles that control breathing, and result in coma. In addition to assessing symptoms, public health practitioners can diagnose cholera by administering a dipstick test on swab or stool samples from the patient.

Cholera has most likely existed since ancient times, traced back to the Ganges River delta of the Indian subcontinent. The name is derived from the Greek word for "bile," or *kholera*, which is from the "yellow bile" of humoral medical theory. Ancient Greeks believed that when yellow bile was out of balance with the other humors, this caused an aggressive or angry disposition. Today, the word for "anger" in romance languages is derived from cholera. The disease of cholera should not be confused with *Cholera morbus,* a term once used to distinguish gastroenteritis or "stomach flu" from cholera.

Cholera was contained within certain geographic regions of India until improvements in transportation and trade infrastructure increased population movement. As people moved into and out of the region, the disease progressed from an endemic problem to pandemic proportions. Repeatedly throughout history, population movements have spread infectious diseases to new, distant locations. Occurrences of cholera throughout much of Asia and Russia are traced to a major outbreak in Bengal, India, in 1817. The disease first arrived in Europe and North America along major shipping and trade routes between 1827 and 1835. The transmission to new areas carried high mortality, killing large numbers of people, especially in urban environments. For much of the 19th century there was no effective remedy for cholera, and the mortality rate was exceptionally high. Cholera is attributed to the deaths of Russian composer Pyotr Tchaikovsky, King Charles X of France, and U.S. president James K. Polk, among others. Subsequent pandemics struck Europe, sub-Saharan Africa, and South America, with the most recent occurring as late as 1961. Instances of cholera decreased in the developed world during the 20th century due to advances in water purification and public health sanitation. However, the disease is still a significant presence in developing countries.

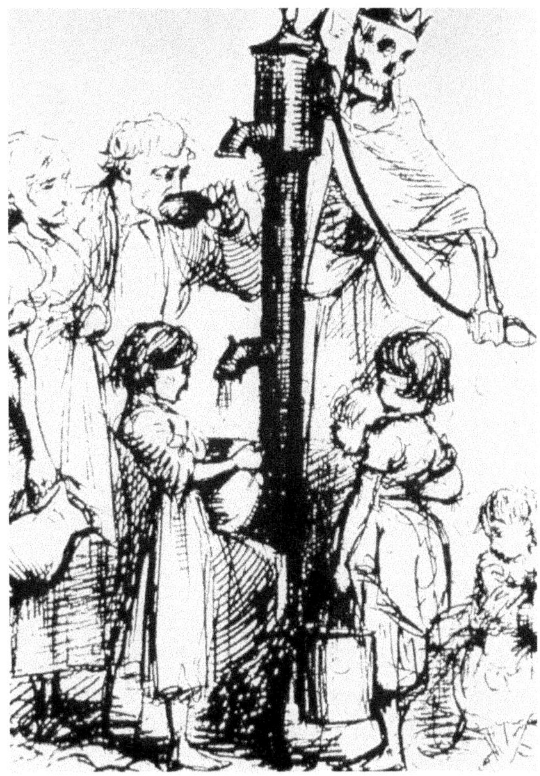

Children drawing contaminated water from the community pump. Despite Snow's evidence that cholera was caused by contaminated water, city officials did little to address the problem. (Centers for Disease Control and Prevention)

Treatment of cholera advanced significantly with the discovery and development of a germ theory in the later half of the 1800s. Before germ theory, people did not know how infections were spread. In 1854, John Snow traced the transmission of cholera to contaminated water and introduced a new field of study known as epidemiology. The bacterium was initially isolated in the same year by Filippo Pacini, an Italian anatomist, and later by the German microbiologist Robert Koch in 1883. Early vaccines were developed to combat cholera by the Spanish physician Jaume Ferran i Clua in 1885 and Russian bacteriologist Waldemar Haffkine in 1892. Despite these efforts, the disease continued to challenge public health systems with high mortality rates. In 1967, Robert Allan Phillips, an American research scientist at Naval Medical Research Unit 2, developed a treatment schedule of rehydration. Phillips later won the prestigious Lasker Award for his discovery.

Today, early rehydration therapy provides critical treatment for those suffering from the effects of cholera or other diseases that produce massive fluid loss. Contemporary cases of cholera can now be treated in a clinical setting with close observation, hydration, and maintenance of healthy levels of electrolytes. In cases of mild dehydration, the patient is encouraged to take oral fluids. With severe cases, the administration of up to 10 percent of the patient's body weight in fluids may be necessary. In such cases, patients must be carefully monitored to ensure that fluids and electrolytes are restored to the appropriate tissues in the body and do not create other electrolyte imbalances that could lead to respiratory failure or cardiac arrest.

With significant advances in treatment already achieved, in recent times the medical and public health communities concentrated on preventative methods and quality of life. The majority of these measures involve effective sanitation and water filtration infrastructures. In developing countries a folded cloth *sari* is recommended as a cheap and effective way to filter drinking water. Proper sterilization and sanitation, when coupled with new developments in vaccines, antibiotics, and hydration/electrolyte therapy, have greatly decreased deadly cases of cholera in the 21st century. Responding to outbreaks of the disease in Haiti, in the early 2000s, the World Health Organization set the goal of eradicating cholera by 2020.

Sean P. Phillips

See also: Ancient World, Public Health in the; Chronic Illness; Environmental Protection Agency; Epidemic; Epidemiology; Genetics; Immigrant Health; Indian Health Service; Infectious Diseases; Koch, Heinrich Hermann Robert; Middle Ages, Public Health in the; National Institutes of Health; Pandemic; Pasteur, Louis; Waterborne Diseases, Winslow, Charles-Edward Amory; World Health Organization

Further Reading

Hamlin, C. (2007). *Cholera: The biography.* Biographies of diseases 2. Oxford, UK: Oxford University Press.

Kudlick, C. J. (1996). *Cholera in post-revolutionary Paris: A cultural history.* Studies on the history of society and culture 25. Berkeley: University of California Press.

Rosenberg, C. E. (1987). *The cholera years: The United States in 1832, 1849, and 1866.* Chicago: University of Chicago Press.

World Health Organization. (2008). *WHO position paper on oral rehydration salts to reduce mortality from cholera.* Retrieved from http://www.who.int/cholera/technical/en/.

CHRONIC ILLNESS

Chronic illnesses are persistent health conditions that last three months or more. They start discretely and progress to more serious problems over time. Sometimes, the terms "chronic illnesses," "chronic diseases," and "noncommunicable diseases" are used interchangeably. The term "chronic disease" refers to the biological problem, such as heart disease, stroke, high blood pressure, cancer, diabetes, asthma, or chronic obstructive pulmonary disease (COPD). The term "chronic illness" refers to the biological disease as well as psychosocial issues related to long-term control and management. Seven of the ten leading causes of death are chronic diseases. Nearly half of all Americans suffer from one or more chronic illnesses, and that number increases to 85 percent for people over the age of 65 (Wiley et al., 2015). Current public health efforts focus on research, prevention, screening, community action, and once a condition is diagnosed, applying best clinical practice guidelines, individual self-management, and coordinating health services. The capacity to manage and treat multiple chronic conditions (MCC) is a significant challenge. The current medical management model of treating each case of disease individually is expensive and allows gaps to occur when each provider focuses on one aspect of the patient, missing the bigger picture. New health care delivery models provide a holistic approach and suggest promise in treating individuals with MCC.

Over the 20th century, advances in science and medicine have fundamentally changed the diseases the vast majority of the population contract. Improved sanitation, better hygiene, and the development of both vaccinations and antibiotics means that infectious diseases, such as diphtheria and smallpox, are no longer the public health threats they once were. The result of these advancements is that Americans are living significantly longer than past generations. Between 1880 and 2010, life expectancy in the United States almost doubled from 39.4 years to 78.8 years (Roser, 2016). The shift from acute illnesses to chronic illnesses meant that medical care also shifted from treating self-limiting communicable diseases to persistent noncommunicable diseases. Although modern medicine has skillfully worked to effectively find cures or eradicate many ailments prevalent over a century ago, chronic illnesses raise other issues. As people live longer, their bodies are more susceptible to multiple chronic illnesses. In 2005, experts speculated that childhood obesity may halt or reverse the upward trend in life expectancy (Olshansky et al.,

2005). Overweight and obese children at risk for heart disease, stroke, and diabetes are at greater risk for premature death.

Early diagnosis of chronic illness is crucial in securing treatment and controlling the complications of any disease. Undiagnosed diabetes can result in blindness, lower extremity amputations, kidney failure, and heart attack. Cancers may metastasize to other organs. High blood pressure can cause stroke or kidney problems. Chronic illnesses are first diagnosed when the patient reports symptoms to a health care provider or abnormal results appear on regular physical examination or screening. A routine sports physical can reveal asthma, epilepsy, congenital cardiac disease, blood abnormalities, or cancer. Primary care providers check blood pressure, blood cell count, and perform numerous screenings to identify chronic conditions. Patients can also screen themselves through testicular self-examination or breast self-examination. Although not as effective as other forms of screening, the female who regularly practices breast self-examination can identify a lump the size of a quarter (0.83 inches), whereas those who do not practice regular self-examination can first identify a lump the size of a half dollar coin (1.42 inches). Mammograms, recommended for women every one to two years after the age of 40, can identify a lump as small as 0.43 inches. Early identification can significantly change the course of the disease. Unfortunately, many Americans do not have access or do not practice regular screening. Only 8 out of 10 women (aged 50–75) report getting a mammogram within the past two years. Less than 4 out of 10 females (aged 13–15) get the HPV vaccine (Johnson, Hayes, Brown, Hoo, & Ethier, 2014).

Once diagnosed, chronic conditions can be challenging to both manage and treat. Diabetics must learn to manage their diet and medications changing many lifelong habits. Twenty-one percent of diabetics do not have their blood sugar under control (Johnson, Hayes, Brown, Hoo, & Ethier, 2014). Individuals with chronic illnesses require many visits to health care providers, pharmacies, and more than one specialist, such as a cardiologist, endocrinologist, or oncologist. Although the primary care physician plays an important role in coordinating care, those with multiple chronic conditions are often required to take on a strong role as their own advocate. Managing multiple visits and treatments can be tiring and frustrating. Many chronic illnesses, particularly diabetes and heart disease, require vast personal lifestyle changes and will get significantly worse if the disease is not managed well or the patient is not compliant with medication and lifestyle changes. Studies have shown that managing chronic illness can be extremely overwhelming and eventually can lead to depression.

The rising costs of managing and treating chronic illnesses is one of the most pressing challenges for health care today. The health insurance system was established to manage acute illnesses with the provider receiving a fee for each encounter or service. Medical expenditures for the average person cost about $4,400 per year. The average patient with Type 2 diabetes costs about $11,700 per year. An estimated 25.8 million people or 8.3 percent of the total population have diabetes

(Moran, Burson, Critchett, & Olla, 2011). Fee-for-service payment structures were established in the early 20th century before chronic illnesses became the leading causes of death. In order to address the rapidly rising costs of health care and improve outcomes, innovative health care delivery models have been introduced. Health insurance companies and policy makers suggest including quality as an aspect of reimbursement. Rather than fee-for-service, health care providers receive an incentive to establish ways in which patients can achieve a better overall outcome. In an effort to reign in steeply rising health care costs, the Patient-Centered Medical Home (PCMH) has emerged as a promising way to manage the large population of chronically ill patients. The PCMH provides multiple, continuous touch points, preventative services, and increased monitoring for disease complications. PCMHs have been shown to reduce emergency room visits, reduce blood glucose levels among diabetics, and achieve overall cost savings with better health outcomes. Although some opponents argue that the cost to reorganize a medical practice is prohibitive, data suggests that long-term savings can be realized through reduced adverse health outcomes and better-quality health care. The need to reengineer medical practices to address the ongoing need for chronic illness management is logical, but implementation costs and existing fee-for-service payment structures, rather than pay for performance pay structures, continue to present challenges.

Prevention of chronic diseases is a primary goal of *Healthy People 2020* and public health efforts. Over the past several decades, multiple programs have been launched to educate people on healthy choices and preventing chronic illnesses. Chronic illnesses have many causes, including genetics, a hereditary predisposition, environmental factors, or can be directly attributed to lifestyle choices. For example, heart disease can be caused in part by many factors, including heredity, a high cholesterol diet, lack of exercise, and smoking, to name just several major risk factors. However, if an individual can reduce risk factors for heart disease by not smoking, exercising regularly, and eating a healthy diet, the individual, even with hereditary factors, may be able to reduce his or her risk or delay the onset of heart disease. Given that chronic disease is often caused by many complex factors, it becomes a challenging public health effort to educate the public about how lifestyle choices may have an effect on one's health later in life. Successful public health campaigns have been launched in an effort to reduce incidences of heart disease and several types of cancer.

Although the prevention, screening, and management of chronic diseases are constantly improving, the rising epidemic of chronic illnesses and the resulting high cost of health care are among the nation's most pressing public health issues. Although prevention is the ultimate goal, the statistics demonstrate that a large sector of our population is suffering from at least one chronic illness. The cost of chronic illness from an economic perspective is great, but the implications for society continue to be a pressing issue as well. Patients, particularly those with more than one chronic illness, struggle to manage lifestyle changes, medications, and health care costs, which often result in overwhelming frustration and depression. If quality outcomes for chronic illnesses are going to continue to be a priority, the health care system must continue to evolve. Payment structures can no longer depend on fee-for-service payment structure alone, since so many chronic illnesses require many touch points with health care staff. The approach to chronic illnesses must continue to be multifaceted—prevention, screening, management, and the continued innovation of health care delivery models will all be necessary as the nation continues to address this crisis.

Diana Bertorelli and Sally Kuykendall

See also: Acute Illnesses; Addictions; Alzheimer's Disease; Beers, Clifford Whittingham; Cancer; Diabetes Mellitus; Heart Disease; Men's Health; Nutrition; Prevention; Roosevelt, Franklin Delano; Social Determinants of Health; Women's Health

Further Reading

Johnson, N. B., Hayes, L. D., Brown, K., Hoo, E. C., & Ethier, K. A. (2014). CDC national health report: leading causes of morbidity and mortality and associated behavioral risk and protective factors—United States, 2005–2013. *Morbidity and Mortality Weekly Report Supplements*, 63(4), 3–27.

Moran, K., Burson, R., Critchett, J., & Olla, P. (2011). Exploring the cost and clinical outcomes of integrating the registered nurse-certified diabetes educator into the patient-centered medical home. *The Diabetes Educator*, 37(6), 780–793. doi:10.1177/0145721711423979

Olshansky, S., Passaro, D., Hershow, R., Layden, J., Carnes, B., Brody, J., Hayflick, L., Butler, R. N., Allison, D. B., & Ludwig, D. (2005). A potential decline in life expectancy in the United States in the 21st century. *New England Journal of Medicine*, 352(11), 1138–1145.

Renedo, A., & Marston, C. (2015). Developing patient-centered care: An ethnographic study of patient perceptions and influence on quality improvement. *BMC Health Services Research*, 15(1), 1–11. doi:10.1186/s12913-015-0770-y

Roser, M. (2016). *Life expectancy.* Retrieved from https://ourworldindata.org/life-expectancy.

Sidorov, J. E. (2008). The patient-centered medical home for chronic illness: Is it ready for prime time? *Health Affairs*, 27(5), 1231–1234. doi:10.1377/hlthaff.27.5.1231

Wiley, J. A., Rittenhouse, D. R., Shortell, S. M., Casalino, L. P., Ramsay, P. P., Bibi, S., & Alexander, J. A. (2015). Managing chronic illness: Physician practices increased the use of care management and medical home processes. *Health Affairs*, 34(1), 77–86. doi:10.1377/hlthaff.2014.0404

CODE OF ETHICS

When people trust health professionals to care for them, they yield power over the body and mind to the caregiver and the health care system. In return, the caregiver, the organization, and the system have a moral responsibility to fulfill the duty of care and not to abuse that power. Violations of trust or abuse of power can seriously damage the reputation of the profession and undermine future trust and relationships. A code of ethics defines the expectations and boundaries of practice in order to protect people and to ensure ongoing trust in the profession. All moral codes analyze the rightness or wrongness of a particular action or decision in policy or practice. The basic ethical principles of *respect for persons*, *beneficence*, and *justice* are common throughout the health professions. Variations appear because of the focus of the discipline. Bioethics is the study of ethical issues created by advances in medical technology and biological sciences. Clinical ethics is the analysis of ethical issues in clinical practice, focusing on individual cases. Research ethics is the protection of human participants in research studies. The main difference between medical or research ethics and public health ethics is that medicine deals with individual patients whereas public health deals with people. The collective nature of public health means that conflicts between human rights and civil liberty may arise. Because conflicts involve populations, ethical dilemmas are addressed in open discussion with key stakeholders and the affected populations. Decision making occurs as a collaborative process following a bottom-up approach rather than the top-down, authoritarian approach.

Moral codes have been a common theme throughout recorded civilization. The Code of Hammurabi (c. 1760 BCE) established standard fees for medical services and consequences for negligence or malpractice. Vaidya's Oath (15th century BCE) urges Hindu physicians to do no harm (maleficence), keep their nails cut short, tell the truth, behave professionally, and to serve vulnerable populations. Health care professionals taking the Hippocratic Oath (c. 400 BCE) promise to perform to the best of their ability, respect patient privacy, and mentor the next generation of health care workers. The Hebrew Oath of Asaph (sixth century CE) emphasizes ethical standards of professional practice, banning sexual relations with patients, adultery, and the use of poison for euthanasia or abortion. The Oath of Sun Simiao (581–682 CE) advised Chinese doctors to treat the patient as they would a close relative. The Seventeen Rules of Enjun list expectations of Japanese doctors, citing devotion to the patient, protecting medical information from misuse, and warning against undue extravagance. In public health history, *The Belmont Report* summarizes the basic ethical principles of *respect for persons* (autonomy), *beneficence* (nonmaleficence), and *justice* (fair distribution of burdens and benefits) (National Commission for the Protection of Human Subjects of Biomedical and Behavioral Research, 1979).

In 2000, graduating students of the Public Health Leadership Institute developed the *Principles of the Ethical Practice of Public Health* (Thomas, Sage, Dillenberg, & Guillory, 2002). The developers identified 12 ethical principles reflecting 14 professional values and beliefs. After refining the document through consensus building, the American Public Health Association formally adopted the Public Health Leadership's *Principles of the Ethical Practice of Public Health*:

1. Public health should address principally the fundamental causes of disease and requirements for health, aiming to prevent adverse health outcomes.
2. Public health should achieve community health in a way that respects the rights of individuals in the community.

3. Public health policies, programs, and priorities should be developed and evaluated through processes that ensure an opportunity for input from community members.
4. Public health should advocate for, or work for the empowerment of, disenfranchised community members, ensuring that the basic resources and conditions necessary for health are accessible to all people in the community.
5. Public health should seek the information needed to implement effective policies and programs that protect and promote health.
6. Public health institutions should provide communities with the information they have that is needed for decisions on policies or programs and should obtain the community's consent for their implementation.
7. Public health institutions should act in a timely manner on the information they have within the resources and the mandate given to them by the public.
8. Public health programs and policies should incorporate a variety of approaches that anticipate and respect diverse values, beliefs, and cultures in the community.
9. Public health programs and policies should be implemented in a manner that most enhances the physical and social environment.
10. Public health institutions should protect the confidentiality of information that can bring harm to an individual or community if made public. Exceptions must be justified on the basis of the high likelihood of significant harm to the individual or others.
11. Public health institutions should ensure the professional competence of their employees.
12. Public health institutions and their employees should engage in collaborations and affiliations in ways that build the public's trust and the institution's effectiveness. (PHLS, 2002)

The principles of ethical practice describe the obligation of the profession to the people that they serve. As a living document, the principles will require ongoing revision to accommodate expanding policy and practice, new technology, and emerging health issues (Lee, Fisher, & Jennings, 2016).

Courses in ethics are offered as basic curriculum in many undergraduate and graduate public health programs. Ethics is the systematic study of morality, and morality is the practice of furthering human good by doing the right thing. Students are taught strategies to ethical decision making: identify the ethical problem, assess the facts, engage stakeholders, analyze underlying values, determine options, and outline the steps to making the decision (Jennings, Kahn, Mastroianni, & Parker, 2003). The case of Mary Mallon demonstrates common ethical dilemmas in public health. Mary Mallon, pejoratively known as Typhoid Mary, was an Irish immigrant who worked as a cook. After several outbreaks of typhoid fever, investigators tracked the source to Mallon revealing the first known asymptomatic carrier of *Salmonella*

Typhi. Uneducated and healthy, Mallon failed to understand how she could be making others ill. She refused to consent to surgery to remove the source of the typhus. To prevent further outbreaks, health officials held Mallon in isolation for three years on North Brother Island in New York. The quarantine raised questions regarding Mallon's individual civil rights. She was released under the agreement that she would no longer work as a cook. After several years of low-paying jobs in laundry, Mallon changed her name and resumed working as a cook. Mallon's employment at the Sloane Hospital for Women resulted in 25 cases of typhoid fever and two deaths. In total, 51 cases of typhoid fever, including three deaths, were traced to Mallon. Still refusing surgery, Mallon was placed back in quarantine on North Brother Island for the remainder of her life. The struggle between protecting public health (beneficence) and individual civil rights (respect for persons) is a common theme in public health. Public health ethics seek collaborative solutions that respect the rights of individuals and communities.

The public health code of ethics ensures that public health professionals act in the best interest of the populations that they serve. Public health professionals are bound by the code of ethics balancing respect for persons, beneficence, and justice. As new fields, practices, and technology emerge, new choices challenging ethical principles will also emerge.

Sally Kuykendall

See also: Administration, Health; *Belmont Report, The*; Core Competencies in Public Health; Ethics in Public Health and Population Health; Greco-Roman Era, Public Health in the; Hippocrates; Mallon, Mary; Public Health Law; Research; Tuskegee Syphilis Study; *Controversies in Public Health:* Controversy 4

Further Reading

Jennings, B., Kahn, J., Mastroianni, A., & Parker, L. S. (Eds.). (2003). *Ethics and public health: Model curriculum.* U.S. Department of Human Services, Association of Schools of Public Health, Hastings Center. Retrieved from http://www.aspph.org/app/uploads/2014/02/EthicsCurriculum.pdf.

Lee, L. M., Fisher, C. B., & Jennings, B. (2016, July). Revising the American Public Health Association's Public Health Code of Ethics. *American Journal of Public Health*, 1198–1199. doi:10.2105/AJPH.2016.303208

National Commission for the Protection of Human Subjects of Biomedical and Behavioral Research. (1979). *The Belmont Report: Ethical principles and guidelines for the protection of human subjects of research.* Bethesda, MD: Author.

Public Health Leadership Society (PHLS). (2002). *Principles of the ethical practice of public health, version 2.2.* Retrieved from https://www.apha.org/~/media/files/pdf/membergroups/ethics_brochure.ashx.

Thomas, J. C., Sage, M., Dillenberg, J., & Guillory, V. J. (2002). A code of ethics for public health. *American Journal of Public Health, 92*(7), 1057–1059. Retrieved from https://www.ncbi.nlm.nih.gov/pmc/articles/PMC1447186/.

COLLABORATIONS

In public health, collaborations are working groups of people from different organizations serving together to prevent or reduce social problems. Many serious public health issues are deeply rooted within communities. One institution, project, or policy cannot fix problems of childhood obesity, heroin addiction, family violence, teen pregnancy, or poverty. Collaborations connect fragmented systems of care, sharing resources, expertise, and information to achieve a common goal. The groups that make up the collaboration often have common missions, yet approach the problem from different perspectives.

Collaborative activities go beyond networking, coordination, and cooperation. Networking occurs when individuals exchange information, a technique common in business practice. Coordination is both the exchange of information and linking of service activities. For example, a public health practitioner providing care to an overweight patient might coordinate services with a nutrition counselor or health educator of a weight management program. Cooperation is the sharing of resources, a technique that is common in social services and rarer in the business world. Collaboration uses all three techniques—networking, coordination, and cooperation—to create and implement a prevention program or intervention activity. Collaborations are highly effective ways to pool resources and optimize unique skills in order to address complex issues. On the other hand, the collaborative process is time intensive, requiring careful planning and oversight. Each organization must donate time, talent, space, or finances to the project. Conflicting interests, poor communication, incongruent values, limited resources, or organizational dysfunction can easily become an obstacle to effective collaboration.

Building an effective collaboration takes time. The major steps are (1) preformation, (2) formation, (3) strategic planning, (4) action, (5) closure or maintenance, and (6) dissemination. During preformation, the initial organizers dialogue with the affected community and key stakeholders around the problem. A needs assessment is used to determine who is impacted by the problem and the severity of the impact. An inventory assessment maps local resources and available expertise. Through the needs and inventory assessments, organizers can identify potential partners to fill specific roles within the collaboration. During the formation phase, the organizers communicate with potential partners to determine willingness and level of interest. Formal collaborations secure letters of commitment that outline specific roles of each member. A natural leader, someone who is invested in the cause and can convene the coalition, typically emerges by this point. During the strategic planning phase, the coalition identifies realistic goals and objectives and brainstorms possible activities. The convener must manage meetings carefully, ensuring that everyone is involved in decision making and remains committed to the project. Individual members must be clear about their own role on the project and set boundaries in terms of what is expected. Overinvestment can burn out members or stretch resources too far, causing people to disengage. Once a plan of action is envisioned, the group develops a timeline of events, identifies staffing needs, and secures funding support. The plan for evaluation takes shape as the group determines impact and outcomes. A logic model is used to define the project, linking activities with intended outcomes. Through strategic planning, coalition members build relationships that are important in moving the project forward. Individual members (people) are what make collaborations successful, not the bricks and mortar of an organization.

The action phase is the implementation and evaluation of the project, when the group manages day-to-day activities of the program or outreach efforts. It is common for groups to come up against problems during this phase. Working within existing systems creates additional, unexpected obstacles. The group can work around or through obstacles using regular meetings to facilitate communication between the individuals and organizations. Evaluations are used to determine whether activities are efficient and effective. Through the evaluation, the group can gain insights in how to improve practices for the future. As the project nears the end of the proposed timeline, the group must assess sustainability, the ability of a project to continue after initial oversight and resources end. In some cases, the collaboration will have successfully developed coordination and cooperation between service organizations and the program will continue without major obstacles. In other cases, the program must end because funding is no longer available, trained staff leave, or the activities are ineffective or poorly attended. The group must develop ways either to continue the efforts or to formally end the project. At this point, experts recommend that each collaborative takes time to acknowledge achievements. Establishing a network of coordinated services for a complex problem is in itself a successful outcome. The final stage is dissemination of the evaluation results. During this stage, evaluation findings and lessons learned are shared with key stakeholders, participants, the public health community, and other researchers. Many groups lose momentum at dissemination. Evaluation results may not show statistical significance or data may be incomplete, creating a reluctance to share results. It is worth remembering Elkhorne's (1967) quote of Thomas Edison, "I have not failed. I've just found 10,000 ways that won't work" (p. 52). In public health, it is just as important to know what does not work as it is to know what works. Dissemination of successes helps to advance efforts in alleviating the health problem. Dissemination of failures helps other collaborations to avoid pitfalls.

In 2006, a group of us established a collaborative to increase physical activity among inner-city children living near our university. We gathered state and local data on childhood obesity, searched the literature on suggested interventions, and surveyed the surrounding area (preformation). Needs and inventory assessments suggested that the community needed a playground. We met with nearby school officials who agreed to allocate land at the local elementary school, a fenced area adjoining the university grounds. The principal arranged a meeting between parents, members of the community, students, teachers, and university faculty. Before a packed auditorium, we presented the playground idea. We were unsure how the community would respond. The playground could be viewed as a public nuisance, creating additional traffic and unwanted visitors in the neighborhood. The community embraced the idea. We listened carefully to concerns of no adult-sized basketball hoops and the gates must be locked at dusk. Parents and grandparents suggested a community-build in order to stretch the limited funds as far as possible. The collaborative developed to include the school principal, district and university legal consultants, a playground design consultant, the school's physical education teacher, university faculty in health services and education, and parent representatives (formation). Over the school year and summer, the collaborative met to plan the playground build (strategic planning). Children drew pictures that were translated to a wish list of equipment. The lawyers nixed the swings, citing safety concerns. The physical education teacher emphasized the need for climbing frames to build upper body strength, an item identified for improvement on annual fitness tests. The chair of the university's art department assisted in developing a color scheme. Before consulting with the community, we expected bright primary colors—reds, blues, and yellows. The community requested browns and greens. Their preference was to mimic the background of trees on the university property. A contractor was hired to oversee construction. One weekend in September was chosen for the build. Advertisements were posted for volunteers in the community, the university, and the school district (action). Equipment was delivered to the worksite. On Friday evening, the men's lacrosse team set up benches and lay out the equipment for easy identification and access. On Saturday, more than 600 volunteers came to the school. Community members stood at the gates, rotating volunteers on the building site. Three skilled construction workers directed volunteers in assembling slides, ladders, climbing frames, and walkways. Additional volunteers painted the library, sorted donated clothing for charity, and organized school supplies. The Parent-Teacher Association served meals and snacks in the cafeteria. The college students were grateful for a home-cooked meal. Intended as a three-day build (Friday evening, Saturday, and Sunday), the playground was completed by Saturday evening. Evaluation results showed no significant difference between average daily step count before and after the playground. There were challenges during the project. Members of the community requested a second playground for children aged three to five years. We were unable to fulfill this request due to lack of funds. Some neighbors used the school wall to play wall ball. They were displaced by the playground. Ensuring that no volunteer was turned away and everyone felt appreciated was an unexpected challenge. Evaluation results were shared with the funder, the school district, and at professional conferences (dissemination). However, the real, unmeasured successes were that children who did not have access to a playground now have access, university alumni report revisiting the playground and proudly saying, "I put that bolt on," and the network established between school, community, and university.

Public health professionals collaborate with staff from hospitals, doctor offices, community agencies, nonprofit organizations, media, academic institutions, and businesses to prevent and reduce multiple public health problems. Combining skills, talents, and resources can achieve outcomes that would not be possible by acting alone or as separate systems. Collaborations can be highly successful tools of empowering communities to resolve complex health issues.

Sally Kuykendall

See also: Community Health; Community Organizing; Evaluation; Intervention; Logic Model; Prevention; RE-AIM (Reach, Effectiveness, Adoption, Implementation, and Maintenance); U.S. Public Health Service; World Health Organization

Further Reading

Association of State and Territorial Dental Directors. (2012). *Handbook on planning, evaluating, and improving collaboration for oral health programs.* Retrieved from http://www.astdd.org/docs/collaboration-evaluation-handbook-final.pdf.

Elkhorne, J. L. (1967). Edison: The fabulous drone. *73 Magazine XLVI*(3), 52–54. Retrieved from http://www.arimi.it/wp-content/73/03_March_1967.pdf.

National Association of County & City Health Officials. (2016). *Pulling together, Section Two: Building collaboration.* Retrieved from http://archived.naccho.org/topics/environmental/pullingtogether/sectiontwo.cfm.

Office of Public Health Scientific Services, Center for Surveillance, Epidemiology, and Laboratory Services, Division of Scientific Education and Professional Development. (2013). *Public health and health care collaboration: The workforce perspective.* Retrieved from http://www.cdc.gov/ophss/csels/dsepd/strategic-workforce-activities/ph-healthcare-collaboration.html.

COMMUNITY HEALTH

Community health is a field of study within public health sciences that focuses on promoting, protecting, and preserving the health of a defined group of people (Green & Ottoson, 1999). The word "community" refers to a group of people who live in the same locality, adhere to similar norms or values, or are bound by common laws or regulations (Green & Ottoson, 1999). The group may share similar experiences, language, or activities. Commonalities create a sense of identity, which transcends into emotional connections and mutual support (McKenzie et al., 2009). A community can also be viewed as a group of people who identify with particular issues, such as cancer survival, physical disability, or survivors of emotional, physical, or sexual abuse (Goodman et al., 2014). Community health programs focus on developing a healthy community, able to access resources and attain quality of life. The process typically consists of organized efforts performed by functional partnerships sharing resources. Common community health agendas are to prevent community violence, promote safety, support mental health, create linkages between community resources and other health resources, or increase access to quality health care. Some partnerships are formed between government and private agencies with the goal of reducing risk factors for disease, reducing the burden of disease, decreasing intentional and unintentional injuries, or promoting wellness (Goodman et al., 2014). Although this description provides a preliminary framework for understanding community health, the definition continues to expand as our understanding and interpretation of both community and health evolve. Experts recommend that future definitions should consider the diversity of communities, how communities connect, and how communities make decisions (Goodman et al., 2014).

Community health programs engage people from different organizations and backgrounds to work together to address the health issues in a community. Members may be from the community of interest, local government, community-based organizations, public health departments, faith-based organizations, universities, or hospitals. Each individual or group provides specialized skills, knowledge, connections, or insights. Frontline support staff typically consist of locally trained volunteers, community health advisers, community health representatives, health advocates, or health promoters who are both members of the target community and members of the community health partnership. Other workers may be public health staff who have crafted close professional ties with the community. Community health professionals are often university graduates with a bachelor's, master's, or doctoral degree in community health and specialization in health education, health promotion, or nutrition. To be effective, all staff must respect the values and culture of the community.

Community health efforts start by formally identifying the community health needs, determining priorities, defining goals, and establishing a common agenda. The group must determine the most effective intervention or prevention activities that will meet project goals. Examples include evidence-based programs or practices, outreach services, education programs, counseling, or advocacy. During program activities, community health workers also have an opportunity to connect members of the community with local health or social services. All community health programs, and especially those receiving grant funding, should include an evaluation component. Community health professionals may develop their own tools or use published instruments to assess program impact and outcomes. Some of the tools used are the Behavioral Risk Factor Surveillance System (BRFSS), Youth Risk Behavior Survey (YRBS), and the National Health and Nutrition Examination Survey (NHANES). Additionally, many different academic disciplines, such as health economics, behavioral sciences, health education, and law, offer measurement tools and expertise to support community health practice (Goodman et al., 2014).

There are multiple organizations and resources designed to support community health partnerships and community health programs. The Centers for Disease

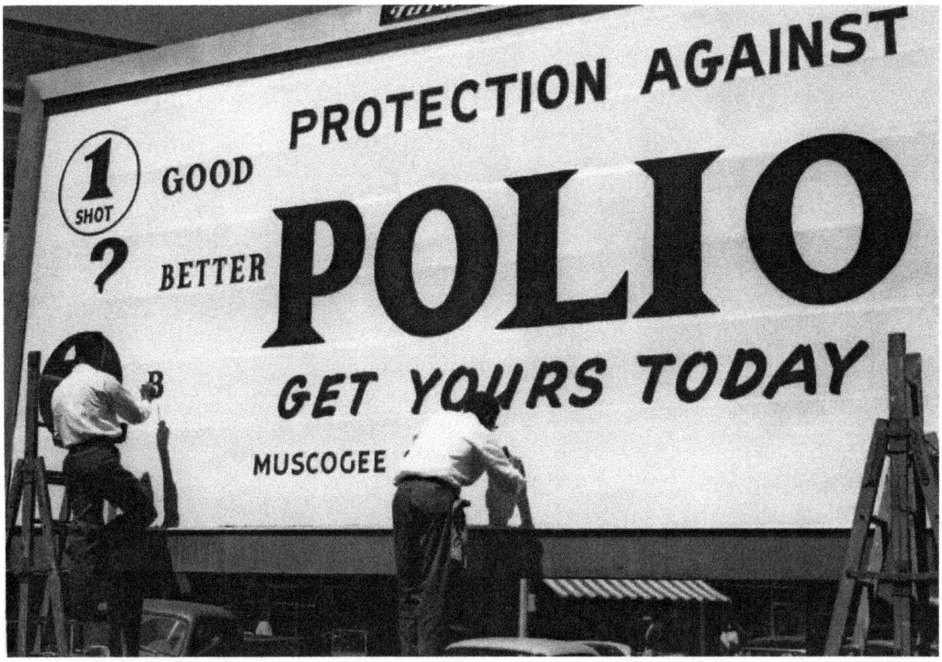
PROTECTION AGAINST
1 SHOT
GOOD
?
BETTER
POLIO
GET YOURS TODAY
MUSCOGEE

Community health workers erect a billboard encouraging residents of Columbus, Georgia, to get vaccinated against polio. Community health programs engage people from different organizations and backgrounds to work together to address the health issues of the community. (Centers for Disease Control and Prevention)

Control and Prevention (CDC) Community Health Program offers resources, best practices, and innovative ideas for groups working toward community health. The resources are designed to strengthen and support community health efforts, especially in the prevention of chronic disease and in the promotion of healthy living (CDC Division of Community Health, 2013). Kaiser Permanente's Community Health Initiatives is an example of a community health program. The Community Health Initiatives developed the HEAL (Healthy Eating Active Living) program, a partnership of community-based organizations, local residents, and Kaiser Permanente. The program is designed to promote healthy eating and active living in local neighborhoods, schools, and workplaces (HEAL Cities, 2017). Community health is an evolving field with many challenges. Future directions must focus on developing methods of data collection that are specifically designed for community health practice. Data collection tools should serve to assess, evaluate, and implement evidence-based principles while also considering cost effectiveness. Some experts suggest the need for better integration between community health practice and other public health disciplines (Goodman et al., 2014).

Community health efforts focus on reducing disease, reducing health disparities, and improving health and wellness. Community health partnerships draw from the combined efforts and knowledge and expertise of multiple agencies and disciplines. The Bureau of Labor Statistics (BLS) predicts that job opportunities in community health will continue to grow over the next decade. Thus, the vision of a healthy community may be attainable.

Victor Okparaeke

See also: Collaborations; Community Organizing; Cultural Competence; Evidence-Based Programs and Practices; Family Planning; Goals and Objectives; Health Education; Healthy Places; Needs Assessment; Population Health; RE-AIM (Reach, Effectiveness, Adoption, Implementation, and Maintenance)

Further Reading

Centers for Disease Control and Prevention (CDC), Division of Community Health. (2013). *A practitioner's guide for advancing health equity: Community strategies for preventing chronic disease.* Atlanta: U.S. Department of Health and Human Services. Retrieved from https://www.cdc.gov/nccdphp/dch/health-equity-guide/index.htm.

Goodman, R. A., Bunnell, R., & Posner, S. F. (2014). What is "community health"? Examining the meaning of an evolving field in public health. *Preventive Medicine*, *67*(Suppl. 1), S58–S61.

Green, L. W., & Ottoson, J. M. (1999). *Community and population health* (5th ed.). New York: McGraw-Hill.

HEAL Cities. (2017). *Healthy eating active living cities campaign.* Retrieved from http://www.healnation.com/.

Kaiser Permanente. (2017). *Community health initiatives.* Retrieved from https://share.kaiserpermanente.org/article/community-health-initiatives-3/.

McKenzie, J. F., Neiger, B. L., & Thackeray, R. (2009). *Planning, implementing, & evaluating health promotion programs: A primer* (5th ed.). New York: Pearson.

COMMUNITY HEALTH CENTERS (CHCs)

Community health centers (CHCs) are public health clinics and medical facilities that provide comprehensive primary and preventative health care to children and adults. Nationwide, approximately 4,000 CHCs provide medical treatment, behavioral health services, oral care, vision care, substance abuse treatment, and pharmacy services to 24 million people (HRSA, 2017). Anyone may attend a CHC. The centers are specifically intended to provide a *medical home* for people with limited access to health care services due to poverty, geographic isolation, homelessness, working as a migrant farmworker, or veteran. Patients pay for treatment and care based on income. CHCs are the front line of public health for many Americans. Physicians, nurses, social workers, podiatrists, dentists, laboratory technicians, pharmacists, health educators, and other health professionals work in CHCs to reduce and prevent disease and improve health outcomes and quality of life for people in the surrounding community. CHCs differ from other health organizations in that they are designed to serve the community. This means that services are tailored to the needs of the community rather than the potential to make money.

CHCs are financed by the Health Resources and Service Administration (HRSA) under the Public Health Service Act. HRSA provides grants to local government, faith-based organizations, universities, or other organizations that manage the center and provide direct care to residents. Each CHC has a board of directors composed of members of the community and public health and medical professionals. The board determines what services are needed and what services will be offered. Localized planning ensures that local needs are being met. Common medical services offered include annual physical examinations, medical care, immunizations, and dental care. Some centers offer specialty services such as HIV/AIDS treatment, sexually transmitted disease screening and treatment, reproductive services, housing support services, psychiatric care, or chronic disease management. For example, the CHC in Eastport, Maine, offers podiatric care, alcohol and substance abuse counseling, physical therapy, and radiology services. The Curry Senior Center in San Francisco, California, offers primary care and preventive services for residents aged 55 and older, delivered by staff fluent in English, Cantonese, Mandarin, Tagalog, Vietnamese, Spanish, or Russian. The ability of centers to personalize care ensures that members of the community receive the care that they need and that resources are used wisely.

The public health accomplishments of CHCs and health center staff are particularly noteworthy. Health care costs of CHC-Medicaid patients are 24 percent less than other patients. In comparison to patients who use other primary care systems, CHC-Medicaid patients have fewer visits (22 percent), less specialty care (33 percent), fewer admissions (25 percent), and lower inpatient care (27 percent) costs (Nocon et al., 2016). Across the nation, 64 percent of diabetic patients have their condition under control. Among CHC patients, 70 percent of diabetics have their condition under control (HRSA, 2017). Fifty-two percent of non-CHC patients diagnosed with high blood pressure have their condition under control, compared to 64 percent of CHC patients diagnosed with high blood pressure. Better patient outcomes are partially related to the fact that providers are able to develop relationships with community members. Good patient-provider relationship enables regular screening, close monitoring of illnesses and progress, and better follow-up. CHCs are able to break down many of the racial, gender, and ethnic barriers that exist in health care. In addition to reducing disease and health disparities, CHCs influence the local economy. When residents are able to access treatment and preventive services, personal health improves and people are able to work. Also, CHCs hire local residents as technicians, health administrators, or health professionals and purchase supplies, which brings jobs to disadvantaged communities.

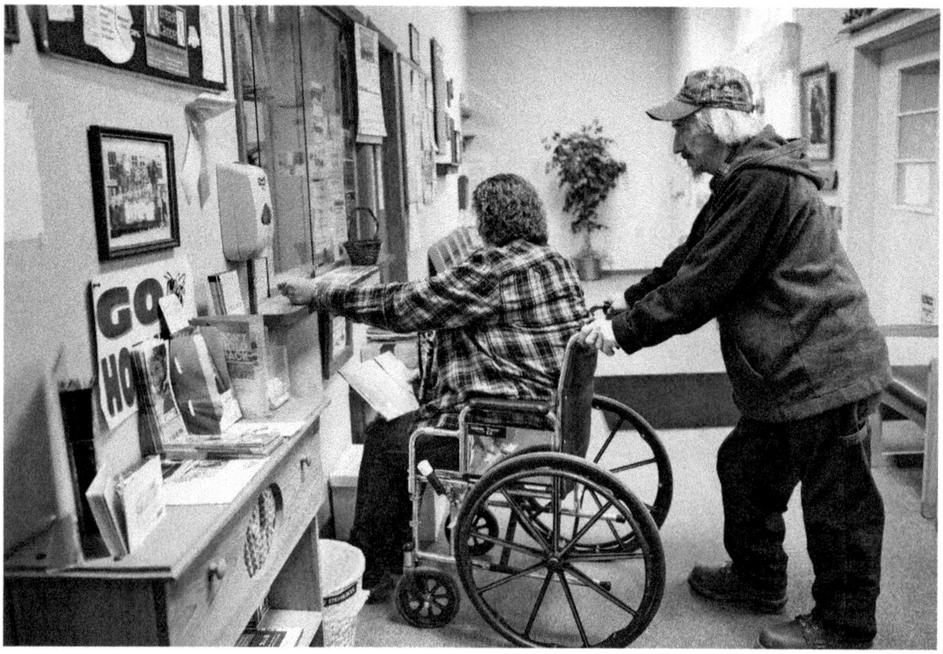

The Community Health Center of Northeastern Wetzel County of West Virginia serves as the medical home for over 4,000 local residents. Doctors, nurses, physician assistants, dentists, and dental hygienists provide medical, dental, and behavioral health services. (Brendan Smialowski/AFP/Getty Images)

CHCs offer medical care and preventive services to people who may not normally be able to access health services. The centers have direct benefits of keeping people healthy and indirect benefits of enhancing the health of the entire community.

Sally Kuykendall

See also: Administration, Health; Association of State and Territorial Health Officials; Community Health; Health Resources and Services Administration; Indian Health Service; Medicaid; Medicine; Population Health; Prevention; State, Local, and Territorial Health Departments; *Controversies in Public Health:* Controversy 3

Further Reading

Essential Services Work Group. (n.d.). *Ten essential services: Purpose and practices of public health.* Atlanta: Centers for Disease Control and Prevention. Retrieved from http://www.cdc.gov/stltpublichealth/hop/pdfs/Ten_Essential_Public_Health_Services_2011-09_508.pdf.

Health Resources & Services Administration (HRSA). (2017). *About the health center program.* Retrieved from https://www.bphc.hrsa.gov/about/index.html.

Institute of Medicine. (1988). *The future of public health.* Washington, DC: National Academies Press. doi:10.17226/1091. Retrieved from http://www.nap.edu/catalog/1091/the-future-of-public-health.

Nocon, R., Lee, S. M., Sharma, R., Ngo-Metger, Q., Mukamel, D. B., Gao, Y., White, L. M., Shi, L., Chin, M. H., Laiteerapong, N., & Huang, E. S. (2016). Health care use and spending for Medicaid enrollees in federally qualified centers versus other primary care settings. *American Journal of Public Health, 106*(11), 1981–1989.

COMMUNITY ORGANIZING

Community organizing is the process of bringing together members of a community in order to address the problems that affect the community. This grassroots approach empowers individuals to solve issues and improve quality of life within their own neighborhoods. The benefit of community organizing is that the people who are affected the most by the problem are invested in finding solutions, and the solutions are likely to continue after the task force disbands. Conversely, community organizing requires certain skills to avoid political pitfalls while attracting, engaging, and sustaining members. Organized leadership, consensus building, and personal investment are critical to achieve the desired goal. Obstacles may arise from changes in community structure, power imbalances, demographics, housing, job demands, and organized activities. Any factor that influences the relationships between neighbors can affect the community's ability to address problems. Bedroom communities, where people work outside of the place they live, lack of interaction with neighbors, overscheduling, and poverty make it difficult to organize a community. In public health, community organizing is used to address many complex issues such as youth violence, childhood obesity, social injustice, and lack of access to health care. Community organizing is a time-tested technique that will continue to evolve as our communities and social groups evolve.

Saul David Alinsky (1909–1972) is considered the father of community organizing. In the 1930s, Alinsky led a series of community efforts to improve living and working conditions in impoverished areas of his hometown Chicago. Less fortunate populations were blocked from improving conditions because powerful stakeholders, businessmen, politicians, and the wealthy had a vested interest in maintaining the status quo. In order to improve the communities, Alinsky and colleagues devised creative ways to empower the powerless, including threatening a fart-in by sympathizers attending a Rochester Philharmonic Orchestra concert. In his 1971 book, *Rules for Radicals,* Alinsky identifies two power groups, organized money and organized people. By organizing people and media sympathy, Alinsky was able to advance civil rights and create economic opportunities for the "have-nots."

Although there are some movements that follow Alinsky's model of shocking people into action, community organizing in public health aims for less militant methods. At the heart of community organizing is organizing for the collective good. The basic steps are (1) formation, (2) maintenance, and (3) institutionalization. During formation, key stakeholders identify the problem or concern; assess local politics, gatekeepers, and power holders; identify, recruit, and organize a task force; identify needs, assets, and obstacles; prioritize goals; and select intervention strategies.

During maintenance, the group initiates the plan of action and evaluates success. In the final step, institutionalizing integrates efforts into existing systems. The Community Organizing for Obesity Prevention in Humboldt Park (Co-Op HP) is an example of community organizing in public health. A 2002–2003 health survey by Sinai Urban Health Institute (SUHI) revealed that Chicago communities had higher rates of obesity in comparison to the rest of the nation, increasing risk for heart disease, diabetes, hypertension, depression, and arthritis. Fifty percent of children in the Humboldt Park community were obese, significantly higher than the national rate of 14 percent (Estarziau, Morales, Rico, Margellos-Anast, Whitman, & Christoffel, 2006). Co-Op HP was formed with financial support from Otho S. A. Sprague Memorial Institute, people power from the Puerto Rican Cultural Center and Centro Sin Fronteras, and technical support from the Consortium to Lower Obesity in Chicago Children (CLOCC) and SUHI. Over the years, many churches, colleges, communities, and nonprofit organizations have joined the effort. The project uses existing resources to provide four interventions: increasing availability and demand for healthy foods, expanding and supporting fitness programs, healthy living, and community development to coordinate health prevention programs. A few of the many outreach and education programs are encouraging store owners to provide a better selection of fresh fruits and vegetables, fitness classes at the YMCA, bilingual wellness programs by the Erie Family Health Center, and cooking classes. The co-op monitors success by tracking quantity and demand for healthy food, participation in fitness programs, eating behaviors, bike lanes and footpaths, and number of organizations advocating health in the community. Co-Op HP demonstrates how existing systems and resources can be leveraged to address the multifactorial problem of obesity.

Underlying community organizing are certain hidden assumptions. Community organizing assumes that people want to solve the problems that affect them and that they are capable of creating sustainable solutions. There may be some issues where people are reluctant to change. Changing diet and integrating physical activity into daily routine may not be desirable for some members of the community. Therefore, it is important that the changes have meaning to the community members. Community organizing assumes that a coordinated approach is more effective than a fragments approach. The coordinated approach requires that people cooperate. This may mean yielding to the needs of the group. The grocery store owners may have a lower margin of profit on fruits and vegetables than they gain on bags of chips or soda pop. Giving up a higher profit for the benefit of the customers' health is something that store owners might struggle with. This is where it may be difficult for community organizers to keep the store owners engaged. Successful community organizing is able to foresee and navigate obstacles and come to consensus on solutions.

Community organizing coordinates existing systems and community members through efforts to improve their own community, health, or quality of life. The technique may be applied to numerous complex health issues that adversely affect communities. And although community organizing can be challenging, juggling multiple systems and people, the results are highly effective and lead to long-term sustainable solutions.

Sally Kuykendall

See also: Collaborations; Community Health; Community Health Centers; Evaluation; Intervention; Logic Model; Obesity; PRECEDE-PROCEED Planning Model; Prevention; RE-AIM (Reach, Effectiveness, Adoption, Implementation, and Maintenance)

Further Reading

Agency for Toxic Substances and Disease Registry, Clinical and Translational Science Awards Consortium, Community Engagement Key Function Committee Task Force on the Principles of Community Engagement. (2011). *Principles of community engagement* (2nd ed.). Department of Health and Human Services. Retrieved from https://www.atsdr.cdc.gov/communityengagement/pdf/PCE_Report_508_FINAL.pdf.

Alinsky, S. (1971). *Rules for radicals: A practical primer for realistic radicals.* New York: Random House.

Estarziau, M., Morales, M., Rico, A., Margellos-Anast, H., Whitman, S., & Christoffel, K. (2006). *Report on the findings and recommendation of the community survey in Humboldt Park: Preventing obesity and improving our health.* Puerto Rican Cultural Center, Centro Sin Fronteras, Sinai Urban Health Institute, Consortium to Lower Obesity in Chicago Children. Retrieved from http://www.sinai.org/sites/default/files/comm%20surv%20in%20HP%20prev%20obesity.pdf.

CORE COMPETENCIES IN PUBLIC HEALTH

The core competencies for public health professionals are the basic skills that every public health professional should possess. The public health workforce is made up of many different people from many different fields. From health administrators to epidemiologists, emergency medical technicians, optometrists, sanitarians, laboratory technicians, animal control workers, pharmacists, policy makers, health educators, researchers, and behavioral health professionals, each worker has unique duties and responsibilities. Where an epidemiologist studies health issues in the community and helps determine priorities, the public health nurse gives direct patient care to alleviate such problems. Individuals work together to create a system of care and prevention. Yet, the breadth and depth of public health practice can be confusing. We don't immediately think of the animal control officer as a public health officer, unless we are experiencing an outbreak of ringworm, rabies, or mad cow disease. Furthermore, when public health efforts are successful, disease and illness *do not occur*. It is hard to measure and appreciate a problem that does not affect us. When we eat at a restaurant, we assume the food was properly stored and prepared, restaurant workers used good handwashing techniques, and the restaurant was clean and passed food safety inspections. If the meal was good and we didn't get nausea or diarrhea after eating, we don't stop to appreciate the fact that we didn't get sick. Public health counts the number of cases of salmonella poisoning. No one counts the number of people who don't get salmonella poisoning. It is hard to measure something that doesn't occur.

When public health is successful, diseases do not occur. Yet, without data and public recognition, funding becomes a problem. In 1988, the Institute of Medicine (IOM) called attention to the political and perceptual issues affecting public health in the United States. The IOM noted that the public health system was suffering from severe underfunding, resulting in outdated tools and materials, and fragmented services. The IOM suggested developing a consensus on the role of public health. The Council on Linkages between Academia and Public Health Practice gathered faculty, experts, and practitioners from 20 different organizations to develop a list of common competencies, which all public health professionals should have. Public health core competencies are classified by eight domains or skill sets:

- Program planning and policy development
- Community dimensions of practice
- Communication
- Cultural competency
- Analytical and assessment
- Public health sciences
- Financial planning and management
- Leadership and systems thinking

The core competencies provide a structure, defining who and what public health is. The Council on Linkages between Academia and Public Health Practice detail each competency by tier. Tier 1 workers, entry level staff, need a working knowledge of each skill set to support optimal patient care. Tier 2, program managers and supervisory staff, need a greater level of expertise. Tier 3, executives, are responsible for the highest level of skill in order to foster a professional culture. The competencies are used by colleges and universities offering degrees in public health or by local health departments building or maintaining a quality workforce. Most importantly, the core competencies allow all public health professionals—from entry level to senior administrators—to understand and appreciate the talents, efforts, and contributions of colleagues to the larger system of care.

Many of the core competencies require an interdisciplinary approach, being able to take information and methods from different fields of study and piece them together to create evidence-based practices. *Program planning skills* require public health practitioners to identify health goals and objectives of a community, plan workable and effective interventions, coordinate activities, evaluate efforts, and suggest next steps. Today's health issues are very complex, requiring multifaceted solutions. One person or one agency alone cannot solve today's convoluted health issues. Problems, such as teen pregnancy, substance abuse, poverty, crime, and violence, have deep roots that need to be addressed from both inside and outside of the affected community. Yet, as the IOM report noted, services are often disjointed. Public health professionals must be able to work within and across government agencies and nonprofit organizations to coordinate resources. Related to program planning are the *community dimensions of practice,* skills that public health professionals need in order to interact with people and organizations in the community. When community data show that teen pregnancy is a problem, the public health professional would seek to coordinate resources from schools, family planning centers, local hospitals, recreational centers, religious institutions, businesses, and others within the community (Huberman, Klaus, & Davis, 2014). Community collaborations can be difficult, particularly if organizations are competing for the same grants or funding streams. To create coordinated systems of care, public health program planners identify the key stakeholders, establish a working group, develop shared vision, create a plan, coordinate, and mobilize services. It is also important to develop a plan to continue services after the initial funding ends. It takes time to get a well-planned program up and running in a community. Starting a program and then having to stop when funding has ended may leave the community in worse condition than when they started. Public health professionals must be competent to work with communities to establish effective, long-term solutions. *Policy development* is one way to ensure long-term, sustainable solutions. Policy development consists of working within government systems to develop laws, regulations, strategies, organizations, and plans to enhance health. Although not every public health professional will develop laws, they should be able to understand and explain how policies on communicable disease surveillance, immunizations, tuberculosis screening, and inspections of schools and day care centers work to prevent the spread of disease. Policy development also helps to determine resource allocation within the federal organizations that make up the Department of Health and Human Services, local and state health departments, and community grants.

Oral and written *communication skills* are necessary to be able to clearly interact with patients, community members, stakeholders, and other professionals. Those providing direct and indirect care must be able to listen and respond appropriately to concerns. Doctors and nurses must listen to patients and patient caregivers, assess symptoms, and discuss proposed treatment plans. Even those who do not give direct care must have good communication skills. Scientists must listen to participants in order to gather accurate information, and administrators must listen to staff in order to develop workable solutions. Clear, brief, and accurate messages are best. The goal is to provide people with the information that they need to make educated decisions. Using a variety of methods (e.g., community speaking, news outlets, e-mails, or posters) ensures wider outreach and greater integration of health ideas into everyday life. *Cultural competency* means recognizing the unique needs, values, social norms, experiences, and beliefs of minority individuals and populations in order to positively influence policies, programs and services. Cultural competency advocates and empowers people regardless of gender, ethnicity, language, age, sexual affiliation, religious preference, ability, and experiences. Although some cultural competency skills, such as language, may be taught, having a diverse public health workforce is one of the most highly effective ways to develop and maintain a culturally competent health center. The health educator who provides parenting classes for teen mothers and fathers must be able to understand the unique needs of teen parents. The experiences of raising a child when one is still finishing high school, living with parents, establishing a career, and/or dating are very different from those who have already finished high school, have their own home, and source of financial support. Furthermore, relationships between health care workers and patients are based on mutual trust and respect. The patient must trust that the health care worker will provide respect, maintain confidentiality, and recommend treatments where the advantages (improved quality of life or reduced disability and death) outweigh disadvantages (cost or inconvenience). Trust develops more easily and quickly when the patient can see that the health care worker has had similar life experiences.

Future generations of health professionals must be able to think critically about health issues in order to refine and improve practices. *Analytical thinking skills* are the ability to recognize reputable sources of information, access data, accurately interpret the results, and come to thoughtful and rational conclusions. Rigorous scientific data allow us to assess where we are in conquering a health problem and what we need to do next. Public health uses facts, discoveries, knowledge, and theories from biology, chemistry, medicine, social and behavioral sciences, psychology, epidemiology, biostatistics, informatics, microbiology, and health administration to build effective practices. *Public health sciences* are the scientific foundations on which public health is practiced. Practitioners must have a functional knowledge of many different disciplines in order to implement effective programs and activities. The program planner working to prevent teen pregnancy needs a working understanding of the community (sociology), teenage brain development (neuropsychology), reproductive health (biology), evidence-based programs (health education), trends in teen pregnancy rates (epidemiology), grant writing, management, and finance (health administration). A well-rounded interdisciplinary education enables health professionals to draw knowledge from a variety of sources, creating a coordinated approach. Knowledge does not end with the awarding of a degree. Health professionals must stay up to date and relevant in their field. Membership in a professional organization, continuing education units, professional conferences, and trade journals are some of the ways that professionals stay up to date. Some organizations provide heavily discounted student memberships in order to encourage the lifelong habit of staying current in the field. The ability to read, understand, and critique health information empowers health care personnel to immediately employ new research findings while dismissing questionable findings. Many public health departments work with scholars from local colleges and universities to study the needs of residents, evaluate efforts, and communicate successes and failures through professional conferences and journals. Professional partnerships can benefit the public health department, the scholar, local communities, and public health in general.

With limited public funding and resources, meeting *Healthy People* goals and objectives is challenging. Skills in *financial planning and management* support programs, advances, and day-to-day activities of local health departments. Financial planning includes the ability to apply for federal, state, or nonprofit organization funding, weigh costs of a program against benefits, and manage contracts and budgets. The health educator offering classes to teen mothers may need to write grants advocating for program funding, come up with a budget for food, supplies, and incentives, manage the budget, and report expenses to program funders. Financial management requires a different skill set than collaborating with community partners or working with patients. Although some public health professionals may never manage budgets, all must understand budget constraints in order to make maximum use of limited public resources. All public health personnel function as managers, either managing patient care, staff, programs, or policies. Each member of the health care team contributes specialized skills and empowers colleagues to also contribute their own skills. *Management* skills encompass supporting teams, honoring different disciplines, motivating team members to work toward organizational goals, performance management, and continuous process improvement. The public health nurse serving a pregnant teen mom who is at risk for gestational diabetes could provide preliminary diet counseling, yet would also refer the young mother to a registered dietician. The nurse recognizes and respects that the registered dietician can provide more detailed, helpful nutritional information, resources, and tools. Public health is carried out through careful resource planning, management, and dedicated partnerships.

Leadership and systems thinking skills are used by all public health workers, from frontline, entry level staff to senior executives. Leadership requires that public health professionals possess a vision of what health looks like for the communities that they serve. All programs, activities, and services are guided by strong ethical standards. Public health professionals are not simply performing a job. Every person, every life, is important, regardless of sexual preference, ethnicity, or socioeconomic status. Public health professionals are not only part of a system of care, they are part of communities where they act as mentors, coaches, advisers, and trainers. Community health workers are often the first ones that family members, friends, neighbors, and colleagues look toward when health concerns arise. Questions are posed that patients may be afraid to ask their own doctor. Making connections between individuals, systems, and communities allows the health professional to critically analyze internal and external factors that may ultimately improve delivery of care.

The core competencies provide clear and measurable outcomes for public health training and professional standards. Schools of public health use the core competencies to plan curricula, and health departments use the core competencies for workforce development. The field of public health is extremely complex with multiple interrelated concepts. As the field develops further and specialization increases, schools will be challenged to fit everything that they need to fit into public health curricula. Although the core competencies were developed as a tool, a way to ensure competency within the field, the core competencies also effect a collegial and collaborative work environment. Public health professionals respect and appreciate the individual expertise and function of each discipline within the larger system of care. The sanitarian who performs health and safety inspections to ensure that the food we eat in a restaurant is properly prepared, stored, and disposed of is just as critical in preventing illness as the physician who diagnoses and treats salmonella.

Sally Kuykendall

See also: Certified in Public Health; Code of Ethics; Cultural Competence; Prevention; *Controversies in Public Health:* Controversy 4

Further Reading

Association of Schools & Programs of Public Health. (2017). Retrieved from http://www.aspph.org/.

Council on Linkages between Academia and Public Health Practice. (2014). *Core competencies for public health professionals.* Retrieved from http://www.phf.org/resourcestools/pages/core_public_health_competencies.aspx.

Huberman, B., Klaus, T., & Davis, L. (2014). *Strategies guided by best practice for community mobilization.* Advocates for Youth. Retrieved from http://advocatesforyouth.org/storage/advfy/documents/Factsheets/strategies%20guided%20by%20best%20practice_8-11-14.pdf.

Institute of Medicine. (1988). *The future of public health.* Washington, DC: National Academies Press. doi:10.17226/1091. Retrieved from http://www.nap.edu/catalog/1091/the-future-of-public-health.

Institute of Medicine. (2002). *Who will keep the public healthy? Educating public health professionals for the 21st century.* Washington, DC: National Academies Press. doi:10.17226/10542. Retrieved from http://www.nap.edu/catalog/10542/who-will-keep-the-public-healthy-educating-public-health-professionals.

CORNELY, PAUL BERTAU (1906–2002)

Dr. Paul B. Cornely was the first person of color to earn a doctoral degree in public health in the U.S. and the first person of color to serve as president of the American Public Health Association (APHA). Born of Afro-Caribbean descent, Dr. Cornely witnessed the injustices, indifference, and apathy of health, education, and social systems toward the struggles of African Americans. He traveled across the nation, investigating and documenting the living and working conditions of African Americans, Latinos, and Native Americans. His lectures, articles, and speeches raised awareness of overt and covert discrimination, which further subjugated racial minorities. Cornely believed in social justice, that no one in society should carry a larger burden of deprivation and hardship than others. With a vision toward voluntary desegregation of hospitals, he founded the Imhotep National Conference. When he realized that those in power would not voluntarily yield their power, he joined and became a leader in the American civil rights movement. Because of the civil rights movement, discrimination based on race or ethnicity is illegal. However, many of Cornely's observations and recommendations continue to apply to health and social services today.

Paul Bertau Cornely was born on March 9, 1906, in the French West Indies to Adrienne (Mellon) and Eleodore Cornely. In 1921, the family immigrated to the states and settled in Detroit. Thriving auto, coal mining, steel, and meatpacking industries attracted two main groups, Poles escaping the Russian invasion in Poland and African Americans escaping poverty in the south. The promise of steady employment and financial opportunity was crushed by the Great Depression (1929–1939). Competition for jobs and resources created tensions between Polish Americans and African Americans, which escalated to frustration, anger, and contempt. Rather than questioning the social systems that created hardship, the two groups argued for preferential treatment. Since the recently immigrated Polish Americans were white, they could blend in better than black Americans. In this tumultuous environment, Cornely earned a BA (1928), an MD (1931), and a DrPH (1934) from the University of Michigan.

Cornely's choice of medical school and internship would have been very limited. With the exceptions of Howard University and Meharry Medical College, medical schools accepted few black students. Segregation meant that white doctors interned at white hospitals and black doctors interned at black hospitals. The conditions of black hospitals were well below health and safety standards. Black hospitals were overcrowded and lacked supplies. In some hospitals, two to three patients shared one bed. Cornely interned at Lincoln Hospital in Durham, North Carolina (1931–1932). Lincoln Hospital was established by African American community leaders who negotiated support from wealthy white donors because blacks worked in close proximity to whites and treating disease among black people would prevent spreading diseases to whites. As an intern, Cornely would have treated patients with heart disease, cancers, respiratory illnesses, tuberculosis, influenza, typhoid fever, renal problems, congenital malformations, and malnutrition. In 1934, Cornely became a naturalized citizen and married Mae Stewart.

After earning his doctorate in public health, Cornely joined Howard University as assistant professor in the Department of Bacteriology, Preventive Medicine, and Public Health. In 1942, he was named chair of the department, and five years later he became medical director of Freedmen's Hospital. At Howard University, Cornely was a prolific researcher and writer. In 1938–1939, Cornely visited historically black colleges to investigate the quality of student health centers, dormitories, cafeterias, showers, libraries, and other campus facilities. The 54 colleges employed 47 part-time physicians, 2 part-time nurses, and 19 full-time nurses to serve the health and medical needs of almost 24,000 students. In cafeterias, Cornely observed unsanitary food preparation, lack of handwashing facilities, cheap foods with poor nutritional value, and use of unpasteurized milk. Dormitories were crowded and lacked basic amenities for personal hygiene or studying. Rooms designed for two students frequently housed three or more students, forcing some students to share beds. Buildings were in disrepair with sewage, plumbing, ventilation, or heating problems. Many rooms had no desks and poor lighting, which meant that students had to perch on the edge of their bed to study. Dormitory regulations requiring lights out at 10, 10:30, or 11 p.m. forced students with after school jobs to study in dimly lit hallways. Female dormitories were in slightly better condition than male dormitories. Males carried the brunt of overcrowding and poor facilities. Cornely made several recommendations to improve student life conditions including raising the rate of student health fees from approximately three dollars to developing a task force of faculty members to address the issues and hiring more health services personnel.

In the 1950s, Cornely became active in the American civil rights movement. With Dr. William Montague Cobb, Cornely planned the Imhotep National Conference on Hospital Integration (1956). The conference was suitably named after the early Egyptian physician, Imhotep, whose name translates as *he comes in peace*. The conference was intended to lead a national discussion on voluntary desegregation of hospitals, giving black patients the right to access care at premier medical institutions. Sponsored by the Council on Medical Education and Hospitals of the National Medical Association, the National Health Committee of the National Association for the Advancement of Colored People (NAACP), and the Medico-Chirugical Society of the District of Columbia, the meeting was held at the neutral location of the Fifteenth Street Presbyterian Church. Sadly, the conference was boycotted by the American Medical Association, American Hospital Association, American Nurses Association, the National Health Council, the U.S. Public Health Service, the American Protestant Hospital Association, and the Catholic Hospital Association. No white medical school, nursing school, or hospital sent an official representative (Byrd & Clayton, 2000). Despite lack of support, Imhotep continued with annual meetings until President Lyndon B. Johnson passed the 1964 Civil Rights Act requiring mandatory desegregation. The conference was both a success and a failure. Despite the boycott by large, influential institutions, the meeting raised public awareness of racial discrimination in health care. White institutional disinterest forced Cobb and Cornely to adopt more aggressive strategies. On August 28, 1963, Cornely attended the March on Washington. With the passage of the Civil Rights Act, President Johnson convened a conference to discuss ways to disband segregated hospitals. All of the formerly reluctant organizations attended.

In 1968, Cornely organized the Black Caucus of Health Workers. The following summer, he toured the country with APHA president Lester Breslow investigating the state of minority health. In Chicago, they observed children playing in abandoned cars surrounded by rotting garbage and broken sewers. In Houston, they met a mother with eight children whose welfare benefits were cut after two of her children participated in a demonstration against hunger. In California, Mexican American agricultural workers reported headaches, dizziness, and sickness after being sprayed with pesticides by crop dusters. In Montana, Native Americans only received benefits during the winter. The assumption was that able-bodied men could find work during the summer. Cornely noted chronic neglect and abuse by government officials—those entrusted and empowered to care for vulnerable populations.

> These visits revealed in dramatic and sometimes shocking fashion that millions of Americans, and particularly ethnic minorities—20 million blacks, five million Mexican-Americans, 400,000 to 500,000 Indians—are being brutalized by those governmental institutions that daily affect their lives; the police department, the welfare bureau, the public employment services, the housing administration and the departments of education, health and recreation. (Cornely, 1970a, p. 354)

Cornely's descriptions provided real life examples of how minorities carry the weight of social and economic burdens. American democracy favors the wealthy and disadvantages the poor. Minorities are at the mercy of the white majority for support, and when support is given it is offered as charity, not as subsidy for the hardships endured by discrimination, poverty, housing, unemployment, and limited access to health care. Because of the investigation, Cornely reported the need to integrate minorities into current political structures, to give minority communities a voice in health care and social services, and expand opportunities for medical training of people of color.

In 1969, Cornely was elected APHA president. As a public health leader, Cornely continued to shed light on the issues of racism in health care. He encouraged redirection and reorientation of research. He called out research studies that concluded an inherent inferiority of blacks, ignoring social determinants of health. He recommended that researchers focus on assets rather than deficiencies. Cornely advocated for cultural sensitivity training of white health care providers and more minority health professionals as leaders in health care. He called on psychiatrists and psychologists to acknowledge the mental health issues caused by racism and discrimination. He advocated to giving voice to black communities in decision making, implementation, planning, and delivery of health services. To ensure health care for all, Cornely advocated replacing the national system of charity medicine with a national system of health care. He believed that the government should support "a man in his home" before "a man on the moon" (Cornely, 2011, p. s163). In 1972, Cornely was awarded APHA's highest honor, the Sedgwick Memorial Medal.

Dr. Paul B. Cornely was a physician, a public health leader and a civil rights activist who highlighted the health and social injustices created by racial discrimination. He observed and called attention to the apathy, insensitivity, and neglect of doctors, nurses, hospitals, and government officials toward the plight of minorities. Although Cornely noted that, "Discrimination and segregation have no place in health," he also had a greater vision for public health (Cornely, 1985, p. 418).

His vision was to address the social determinants of health to support quality of life for *all* people.

Sally Kuykendall

See also: American Medical Association; American Public Health Association; Health Care Disparities; Health Disparities; Indian Health Service; Social Determinants of Health; U.S. Public Health Service

Further Reading

Byrd, W. M., & Clayton, L. A. (2000). *An American health dilemma: A medical history of African Americans and the problem of race: Beginnings to 1900.* New York: Routledge.

Cornely, P. B. (1949). Nature and extent of health education among Negroes. *Journal of Negro Education, 18*(3), 370–376.

Cornely, P. B. (1970a). Community participation and control: A possible answer to racism in health. *Milbank Memorial Fund Quarterly, 48*(2), 347.

Cornely, P. B. (1970b). The Role of Public Health Associations. *Canadian Journal of Public Health/Revue Canadienne de Sante'e Publique, 61*(6), 463.

Cornely, P. B. (1976). Racism: The ever-present hidden barrier to health in our society. *American Journal of Public Health, 66,* 246–247.

Cornely, P. B. (1985). Review: Crippling a nation: Health in apartheid South Africa by Aziza Seedat. *Journal of Public Health Policy, 6*(3), 415–418.

Cornely, P. B. (2011). The health status of the Negro today and in the future. *American Journal of Public Health, 101*(Suppl. 1), S161–S163.

COUNCIL ON EDUCATION FOR PUBLIC HEALTH (CEPH)

The Council on Education for Public Health (CEPH) is an agency that reviews the teaching, research, and service efforts of schools and programs in public health and accredits those schools and programs that meet the documented standards. CEPH reviews both the process (admissions, classes, and practical experiences) and the outcomes (alumni satisfaction and job placement) of the education offered by each school or program. Attaining CEPH accreditation is initially a three-year process followed by regular reviews to ensure ongoing compliance to the accreditation criteria. Although the criteria for reviewing programs and schools are slightly different, in general CEPH looks at whether the curriculum teaches the core competencies needed to become proficient in public health, recruits, retains, and supports qualified faculty, has the fiscal resources to support the educational operations, and integrates public health values into the academic experience. CEPH accreditation is a mark of excellence and means that the school or program adequately prepares graduates to work in the field. Accreditation is particularly important in professional fields where people trust others with their lives.

Higher education is a major investment of time and finances. The U.S. Department of Education (DOE) and the Council for Higher Education Accreditation

(CHEA) approve regional organizations to review and accredit the more than 23,700 degree-granting higher education programs in the United States. Accreditation is a sign that the education is a quality investment. The federal government, some state governments, and many employers will only grant scholarships or loans to students attending accredited colleges, universities, or institutions, and some federal research grants are restricted to accredited institutions only. It is important to note that the regional accrediting organizations accredit all of the programs in an institution and are not program specific. CEPH is the only agency recognized by the Department of Education to accredit public health programs and schools. This means that a program or school may have regional accreditation without CEPH accreditation. CEPH reviews public health programs leading to bachelor's, master's in public health (MPH), doctor of philosophy (PhD), or doctor of public health (DrPH) degrees. Some public health fellowships, scholarships, and job opportunities are limited to students attending CEPH-accredited schools and programs.

Not everyone is a good fit with the field of public health, and it would be an injustice to the individual and other students in the program to accept students who are unable to be successful in a program. To ensure that the program or school recruits and selects individuals who are capable of developing professional competencies in public health, CEPH reviews recruitment materials, recruitment policies, and admissions requirements. Each school provides data on number of applicants, accepted students, enrolled students, and graduation rates. By reviewing recruitment and admissions policies, CEPH provides a level of consumer protection. Students are assured that they are not attending a diploma mill, and the institution follows best practices in selecting students who will benefit from the educational experience and will be able to secure a job after graduation.

The CEPH-accredited bachelor's degree in public health typically requires four years of full-time study (120 credit units) and includes courses outside the major. The CEPH-accredited MPH requires at least 42 credit hours, which is equivalent to two and a half years of full-time study. (Full-time graduate study is nine credits per semester.) Core curricula include biostatistics, environmental health sciences, epidemiology, health services administration, and social and behavioral health sciences and the cross-cutting competencies of communication and informatics, diversity and culture, leadership, public health biology, professionalism, program planning, and systems thinking. Public health programs provide a one-semester practicum experience where the student plans and implements a public health activity. The practicum experience is intended to bring concepts together and reinforce and apply knowledge from individual courses.

Beyond the curriculum, CEPH ensures that programs and schools have systems in place to support quality education. CEPH reviews the strength of academic advising and career counseling. Part of the accreditation process requires that schools or programs survey past graduates to assess satisfaction with the education and support services. Institutions must also have an adequate number of professors to teach in the programs, and the faculty must have the necessary expertise. The academic system is unique in that faculty are partners in the governance of the university or college rather than simply employees. Teaching faculty have a responsibility to provide quality teaching, engage in novel research, and provide service that will promote the good of the community. These activities allow faculty to maintain expertise in their field, which ultimately supports student learning. By maintaining professional connections with government health authorities, public health clinics, hospitals and local communities, academic institutions are able to offer practical and relevant learning activities to students of public health.

CEPH accreditation is a sign that a school or program provides excellent preparation for public health practice. By selecting a CEPH-accredited program or school, students are assured a quality education by qualified professors. Successful completion of the CEPH-accredited program or school ensures that the student is prepared to function in the public health workforce.

Sally Kuykendall

See also: Certified in Public Health; Core Competencies in Public Health; Degrees in Public Health

Further Reading

Council for Higher Education Accreditation. (2016). Retrieved from http://www.chea.org/.
Council on Education for Public Health. (2016). Retrieved from http://ceph.org/.

CULTURAL COMPETENCE

Culture influences lifestyle, attitudes toward health and wellness, health behaviors, and perceptions of health care systems and providers. Differences in language, values, and habits between the patient and the provider can lead to misunderstandings that impact quality of life and health outcomes. Public health professionals are challenged to think beyond their own personal values and experiences in order to work effectively with patients, family members, and other health care or social service providers. Cultural competence is the ability to understand and value another culture and incorporate that culture's beliefs, perceptions, and attitudes into practice. Experts define cultural competence as, "a set of congruent behaviors, attitudes, and policies that come together in a system, agency or among professionals and enable that system, agency, or those professionals to work effectively in cross-cultural situations" (Cross et al., 1989). Since public health works with people and communities of diverse cultures, professionals are responsible for developing and maintaining cultural competence of the communities that they serve. Strategies to achieve cultural competence include professional trainings, fostering a climate of respect within the workplace, representation by members of the community, and long-term commitment to cultural competence by the agency or system.

Culture is defined as a "structure of behaviors, ideas, attitudes, values, habits, beliefs, customs, language, rituals, ceremonies, and practices of a particular group of people that provides them with a general design for living and patterns for interpreting behavior" (Annie E. Casey Foundation, 2003). Many of the leading causes of death in the United States, such as heart disease, stroke, cancer, and diabetes, are related to lifestyle and culture. Differences in culture between patient and health care provider can lead to harmful stereotypes, language barriers, or delays in disease detection, screening, and treatment compliance. The Office of Minority Health (2016) reports numerous health disparities based on race and ethnicity. African Americans have higher infant mortality, heart disease mortality, diabetes, HIV/AIDS, and homicide in comparison to non-Hispanic whites. Latino Americans have higher rates of tuberculosis, diabetes, obesity, hypertension, and low birth weight infants. Asian and Pacific Islander Americans have higher rates of cervical cancer, tuberculosis, and hepatitis. The connections between lifestyle, culture, and health outcomes are important in that they allow public health professionals to target negative behaviors and improve health status.

At the individual level, cultural competence is displayed as the ability to reflect on one's own culture and the impact it has on others; the ability to value differences and similarities among all people; the ability to respond effectively to cultural differences; the ability to adapt services and service delivery to match community or client needs; and the ability to sustain cultural competence within the institution (Denboba, 1993). Cultural competence training is a tool that encourages health care providers to examine their own cultural beliefs; to identify values, attitudes, and assumptions that pose barriers to screening, diagnosis, or treatment of patients of various cultures; and to practice framing effective messages. Dogra, Giordano, and France (2007) note that cultural competency training is not as much about expertise in a particular culture as it is about dealing with uncertainty. A list of dos and don'ts may be an early step toward cultural competence. However, such a list will not apply to every person of that culture or every situation.

Organizational strategies to support cultural competence include providing foreign language or sign language interpreter services, recruiting and retaining staff with shared customs, coordinating care with traditional healers, developing culturally competent health communication tools, and including the family or significant community members in patient care (Brach & Fraser, 2000). Many large public health departments employ professional medical interpreters to assist in patient-provider communication. Medical interpreters adhere to a code of ethics that respects patient confidentiality and ensures transparency, accuracy, and completeness (no adding, omitting, or substituting) in translation. Interpreters use specific techniques such as asking the patient and provider to speak directly to one another (using the first person), positioning themselves equidistant from provider and patient yet out of sight of both, and gathering feedback to ensure the correct message was received. Whenever possible, public health clinics create and use language translations of patient education forms, intake forms, consent forms, treatment instructions, discharge instructions, Patient Bill of Rights, privacy notices, and public service announcements. Some public health departments in large cities are prepared to handle up to 500 different dialects! Another common technique is for health centers to recruit and retain personnel from the same culture as the patient population. However, it is important to note that common origin does not ensure shared language, values, or beliefs. Differences may still exist due to social class, religious practices, or education.

Cultural competence is an asset to the individual public health professional and public health organizations. Through cultural competent care, health care providers, patients, and members of the community can work together to reduce preventable diseases and promote early diagnosis and treatment. Although there are many strategies to achieve cultural competence, the primary foundation is willingness to respect people's similarities and differences and an earnest desire to help and support one another.

Sally Kuykendall

See also: Code of Ethics; Core Competencies in Public Health; Health Care Disparities; Health Communication; Health Disparities; Indian Health Service; Social Ecological Model

Further Reading

Annie E. Casey Foundation/AED Center on AIDS & Community Health. (2003). Cultural Competency. *2003 Community Health Summit Toolkit.* Author.

Brach, C., & Fraser, I. (2000). Can cultural competency reduce racial and ethnic health disparities? A review and conceptual model. *Medical Care Research and Review, 57*(Suppl. 1), 181–217.

Cross, T., Bazron, B., Dennis, K., & Isaacs, M. (1989). *Towards a culturally competent system of care* (Vol. 1). Washington, DC: Georgetown University Child Development Center, CASSP Technical Assistance Center.

Denboba, D. (1993). *MCHB/DSCSHCN Guidance for competitive applications, maternal and child health improvement projects for children with special health care needs.* U.S. Department of Health and Human Services, Health Services and Resources Administration.

Dogra, N., Giordano, J., & France, N. (2007). Cultural diversity teaching and issues of uncertainty: The findings of a qualitative study. *BMC Medical Education, 7.*

Johnson, R. L., Saha, S., Arbelaez, J. J., Beach, M. C., & Cooper, L. A. (2004). Racial and ethnic differences in patient perceptions of bias and cultural competence in health care. *Journal of General Internal Medicine, 19,* 101–110.

Office of Minority Health. (2016). *Minority population profiles.* Retrieved from http://minorityhealth.hhs.gov/omh/browse.aspx?lvl=2&lvlid=26.

CUTTER INCIDENT, THE

Throughout the early half of the 20th century, mid-August to mid-September was a time of fear and dread. It was poliomyelitis season, a time when the highly infectious virus emerged, unabated and reaping havoc in communities. The deadly virus attacked the nervous system causing motor paralysis within hours. Children would complain of headache, nausea, or fatigue at bedtime and wake up paralyzed. Five to ten percent of polio victims died due to respiratory paralysis (WHO, 2016). Survivors were doomed to life in an iron lung. In 1953, the year prior to Salk's large-scale polio vaccine trials, polio attacked 35,592 people in the United States, resulting in 1,450 deaths and 15,648 cases of permanent paralysis (Freyche & Payne, 1956). Young children of middle to high socioeconomic status families were the most susceptible because they were the least likely to have been exposed to the milder strains of polio earlier in life. When Salk's vaccine was pronounced "safe, effective, and potent," church bells rang and air raid sirens shrieked. However, the joy was short-lived. Within a few weeks of the start of the nation's mass immunization campaign, six children immunized with vaccine from Cutter Laboratories were paralyzed. The event created confusion, fear, and distrust and exposed weaknesses in the overly enthusiastic research and government program. Although Cutter's vaccines met government safety standards, the company was found liable without fault. Since vaccines were sold to public health agencies and provided very low profit margins, pharmaceutical companies responded by shying away from the development and manufacture of vaccines. To encourage vaccine manufacture, the federal government created the National Vaccine Injury Compensation Program. The program compensates people who become ill or injured as a result of vaccination and ensures that infectious diseases, such as polio, are kept under control.

The factors that created the Cutter Incident started long before Cutter manufactured their first batch of polio vaccine. Preventing poliomyelitis was a global priority. The National Foundation for Infantile Paralysis, founded by President Franklin D. Roosevelt, funded multiple vaccine development studies. Albert Sabin's polio vaccine contained attenuated forms of all three polio serotypes while Jonas Salk used the deactivated Type 1 (Mahoney) poliovirus. The Mahoney serotype is the most deadly of the poliovirus strains. Salk's logic was that the deadliest strain would produce more antibodies than the less virulent serotypes. Salk's vaccine was successfully field tested on 1.8 million schoolchildren and adults. On April 12, 1955, Dr. Thomas Francis, Jr., director of the Poliomyelitis Vaccine Evaluation Center at the University of Michigan School of Public Health, announced to nearly 200 journalists and 500 scientists that Salk's vaccine was 60 to 90 percent effective. In preparation for a nationwide mass immunization campaign, five pharmaceutical companies were licensed to manufacture the vaccine. All of the companies had difficulty inactivating the Mahoney strain.

In mid-April, approximately 400,000 people, mostly children, were inoculated with vaccine manufactured by Cutter Laboratories of Berkeley, California. Cutter was a small, family-owned business who had manufactured vaccines for anthrax and swine fever. On April 24, the first victim was admitted to Michael Reese Hospital in Chicago with paralysis of both legs. The infant had been immunized with the Cutter vaccine on April 16. By April 27, five additional cases were reported, and Surgeon General Dr. Leonard A. Scheele directed Cutter Laboratories to recall

all of their vaccines. A committee of polio experts was established to investigate and determine if the cases were caused by community exposure or the vaccine. As more cases were reported, the answer became clear. Batches of the Cutter vaccine as well as batches from some of the other laboratories contained live polio virus. Yet, Cutter's product had passed the government safety tests. The disaster revealed serious deficits in manufacturing and safety testing. On May 5, the surgeon general ordered a complete halt to the polio immunization program. Governments throughout the world also put their immunization programs on hold. On May 27, the committee announced new safety standards. The time period for deactivation of the live virus was extended. Larger samples were used for testing of live virus. Batches were tested multiple times until at least two successive negative tests were achieved, and batches were tested an additional time after bottling to ensure against cross-contamination within the factory. The government resumed the polio vaccination program in the fall of 1955.

In 1957, the family of five-year-old Anne Gottsdanker sued Cutter Laboratories for negligence and breach of implied warranty. The live virus administered by vaccine tended to attack the extremity where the person received the injection. Anne suffered permanent paralysis of her right leg. The court found Cutter Laboratories not guilty of negligence. The company had followed government safety precautions. However, they were guilty of breach of implied warranty because the vaccine was labeled "inactivated" virus when, in fact, it contained live virus. The legal precedent of *liability without fault* was a threat to public health. Pharmaceutical companies were reluctant to manufacture vaccines. Companies shied away from manufacturing vaccines, prices skyrocketed, and vaccine shortages resulted. In 1986, the federal government created the National Vaccine Injury Compensation Program to ensure that people who suffer from illness or injury due to a vaccination are compensated quickly and fairly and that pharmaceutical companies manufacturing products intended to benefit public health are not penalized for their efforts.

The Cutter vaccinations are estimated to have caused 40,000 cases of polio, including 200 cases of paralysis and 10 deaths (Fitzpatrick, 2006). Vaccine-induced cases of polio created an epidemic exposing family and community members to the virus, and the pause in the national immunization campaign left children vulnerable to the polio epidemic of 1955. Furthermore, the incident damaged the reputation of American vaccine manufacturers. Today, the government carefully monitors vaccine manufacturers to ensure public safety and vaccine efficacy. As a result, diseases such as polio, diphtheria, and smallpox are no longer the public threat they once were.

Sally Kuykendall

See also: Infectious Diseases; Polio; Roosevelt, Franklin Delano; Salk, Jonas; Vaccines; *Controversies in Public Health:* Controversy 3

Further Reading

Fitzpatrick, M. (2006). The Cutter Incident: How America's first polio vaccine led to a growing vaccine crisis. *Journal of the Royal Society of Medicine*, *99*(3), 156.

Freyche, M. J., & Payne, A. M. (1956). Poliomyelitis in 1954. *Bulletin of the World Health Organization*, *15*(1–2), 43–121.

Nathanson, N., & Langmuir, A. D. (1963). The Cutter Incident. Poliomyelitis following formaldehyde-inactivated poliovirus vaccination in the United States during the spring of 1955. II. Relationship of poliomyelitis to Cutter vaccine. *American Journal of Hygiene*, *78*, 29–60.

Offit, P. A. (2005). *The Cutter Incident: How America's first polio vaccine led to the growing vaccine crisis*. New Haven, CT: Yale University Press.

Oshinsky, D. (2006). *Polio: An American story*. New York: Oxford University Press.

World Health Organization (WHO). (2016). *Poliomyelitis*. Retrieved from http://www.who.int/topics/poliomyelitis/en/.

D

DEAN, HENRY TRENDLEY (1893–1962)

Henry Trendley Dean was a dentist who discovered fluoridation and improved oral health for millions of people. "Bud" Dean was born in Winstanley Park, Illinois, and grew up in St. Louis. After graduating from St. Louis School of Dentistry in 1916, he established his own dental practice. Dentistry was still developing as a medical profession. The toothbrush had not been invented (variations existed, but the first modern, nylon toothbrush came along in 1938). Almost everyone had cavities. Dentists assessed a patient's oral health by counting the number of decayed, missing, or filled teeth (DMFT). The lower the DMFT count, the better the oral health.

After a year in private practice, Dean joined the army. The army needed dentists to keep soldiers healthy and on the front lines. Missing or loose teeth meant that a soldier could not chew food properly, which could lead to malnutrition, fatigue, and decreased ability to fight infectious diseases. The soldier who succumbs to infection could pass the disease to other soldiers, disabling an entire military unit. Front teeth are particularly important for pronouncing words with the sounds *f*, *th*, and *v*. The inability to communicate clearly during military operations could jeopardize lives. During the draft for World War I, 24 out of 1,000 men were rejected because they did not have at least six opposing teeth—the minimum number of teeth considered necessary to chew food (Britten & Perrott, 1941). Soldiers' oral health was further aggravated by a condition known as trench mouth. Trench mouth or acute necrotizing ulcerative gingivitis (ANUG) is an infection of the mouth that causes ulcers and gum deterioration and can result in tooth loss. ANUG is caused by poor oral hygiene (not being able to regularly brush one's teeth), smoking, stress, and malnutrition. As a military dentist, Dean developed a program of oral hygiene for soldiers in the trenches. The program was used throughout World War II. After World War I, Dean returned to private practice and married Ruth Martha McEvoy. However, he did not stay in private practice for very long. By 1921, he joined the U.S. Public Health Service as acting assistant dental surgeon.

Even before Dean considered going to dental school, another dentist in Colorado was laying the foundation for one of the greatest achievements in public health history. In 1901, Dr. Frederick S. McKay graduated from dental school at University of Pennsylvania and moved west. Establishing a private dental practice in Colorado Springs, McKay was surprised to see that most of his patients had strangely colored teeth, the color of brown chocolate. McKay called the abnormality *Colorado brown stain*. He tried to convince other local dentists to study the problem but none were concerned. So, he developed his own field study, tracing the affected area to Pikes Peak watershed. In 1909, McKay presented his findings to other professionals at a dental conference. His presentation aroused the curiosity of Dr. Green Vardiman Black, the preeminent dental expert of the time. McKay and Black joined together to study the problem that Black renamed *mottled enamel*. Although Black died in 1915, their findings were not published until 1916. Mottled enamel seemed to be more severe among children who had recently developed their second set of teeth *and* appeared highly resistant to cavities. The idea that pitted enamel was less resistant to cavities was completely contrary to logic and expert opinion. Most dentists assumed that pitted enamel would increase risk of cavities. However, McKay and Black's findings were quickly validated by other dentists working in areas with mottled enamel. In 1923, McKay was invited to Oakley, Idaho, to investigate cases of mottled enamel. McKay suspected the local water source. However, when he tested the water, he found nothing unusual. He encouraged Oakley residents to use another water source, and within a few years children started having white teeth.

In 1926, Dr. F. L. Robertson, a dentist practicing in Benton, Arkansas, asked public health officials to investigate cases of mottled enamel in the nearby town of Bauxite. Bauxite was a corporate town of the Aluminum Company of America (ALCOA). When the public health service did not respond, the superintendent of the mining company contacted McKay. McKay and Grover Kempf of the Bureau of Child Hygiene investigated the problem and found 100 percent of children afflicted with mottled teeth. ALCOA's chief chemist Harry Van Osdall Churchill was concerned that ALCOA would be blamed for the problem and started his own investigation. ALCOA laboratory attained and tested a sample of Bauxite's water supply using more sophisticated technology than McKay had access to. Analysis revealed high levels of fluoride. Churchill contacted McKay, offering to test samples from other affected towns. Water from areas where mottled enamel was endemic all tested high for fluoride.

Pressured by McKay, Robertson, and others, the National Institute of Health (NIH) hired Dean to investigate mottled enamel in 1931. Dean approached the problem in the same way that he had addressed trench mouth, as an infectious disease. He searched medical reports from around the world, later recalling, "Many times, findings, long buried in the literature and apparently unrelated to oral disease were found on close study to be of unrealized value" (Dean, 1953, p. 705). He found clues from dentists in Japan, Argentina, and England. Based on the literature, Dean devised an epidemiological study. He identified areas where mottled teeth occurred and gathered a team of chemists, dentists, biologists, and engineers. The research team analyzed water samples for hardness and fluoride. Dentists performed hundreds of oral examinations, inspecting and reporting on the teeth of children. Results confirmed what McKay and others had observed. Children with mottled enamel had fewer cavities. In Bruneau, Idaho, 33 percent of children with mottled teeth had cavities compared to 64 percent of children with normal teeth (Dean, 1938).

At Pima Indian School, 58 percent of children with mottled enamel had cavities compared to 81 percent with normal teeth. Overall, children with mottled teeth were five times more likely to be cavity-free than children with normal teeth.

Dean had an idea. If fluoride made teeth resistant to cavities, then adding small amounts of fluoride to local water supplies should reduce cavities. He renamed mottled enamel *fluorosis* and set a new goal of identifying therapeutic levels of fluorine, levels that protect against cavities yet do not cause fluorosis. In order to proceed, dentists needed a more refined way to measure oral health than the crude DMFT scale. Dean developed the Fluorosis Index. The Fluorosis Index measures the severity of tooth discoloration and pitting. Comparing degree of fluorosis with fluoride levels in the local water supply, the researchers identified the therapeutic level of 1 ppm (part per million) of fluoride. The next step was to pilot test water fluoridation as a public health program. In 1945, Grand Rapids, Michigan, fluoridated their public water supply. Over the next 15 years, public health dentists and researchers monitored the teeth of approximately 30,000 children. The pilot was a success. Caries rates in Grand Rapids dropped by 60 percent after water fluoridation, and there were no adverse effects (Dean, 1953).

Dean modeled public health in practice. He recognized and respected the reports and observations from clinicians, developed an epidemiological study, drew conclusions from the study findings and translated the research findings into public health practice. In 1945, Dean became director of dental research at the NIH and from 1948 to 1953, he served as director of National Institute of Dental Research where he worked to bring water fluoridation to towns and communities across the country. He also integrated other aspects of dental care into his work, advocating for diets low in starch and sugar. In 1952, the American Public Health Association recognized McKay and Dean for their pioneering studies and contributions to disease control with the prestigious Lasker Award. By 1953, fluoridation was being used in 427 communities, benefiting 8.5 million people (Dean, 1953). Henry Trendley Dean died in 1962 from emphysema complicated by asthma.

Dean's intuition, logic, perseverance, and never-ending quest for ways to improve public health embody the spirit of translational research. Dean saw a problem, listened to others, examined the facts, and made connections. Although dental caries, gingivitis, and tooth loss still exist today, they are not the scourge that they once were. Therapeutic fluoride in water, toothpaste, mouthwash, and dental practices allow many people to enjoy healthy teeth, nutritious meals, and bright smiles. Dean's efforts in developing water fluoridation are recognized as one of the greatest public health advancements of the 20th century.

Sally Kuykendall

See also: Epidemic; Epidemiology; Fluoridation; Oral Health; Population Health; Research; Veterans' Health

Further Reading

Britten, R. H., & Perrott, G. St. J. (1941). Summary of physical findings on men drafted in the world war. *Public Health Reports (1896–1970)*, *56*(2), 41.

Centers for Disease Control and Prevention. (1999). Achievements in public health, 1900–1999: Fluoridation of drinking water to prevent dental caries. *Morbidity and Mortality Weekly Report, 48*(41), 933–940. Retrieved from https://www.cdc.gov/mmwr/preview/mmwrhtml/mm4841a1.htm.

Centers for Disease Control and Prevention. (1999). H. Trendley Dean, D.D.S. *Morbidity and Mortality Weekly Report, 48*(41), 935. Retrieved from https://www.cdc.gov/mmwr/preview/mmwrhtml/mm4841bx.htm.

Dean, H. T. (1938). Endemic fluorosis and its relation to dental caries. *Public Health Reports*, *53*(33), 1443–1452.

Dean, H. T. (1953). Some reflections on the epidemiology of fluorine and dental health. *American Journal of Public Health*, *43*, 704–709.

Dean, H. T., & McKay, F. S. (1939). Production of mottled enamel halted by a change in common water supply. *American Journal of Public Health, 29*, 590–596.

Mottled teeth. (1940). *Time*, *35*, 40.

National Institute of Dental and Craniofacial Research. (2014). *The story of fluoridation.* Retrieved from https://www.nidcr.nih.gov/OralHealth/Topics/Fluoride/TheStoryofFluoridation.htm.

DEGREES IN PUBLIC HEALTH

Preparation for a career in public health is achieved through a variety of undergraduate and graduate degree programs in public health, health administration, health policy, or health services. Different jobs require different academic preparation, and while it is helpful to know which area of public health one wishes to pursue, not knowing is not a major disadvantage. Public health professionals come from a wide variety of backgrounds, and an undergraduate degree in public health is not necessary for graduate study. An undergraduate degree in math can be used to craft expertise in biostatistics or epidemiology. A foundational degree in sociology, psychology, or anthropology is helpful in behavioral health or community health practice. Communications majors may pursue careers in health communications. Business majors can apply their skills in health administration. Political science majors can find fulfilling positions in health policy. Biology, chemistry, physics, and engineering majors can use their analytical skills in public health research. Undergraduate preparation in a field other than public health strengthens public health practice by drawing on the knowledge and skills of other disciplines.

The Council on Education for Public Health (CEPH) is an independent agency approved by the U.S. Department of Education to review and accredit schools and programs in public health. CEPH reviews public health programs to determine whether the training meets standards of quality. Accreditation is a rigorous process. Programs are assessed on ability to teach students the core competencies of public health as well as any relevant specialty areas, integration of experiential learning into the program, engagement of students in learning and community service, support for qualified faculty who are recognized experts in the field, and successes of students after graduation. CEPH accreditation demonstrates that the school or program has met and continues to meet high standards in teaching, research, and service. The Association of Schools and Programs of Public Health (ASPPH) is the primary organization representing accredited public health schools and programs. ASPPH advances the field of public health by educating the general public on the role of public health, by helping students interested in public health navigate complex academic systems, promoting evidence-based practices, and advocating for public policies that strengthen public health education and research.

Many different types of programs and degrees can lead to careers in public health. A minimum of a bachelor's degree is required for entry level positions in occupational or industrial hygiene, health and safety inspection, environmental health, community health, and health administration. Undergraduate degrees are four-year degrees in public health earning the bachelor of science (BS), bachelor of arts (BA), or bachelor of science in public health (BSPH). Graduate degrees tend to be more common, as these allow the student to develop an area of specialization. Some of the many public health specialties are behavioral health, biostatistics, chronic illnesses, community health, dental health, environmental health, epidemiology, food safety, genetics, global health, health administration, economics, health education, policy, research, infectious diseases, health information management, maternal and child health, nutrition, occupational health, population health, emergency preparedness and response, tropical medicine, veterinary medicine, and women's health (ASPPH, 2016). The master of public health (MPH), master of health administration (MHA), master of science (MS), and master of health sciences (MHS) require two-year, full-time study, leading to job opportunities in hospitals, health departments, international, state and federal agencies, community organizations, and managed care organizations. The MPH degree is a highly desirable degree. Many established doctors, nurses, dentists, pharmacists, statisticians, and environmental scientists go back to school to earn their MPH degree. Early career students are encouraged to consider dual degree programs, obtaining the MPH degree simultaneously with a clinical or other degree. Common dual degree programs are medicine (MD/MPH), law (JD/MPH), nursing (MSN/MPH), business (MBA/MPH), pharmacy (PharmD/MPH), physical therapy (DPT/MPH), and social work (MSW/MPH). Doctoral degrees in public health are advanced graduate degrees, requiring a doctoral dissertation to prepare for positions in research, teaching, or leadership. Doctoral degrees include the doctor of philosophy (PhD), doctor of science (ScD), and doctor of public health (DrPH). The Delta Omega Honorary Society in Public Health is the national honor society recognizing excellence by students and faculty in the field of public health.

The field of public health is increasing rapidly. As the population ages and new specialties in health and medicine emerge, more qualified professionals will be needed to meet the growing demands. The many different pathways allow the individual to craft a unique niche providing important contributions to the field.

Sally Kuykendall

See also: Administration, Health; Core Competencies in Public Health; Council on Education for Public Health

Further Reading

Association of Schools and Programs of Public Health (ASPPH). (2016). Retrieved from http://www.aspph.org/.

Careers in public health.net. (2016). Retrieved from http://www.careersinpublichealth.net/.

Council on Education for Public Health. (2016). Retrieved from http://ceph.org/.

Delta Omega Honorary Society in Public Health. (2016). Retrieved from http://www.deltaomega.org/index.cfm.

Public health degrees.org. (2016). Retrieved from http://www.publichealthdegrees.org/.

DIABETES MELLITUS

Diabetes mellitus is a chronic disease where the body is either unable to produce or to properly manage insulin, the hormone that converts glucose (sugar) from food and drink into energy. The inability to use glucose results in high levels of sugar circulating in the bloodstream, which interferes with functions. The body is forced to divert protein from critical organ functions for use as energy. Approximately 29 million Americans are diabetic and 86 million are prediabetic, at risk for developing diabetes within the next 10 years. In many cases, diabetes comes on slowly and the person is not aware of the problem. An estimated 25 percent of diabetics and 90 percent of prediabetics are undiagnosed. Late diagnosis and treatment can lead to many health issues, such as amputations of the toes, feet and legs, heart disease, stroke, kidney failure, and blindness. Diabetes causes over 76,000 deaths per year and is the seventh leading cause of death in the United States. Despite advances in diabetes prevention and treatment, diabetes is likely to increase as obesity increases and young children of minority ethnicities may end up carrying much of the burden of disease. Public health efforts to reduce diabetes focus on four disease transition points: (1) primary prevention, (2) medical screening for early diagnosis, (3) better access to care, and (4) improved quality of care for people living with diabetes. Twenty *Healthy People 2020* objectives deal specifically with diabetes and diabetes-related care, an indication of how important this problem is in moving the nation toward health and wellness.

When we eat fruits, vegetables, nuts, seeds, dairy products, rice, pasta, or sweets, carbohydrates in these foods are converted into glucose (sugar). Glucose is a great source of energy because it can be easily utilized by the body. Insulin helps glucose to enter the cell thereby providing energy for cell structure, function, and maintenance. Diabetics either do not make enough insulin (Type 1) or can't use the insulin that is produced (Type 2). If the cells cannot take in glucose, sugar stays in the bloodstream. High blood sugar levels pull fluid out of the cell through osmosis, upsetting fluid-electrolyte and acid-base balances. The kidneys will eventually spill some of the excess sugar. However, the person will suffer health consequences because of high blood sugar, depletion of protein, and electrolyte imbalances. Characteristic symptoms are frequent urination, polydipsia (excessive thirst), hunger, weight loss, fatigue, numbness, or tingling of the hands or feet, changes in vision, dry skin, and sores that take longer to heal than expected. The symptoms may be subtle at first as the body tries to compensate for the malfunction. By the time the person seeks medical advice, irreversible organ damage may occur.

Primary prevention is the technique of stopping a health problem before it occurs. There are currently no known causes of Type 1 diabetes. Therefore, no programs or mechanisms exist to prevent Type 1 diabetes. Type 2 diabetes accounts for 90 to 95 percent of cases of diabetes and is highly preventable. Risk factors are overweight and obesity, physical inactivity, family history, age (45 years and older), and history of gestational diabetes (diabetes while pregnant). African Americans, Hispanic/Latino Americans, Native Americans, Pacific Islanders, and Asian Americans are at higher risk in comparison to Caucasian Americans. The American Diabetes Association provides a risk test (available at http://www.diabetes.org/are-you-at-risk/diabetes-risk-test/). In 2016, the Centers for Disease Control and Prevention (CDC), American Diabetes Association, American Medical Association, and the Ad Council partnered to develop the first national prediabetes awareness campaign. Public service announcements encourage people to check out their risk for prediabetes at DoIHavePrediabetes.org. Knowing one's risk helps people to make educated decisions about their health rather than waiting for warning signs to occur.

For anyone, and especially people who are at risk for diabetes, engaging in at least 30 minutes of physical activity most days of the week (60 minutes for children) and maintaining a healthy weight are ideal ways to prevent onset. Reducing the amount of fat and calories in the diet helps to maintain a healthy weight. Diet and exercise can help people with prediabetes to halve their risk of developing the disease, and the benefits are multifold in that these lifestyle changes will also reduce risk of cardiovascular disease, high blood pressure, stroke, some forms of cancer, and many other obesity-related diseases. The National Diabetes Prevention Program (DPP) is a national partnership of evidence-based programs with the goal of reducing diabetes and prediabetes. In order to be designated as a National DPP, the program must use an approved curriculum, offer a minimum of 16 sessions over the first six months taught by trained lifestyle coaches, offer access to a diabetes prevention coordinator, and monitor program effectiveness through participant weight loss and physical activity levels. National DPPs are located within communities throughout the country. The CDC offers a searchable database of available programs (https://www.cdc.gov/diabetes/prevention/index.html).

Screening and early diagnosis are critical to ensure effective disease maintenance. Uncontrolled diabetes can lead to serious health complications of heart disease, blindness, kidney failure, neuropathy, susceptibility to infections, atherosclerosis, and lower extremity amputations. Diabetes is diagnosed through several different laboratory tests. The blood test A1C measures average blood glucose over the past two to three months. Normal range is less than 5.7 percent. An A1C of 5.7 to 6.4 percent on two separate occasions indicates prediabetes, and an A1C of 6.5 percent or higher on two separate occasions indicates diabetes. *Healthy People 2020* objective D-1 is to reduce the rate of new cases of diabetes from 8 per 1,000 people (2006–2008) to 7.2 per 1,000 people. The United States is making good progress toward this goal. In 2012–2014, incidence rates decreased to 6.7 per 1,000. Rates among people on public insurance decreased from 17.2 per 1,000 to 11.5 per 1,000. Further efforts are needed for populations with high incidence rates, people with less than a high school diploma (incidence rate = 12.9/1,000), living at 100 percent below the poverty line (incidence rate = 12.3/1,000), and living with disabilities (incidence rate = 23/1,000). The Prevent Diabetes STAT Screen/Test/Act Today Program is a partnership between the American Medical Association and the CDC, which supports physicians, health care providers, and patients with resources for best practices guidelines in screening and referral.

Access to health services is important to provide early and effective control of diabetes and to prevent complications. In 2010, 1 out of every 5 Americans did not have medical insurance and 1 out of 10 people did not have access to medical care, dental care, or prescription medicines (Office of Disease Prevention and Health Promotion, n.d.). Access to services means that people with prediabetes or diabetes are able to get to a location where health services are offered, obtain services from that health system, and meet with a qualified provider for treatment, care, and health education. The Patient Protection and Affordable Care Act was enacted to close the gap between insured and uninsured by providing health insurance coverage to all Americans.

The goal of diabetes treatment and management is to maintain normal blood glucose levels while avoiding hyperglycemia and hypoglycemia. Successful management requires changing lifetime habits of diet and exercise, calculating calories, monitoring blood sugar, insulin, or medication, and prevention of complications through good skin care and careful selection of footwear. Infections, stress, menstruation, alcohol, and eating disorders can all interfere with successful management. Because blood sugar varies so much throughout the day, managing the disease is a constant process. Primary responsibility falls on the individual and his or her family. This means the patient and their loved ones must have the knowledge and skills to adequately manage the disease and be able to work with various health care providers to coordinate care. Teaching people to manage their disease takes time. However, the rewards are great. Currently, an estimated 20 percent of all health care spending is related to diabetes. Empowering people with diabetes can reduce health care costs and decrease the number of people with lower extremity amputations, kidney failure, and blindness.

The CDC partners with local, state, and territorial health departments to track trends in diabetes in order to provide evidence-based prevention, offer effective treatments, and support improved quality of care. Because Type 2 diabetes overlaps with many other chronic diseases, efforts to reduce diabetes fall within the purview of the National Center for Chronic Disease Prevention and Health Promotion (NCCDPHP). The NCCDPHP oversees efforts to prevent or delay diabetes onset through surveillance, environmental approaches, system interventions, and community-based programs. Researchers are studying triggers for Type 1 diabetes and are actively searching for new ways to prevent and treat both types of diabetes. Techniques, such as pancreas and islet cell transplantations, offer promise for future generations.

An estimated one in three individuals is living with prediabetes, and the majority of these individuals do not know that they are at risk for this life-changing disease. Preventing diabetes is critical to reducing health care costs and improving quality and length of life for many Americans. Diabetes prevention can be achieved through increased public awareness of the disease, awareness of one's own individual risk level, lifestyle changes, and effective, coordinated efforts in self-management and clinical management.

Sally Kuykendall

See also: Body Mass Index; Chronic Illness; Disability; Health Disparities; Healthy Places; Heart Disease; Heart Truth® (Red Dress) Campaign, The; Hypertension; Men's Health; National Heart, Lung, and Blood Institute; Nutrition; Obesity; Physical Activity; Prevention

Further Reading

American Diabetes Association. (2017). Retrieved from http://www.diabetes.org/.

Centers for Disease Control and Prevention. (2016). National Diabetes Prevention Program. U.S. Department of Health and Human Services. Retrieved from https://www.cdc.gov/diabetes/prevention/index.html.

Office of Disease Prevention and Health Promotion. (n.d.). *Healthy People 2020: Access to health services.* Retrieved from https://www.healthypeople.gov/2020/data-search/Search-the-Data#topic-area=3495.

Office of Disease Prevention and Health Promotion. (n.d.). *Healthy People 2020: Diabetes.* Retrieved from https://www.healthypeople.gov/2020/topics-objectives/topic/diabetes.

Prevent Diabetes STAT. (2017). Retrieved from http://www.ama-assn.org/sub/prevent-diabetes-stat/index.html.

DIFFUSION OF INNOVATIONS THEORY

Diffusion of innovations theory describes how consumers accept and embrace new technology, information, or lifestyle practices. The theory applies to public health because it explains why and how people adopt health advancements in the form of products, attitudes, or behaviors. According to the theory, people respond to a new product or innovation in five progressive stages: initial exposure, piqued interest, decision to try, pilot usage, and final adoption (Kaminski, 2011). The stages progress at different rates. The initial stages depend on where and how people get information and the value that they subscribe to that source. The decision to use stage is based on the individual's willingness to take risks and navigate unfamiliar systems. People are more likely to embrace innovations that are easy to use, easy to undo (if the product fails), and seem superior to current alternative options. Rate of adoption within a population is represented as either a bell-shaped or S-shaped curve. As more people use the product or innovation, the curve rises. Diffusion of innovations theory helps public health practitioners to understand why and how people adopt new behaviors and the best ways to market novel health-enhancing technology or practices.

French criminologist and social psychologist Jean-Gabriel De Tarde (1843–1904) was the first person to propose that beliefs and actions are passed from person to person and replicated within a community. As magistrate in Dordogne, France, Tarde estimated that 99 percent of the defendants appearing in his courtroom were simply imitating other criminals. Although the defendants might add a few personal adaptations to their crime, only about 1 defendant out of 100 had an original idea. Tarde's theory was revisited in 1943 when two Iowa sociologists studied farmers' adoption and use of a new hybrid seed corn (Ryan & Gross, 1943). The new hybrid seed yielded larger crops and was more drought resistant. Yet, the researchers found a five-year gap between when the farmers first learned of the new seed and they actually started using the seed. Although salesmen were important in introducing the new product, word of mouth between the farmers and visible proof were more important. The researchers mapped adoption of the hybrid seed and found that the majority of farmers did not start using the corn until they saw other farmers successfully using the product. The son of one of those Iowa farmers was five-year-old Everett "Ev" M. Rogers (Singhal, 2005). Although Ev's father loved new farm machines, he was reluctant to tinker with biology. In 1936, Mr. Rogers's corn field suffered from a terrible drought while the drought-resistant hybrid corn in a neighboring field stood tall. Mr. Rogers started using the hybrid corn seed and Everett Rogers grew up, went to college, and became the world's leading expert on diffusion of innovations!

Rogers (2003) divided adopters into five categories: innovators, early adopters, early majority, late majority, and laggards. Innovators account for approximately 2.5 percent of the overall population. As the first group to try a new product or idea, these are the people standing in line overnight when the latest technology is due to be released for sale. Innovators get their information from multiple sources. They know about new technology before it comes on the market. Innovators have disposable income that allows them to take risks. The next group, early adopters, account for 13.5 percent of the population. Early adopters tend to be popular social leaders. They also have disposable income that allows for risks. However, they are slightly more cautious than innovators because they want to maintain credibility and social prestige. Early majority adopters compose 34 percent of the population.

This group makes careful, deliberate decisions but only after consulting with their wide social network. On the downward slope of the curve are the late majority adopters. Composing another 34 percent of the population, late majority adopters value traditional methods or technology. They tend to be skeptical of new products and believe they have less disposable income. Everett Rogers's father would be a late majority adopter with respect to the hybrid corn. The last group, laggards, make up the remaining 16 percent of the population. Laggards get the majority of their information from neighbors and friends, have no desire to influence others to try a new product, and believe that they have less disposable income. Not every idea or product reaches full dissemination. In some cases, failed diffusion occurs. Inherent weaknesses in the product, competition with alternative products, or lack of awareness of the new technology or idea can prevent the innovation from reaching critical mass saturation.

Diffusion of innovations theory is helpful to understand how and why people embrace medical breakthroughs, such as robotic limbs, new vaccines, gene therapy, wearable health sensors, or disease screening tests. Public health practitioners can use the model to help reduce reluctance to novel health-enhancing behaviors. For example, more public health groups are using social media to encourage evacuation during hurricanes, healthy eating, exercise, or screening for breast cancer. On the other end of the spectrum, the theory also shows how social networking and marketing can influence unhealthy choices. Human beings are social creatures who may forgo values or adopt outrageous behaviors in order to feel accepted by others. This means that social networking is an easy venue for unscrupulous marketers. For example, in 1969, the tobacco companies intentionally misled people into disbelieving that smoking is harmful to health. The industry purposely disseminated misinformation in order to sell cigarettes. Cases such as this highlight the lack of control on marketing and how easy it is to plant misinformation. Public health organizations and professionals must remain vigilant for new products, ideas, and trends designed to mislead people into buying and using harmful products. In an effort to stay ahead of trends and educate people, the Centers for Disease Control and Prevention, Substance Abuse and Mental Health Services Administration, National Institute on Drug Abuse, National Cancer Institute, and many nonprofit organizations offer free online fact sheets to provide accurate information and dispel myths, hoaxes, and marketing shams.

Diffusion of innovations theory is a framework used to describe how people adopt novel technology and ideas. The model applies to a wide range of circumstances and can be used by public health practitioners to disseminate health-enhancing ideas and products. A limitation of the model is that not all ideas and products are worthy of adoption. Public health practitioners must work to dispel misinformation and encourage products, practices, and beliefs that improve quality and length of life for all people.

Sally Kuykendall

See also: Epidemic; Epidemiology; Fluoridation; Health Communication; Health Education; Oral Health

Further Reading

Glanz, K., Lewis, F. M., & Rimer, B. K. (Eds). (1997). *Health behavior and health education: Theory, research, and practice* (2nd ed.). San Francisco: Jossey-Bass.

Kaminski, J. (2011). Diffusion of innovation theory. *Canadian Journal of Nursing Informatics,* 6(2). Theory in nursing informatics column. Retrieved from http://cjni.net/journal/?p=1444.

National Cancer Institute. (2005). *Theory at a glance: A guide for health promotion practice* (2nd ed.). NIH Publication Number 05-3896.

Rogers, E. (2003). *Diffusion of innovations* (5th ed.). New York: Free Press.

Ryan, B., & Gross, N. C. (1943). The diffusion of hybrid seed corn in two Iowa communities. *Rural Sociology*, *8*(1), 15–24.

Singhal, A. (2005). Forum: The life and work of Everett Rogers—Some personal reflections. *Journal of Health Communication*, *10*(4), 285–288. doi:10.1080/10810730590949978

DISABILITY

The term "disability" encompasses many different physical, mental, emotional, and social impairments or limitations. The Centers for Disease Control and Prevention ([CDC], 2017) define disability as "any condition of body or mind (impairment) that makes it difficult for the person with the condition to do certain activities (activity limitation) and interact with the world around them (participation restrictions)." There are many different types of disabilities. The most common involve hearing, vision, cognition, communication, and social, emotional, or physical function. Despite differences, people with disabilities (PWD) are related by common social experiences, risk factors, and health challenges. PWD experience numerous obstacles when accessing health, education, job, and community services. As a result, PWD have significantly lower educational achievement, socioeconomic status, quality of life, and health. Some public health experts purport that *dis*-ability is a socially constructed condition rather than a medical condition. If society adequately considered the needs of PWD when designing the built environment and social systems, disabilities would not exist. Nationally, an estimated 37 to 57 million people live with a disability (CDC, 2017). The World Health Organization (WHO) and World Bank *World Report on Disability* (2011) presents a global picture of the problem and offers recommendations for policy makers, health care, education, and employment professionals.

The onset of a disability may occur suddenly, intermittently, or progressively. Causes include genetic disorders (sickle cell disease), chromosomal disorders (Down syndrome), in utero exposure to drugs, alcohol, or infections (fetal alcohol syndrome), developmental disorders (autism spectrum disorder), injury (spinal cord injury), or chronic or acute diseases (complications of diabetes). The National Health Interview Survey compares health behaviors and outcomes of PWD and people without disabilities. PWD have higher rates of smoking, substance abuse, and depression. For example, among adults, 25 percent with disabilities smoke cigarettes and 17 percent without disabilities smoke cigarettes (CDC, 2017). PWD face multiple obstacles in maintaining healthy weight. Such obstacles include pain, fatigue, activity limitations, and difficulty chewing or swallowing, side effects of prescription medication leading to weight gain, limited access to healthy food choices, or limited access to recreational areas. As a result, adults with disabilities have three times higher risk of heart disease, stroke, diabetes, or cancer in comparison to adults without disabilities (CDC, 2017). Hypertension is also more common among PWD (34 percent) in comparison to people without disabilities (27 percent) (CDC, 2017). To aggravate the problem, PWD are often reluctant to seek medical treatment and preventive services. Negative attitudes by health care providers, lack of services, difficulty accessing and navigating services, or policies and systems that fail to respect the individual delay or obstruct needed care. The problem is likely to get worse. The WHO reports that disabilities are increasing at a faster rate than previously estimated due to the aging population and the increase in chronic health problems. Women, the elderly, and people living in poverty carry a disproportionate share of the burden of disability.

Social scientists purport that disability is not a medical condition. Ability or inability is defined by society where people who can access buildings and communities are considered able-bodied and people who cannot access are considered disabled. If shops, schools, factories, public transportation, sidewalks, buildings, and household items were designed and constructed to accommodate PWD, barriers would no longer exist, and everyone would be *abled*. The WHO (2017) defines three levels of disability: impairment, limitation in activity, and restriction in participation. *Impairment* refers to defects or injuries to body structure or function, including mental faculties. *Activity limitation* refers to difficulty in independently performing personal activities of daily living. *Participation restriction* refers to limitations on engagement in social, recreational, or occupational activities. These levels provide a common language to assess needs and identify appropriate accommodations. In general, the WHO and the World Bank recommend the following practices and policies to reduce health disparities and improve quality of life for PWD:

1. Adopt a national plan that maximizes and coordinates services for PWD.
2. Include PWD in planning policies and services.
3. Use mainstreaming to provide equal access to quality educational, health, employment, and social services.
4. Provide adequate funding for public services.
5. Offer rehabilitation services and vocational training that promote independence.
6. Train engineers, architects, and designers to integrate the needs of PWD in the design, development, and construction stages of projects.
7. Deconstruct public myths and misconceptions that stigmatize PWD.
8. Support further epidemiological research on the impact of disabilities.
9. Identify ways to reduce social barriers. (WHO and World Bank, 2011)

Some of the recommendations do not require additional resources and will greatly improve communities by increasing diversity, social justice, and human resources. The introduction to the WHO–World Bank report is written by world-renowned physicist Dr. Stephen Hawking. At the age of 21, Hawking was diagnosed with amyotrophic lateral sclerosis (ALS), also known as Lou Gehrig's disease. ALS affects the motor neurons, resulting in muscle paralysis and difficulty speaking, swallowing, and breathing. There is no known cure. Completely paralyzed, Hawking notes his good fortune in that he benefits from the best medical care in the world, personal care assistants, and advanced assistive technology. Yet, not everyone is as fortunate. Hawking advocates on behalf of the less fortunate,

> In fact we have a moral duty to remove barriers to participation, and to invest sufficient funding and expertise to unlock the vast potential of people with disabilities. Governments throughout the world can no longer overlook the hundreds of millions of people with disabilities who are denied access to health, rehabilitation, support, education, and employment, and never get the chance to shine. (WHO and World Bank, 2011, p. 3)

History provides numerous examples of people who, with appropriate support, overcame physical and mental challenges to achieve incredible accomplishments.

In *The Future of Public's Health,* the Institute of Medicine (2003, pp. 179–180) notes, "When people are healthy, they are better able to work, learn, build a good life, and contribute to society." PWD have much to contribute to society and want to be a part of society. However, systemic, structural, and social barriers must be removed so that PWD can become fully functioning in society.

Sally Kuykendall

See also: Americans with Disabilities Act; Behavioral Health; Birth Defects; Disability Movement; Greco-Roman Era, Public Health in the; Health; Health Disparities; National Center for Injury Prevention and Control; National Institutes of Health; Obesity; Prevention; Roosevelt, Franklin Delano; Social Determinants of Health; Social Security Act; Spiritual Health

Further Reading

Centers for Disease Control and Prevention. (2017). *Disability and health.* Retrieved from https://www.cdc.gov/ncbddd/disabilityandhealth/index.html.

Institute of Medicine. (2003). *The future of the public's health in the 21st century.* Washington, DC: National Academies Press.

World Health Organization. (2017). *Disability and rehabilitation.* Retrieved from http://www.who.int/disabilities/en/.

World Health Organization and World Bank. (2011). *World report on disability.* Switzerland: World Health Organization. Retrieved from http://www.who.int/disabilities/world_report/2011/en/.

DISABILITY MOVEMENT

Over 53 million people in the United States, one in five adults, have at least one form of disability (Prevalence, 2015). Aside from the primary health issue, people living with disabilities have poorer overall health than those without disabilities. In the past, people with disabilities were segregated in special schools or residential facilities. More recently, attitudes have shifted toward an inclusionary model. This perspective is referred to as the social model of disability. Accessibility policies now target environmental and societal factors that hinder access and equality, rather than purely medical or physical barriers (World Health Organization, 2011). The disability movement is a global movement to secure equal rights and opportunities for people with disabilities. The modern disability movement centers on improving accessibility and equality and therefore enhancing opportunities for and the public health of people living with disabilities.

Ed Roberts (1939–1995) is considered the father of the independent living movement, the start of the disability movement. Roberts was a healthy, young man who enjoyed baseball until he was stricken by polio at age 14. The infection left him completely paralyzed except for two fingers and a few toes. Dependent on his iron lung ventilator, Roberts attended school via telephone. When he grew strong enough to come off the ventilator for a few hours, his mother insisted that he attend school for one day a week. Roberts was embarrassed and worried about the transition. He quickly realized that the other students did not judge him and were simply curious to meet the classmate whom they had talked with but had never seen. Roberts embraced the attention. When it came time to graduate, a school administrator tried to deny his diploma on the grounds that Roberts did not complete the required physical education courses. Mrs. Roberts, a union activist, stepped in to advocate for her son. When she was rebuffed, she contacted the media who pressured the school to count physical therapy as the physical education requirement. After graduation, Roberts decided to attend community college. He should have been eligible for a grant from the California Department of Rehabilitation. The department refused him on the grounds that Roberts would never be able to hold a job. Again, Roberts used the power of the press and the Department of Rehabilitation reconsidered their decision.

After community college, Roberts transferred to University of California at Berkeley. He lived in the student infirmary because it was the only habitable structure that could hold his iron lung. As the news spread of a wheelchair-bound student at Berkeley, other quadriplegic students applied, were accepted, and moved into the makeshift dormitory. The "rolling quads" enjoyed college life with the exception that their fragile wheelchairs kept breaking down. They started improvising their wheelchairs so that they could explore the city. When community members with disabilities saw the more durable wheelchairs, they also wanted them. Able-bodied friends and family members and disabled people from the community joined the group and the Center for Independent Living was formed. Roberts eventually became the director of the California Department of Rehabilitation, the same organization that told him that he would never be able to hold a job. Roberts was instrumental in starting the disability movement and advocating for equal access and opportunities for people with disabilities in the United States.

In 1990, Congress, under advisement from the organization now known as the National Council on Disability, passed the Americans with Disabilities Act (ADA), which protects people with disabilities against discrimination in public services and accommodations, as well as employment. The ADA affords similar protections to the Civil Rights Act of 1964, with the notable exception that the ADA requires employers to make reasonable accommodations for employees with disabilities. The bill was signed into law by President George H. W. Bush on July 26, 1990 (Equal Employment Opportunity Commission, n.d.). Although critics of the ADA claim that it has negatively impacted the employment rate for people with disabilities, citing the expenses for businesses hiring people with disabilities, no link has been found (Picker, n.d.).

The modern social model of disability focuses on the barriers to accessibility created by society. This model puts the responsibility of social change on society, rather than the individual. Changes this model puts forward include altering society's attitude toward people with disabilities, Affirmative Action, and accessible physical infrastructure. This model also posits that attempts to "fix" individuals with disabilities are, in fact, discriminatory. The benefits of the social model include broad improvements to infrastructure and social norms that all people benefit from. Some of the more notable improvements include widespread installation of automatic doors, curb cuts, and the movement to change the terms and words that are used to describe people with disabilities.

Experts in the field argue that disability is constructed by society. If architects, builders, city planners, and other policy makers considered people who have physical, visual, hearing, or cognitive impairment when planning and building workplaces, schools, recreational areas, and public spaces, there would be no disability. The World Health Organization (WHO) identifies three major societal barriers created by ableism, discrimination against people with disabilities. The first is the most visible: environmental barriers. These can vary based on the community. In general, barriers that limit inclusion create disability. Such barriers can be natural or artificial and include places inaccessible to those with physical disabilities (lacking wheelchair access) or intellectual/sensory disabilities (lacking appropriate signage). The next set of barriers are attitudinal, or barriers created by people who are incapable of seeing people with disabilities as anything other than the disability. Attitudinal barriers contribute to all others and lead to discrimination, bullying, and segregation. In some cultures, disabilities are seen as a form of divine punishment. Frequently, for children with disabilities, the fear of bullying is as real an issue as the bullying itself. The final set of barriers is institutional barriers, which include laws and practices that actively discriminate against people with disabilities. Although the ADA has proven to be a positive force in American politics, there are still issues to be addressed in American government with regard to accessibility (World Health Organization, 2011).

Public health advocates for people with disabilities by recognizing societal obstacles and working to educate and eliminate obstacles. The *2005 Surgeon General's Call to Action to Improve the Health and Wellness of Persons with Disabilities* recommends supporting people with disabilities by recognizing and considering the whole person, not just the disability; speaking directly with the person with the disability, rather than a family member of third party; speaking in age appropriate language (do not speak to disabled adults as if they are children); offer assistance but do not assume help is required; allow additional time for the person with the disability to speak or act; recognize what the person can do, not what he or she cannot do; and recognize the obstacles to work, education, health care, and social activities can be more frustrating than the actual disability. Anyone can have a disability. It is up to others in society to ensure that physical or cognitive restrictions do not exclude people from enjoying a happy, healthy, full life.

Mark Black and Sally Kuykendall

See also: Americans with Disabilities Act; Attention-Deficit/Hyperactivity Disorder; Birth Defects; Health Disparities; Roosevelt, Franklin Delano; Social Determinants of Health

Further Reading

Equal Employment Opportunity Commission. (n.d.). *The Americans with Disabilities Act of 1990.* Retrieved from https://www.eeoc.gov/eeoc/history/35th/1990s/ada.html.

Majer, I. M., Nusselder, W. J., Mackenbach, J. P., Klijs, B., & van Baal, P. H. (2011). Mortality risk associated with disability: A population-based record linkage study. *American Journal of Public Health, 101*(12), e9. doi:10.2105/AJPH.2011.300361

Picker, L. (n.d.). *Did the ADA reduce employment of the disabled?* The National Bureau of Economic Research. Retrieved from http://www.nber.org/digest/nov04/w10528.html.

Prevalence of Disability and Disability Type among Adults—United States, 2013. (Cover story). (2015). *Morbidity and Mortality Weekly Report*, 64(29), 777–783.

U.S. Code Title 42, Chapter 126. *Equal opportunity for individuals with disabilities.* Legal Information Institute: Cornell Law School. Retrieved from https://www.law.cornell.edu/uscode/text/42/chapter-126.

U.S. Department of Health and Human Services. (2005). *The 2005 surgeon general's call to action to improve the health and wellness of persons with disabilities: Calling you to action.* U.S. Department of Health and Human Services, Office of the Surgeon General. Retrieved from https://www.cdc.gov/ncbddd/disabilityandhealth/pdf/whatitmeanstoyou508.pdf.

World Health Organization. (2011). *World report on disability.* Geneva: Author. Retrieved from http://www.who.int/disabilities/world_report/2011/report.pdf.

DISEASE

Diseases are pathological conditions characterized by abnormal structure or function in the human body. Major diseases include cardiovascular disease (CVD), a group of conditions resulting from structural damage to the heart or circulatory system; chronic obstructive pulmonary disease (COPD), a disease that affects the bronchi and alveoli impairing the body's ability to oxygenate body tissues; and infectious diseases, conditions resulting from pathogenic organisms. The word *disease* blends the Latin prefix *dis-*, which means "opposite" or "reverse of" with the Anglo-Norman word *ese* (*ease*), meaning "freedom from pain" or "freedom from concern." Based on the root words, *dis-ease* means "the opposite of pain-free or anxiety-free." A logical conclusion would suppose that disease is the opposite of the World Health Organization (WHO, 1946) definition of health, "a state of complete physical, mental and social well-being and not merely the absence of disease or infirmity." Defining disease as the opposite of health means that anything that interferes with biological, emotional, social, or spiritual well-being would and should be classified as disease. Under this definition, anger, greed, bullying, and racism would be considered diseases. Scholars point out that the working definition of disease is context-dependent and changes over time (Scully, 2004). It is important to have a clear definition so that people experiencing health problems are able to access treatment and so that health and medical professionals do not diagnose, medicate, or treat people for behaviors that are not pathological.

Distinguishing between health and disease is a challenge because there is so much that we do not know about the human body. Medical practice is highly dependent on technology and science. For example, the invention of magnetic resonance imaging (MRI) allowed scientists to visualize human brain development and structure in ways that were not possible previously. The ability to scan the living brain refutes the idea that addiction is caused by moral turpitude. We now know that addiction is a dysfunction of neurotransmitters, and adolescents are at higher risk due to unique brain structure and development (National Institute on Drug Abuse, 2015). Even when medicine does possess the technology to examine and define illnesses, society may not recognize or understand a pathological condition as such. Osteoporosis, a weakening of the bone tissue, was once thought to be a normal part of aging. In 1994, the WHO officially recognized osteoporosis as a disease. Classification as a disease means that community agencies offering osteoporosis prevention programs can request grant or government funding, and health insurers will cover access to diagnostic tests and treatment.

The classification of an entity as a disease state is also determined by social values. Homosexuality is an example of how a behavior was at first considered natural, became classified as a disease, and then became depathologized. The art and literature of ancient civilizations suggest that same-gender sexual preferences existed across cultures throughout recorded history. Indigenous North Americans revered the healers, artists, and leaders who exhibited both male and female qualities. "Two-spirits" were viewed as a third or fourth gender rather than a combination of male and female. In Plato's *Symposium* (385–370 BCE), the ancient Greek philosopher theorizes on the nature and purpose of love. This literary work provides insights into Greek life. Homosexuality is featured as an innate and natural sexual attraction. Early Christians were among the first to disapprove of men who had sex with men. Women who had sex with women were ignored. Early U.S. laws, originating in the Plymouth Colony, reflected Puritan values. The colonists feared punishment by God and implemented laws that they believed would placate an angry and vengeful God. Treason, murder, witchcraft, arson, sodomy, rape, bestiality, and adultery were punishable by death (Crompton, 1976). In 1886, the Austro-German psychiatrist Richard von Krafft-Ebing portrayed homosexuality as a mental disorder in his book *Psychopathia Sexualis*. Classifying homosexuality as a disease created the misbelief that homosexuality could be cured. Social misperceptions, hatred, and rejection of homosexuals were furthered under Hitler's fascism. By the 1950s, a series of major research studies investigating human sexuality found that same-sex attraction and practices were more common than people believed. In 1973, the American Psychiatric Association (APA) removed the listing of homosexuality as a psychiatric illness in the *Diagnostic and Statistical Manual of Mental Disorders* (*DSM*). Despite the fact that medical and psychiatric professionals no longer consider homosexuality as a disease, the idea that same-gender sexual preference is curable lingers. Such misperceptions ostracize and harm LGBTQ individuals. From an ethical perspective, it is important that diseases are correctly classified as diseases and minority characteristics are not misclassified as disease.

Physical and mental health diseases may be categorized as acute or chronic. Acute diseases are health problems in which symptoms come on suddenly, within hours or days, and the person recovers fairly quickly, usually within days to weeks. Examples of acute diseases are the common cold, food poisoning, sprains, strains, or traumatic injuries. Chronic diseases are persistent health conditions, lasting three months or more, which start discretely and progress to more serious problems over time. Examples of chronic diseases are CVD, high blood pressure, cancer, diabetes, asthma, or COPD. Both acute and chronic diseases are diagnosed through routine medical examinations, screenings, or when patients report symptoms to their health care providers. For example, the person with asthma may complain of shortness of breath or wheezing. Disease management is a coordinated and systematic approach of treating and controlling the disease. It is important that people suffering from asthma take medication as prescribed so that symptoms do not interfere with work, recreational activities, or sleep. Regularly cleaning of indoor living spaces to minimize dust, molds, and pet dander can prevent asthma attacks. In addition to early diagnosis and disease management, public health works to prevent disease. The Environmental Protection Agency provides guidelines on cleaning up after hurricanes and floods to prevent mold spores, and the Air Pollution and Respiratory Health Branch of the Centers for Disease Control combats environmentally related respiratory diseases through surveillance, dissemination of information on effective interventions, and by encouraging local collaborations to develop, implement, and evaluate asthma control programs.

Diseases are a medical classification that refers to a biological, social, or psychological condition, which creates malfunctioning of the human body. The classification of a condition as a disease raises policy and ethical questions, regarding social values, insurance reimbursement, and the ability of health care to diagnose and treat the condition. Is a condition truly a physical or psychological malfunction or merely a reflection of social norms and values? As science and technology advance, public health and medical professionals are challenged to determine whether a condition is actually a disease or is instead, an unfamiliar attribute. Society must also guard against the fabrication of diseases as for-profit health care groups or pharmaceutical companies encourage or manufacture new diagnoses in order to create a market for treatment.

Sally Kuykendall

See also: Acute Illnesses; Behavioral Health; Chronic Illness; Disability; Health; Heart Disease; Infectious Diseases; Intervention; Middle Ages, Public Health in the; Prevention; Public Health in the United States, History of; Spiritual Health; Waterborne Diseases

Further Reading

Centers for Disease Control and Prevention. (2016). *Asthma.* Retrieved from https://www.cdc.gov/asthma/.

Crompton, L. (1976). Homosexuals and the death penalty in colonial America. *Journal of Homosexuality, 1*(3), 277–293. Retrieved from http://citeseerx.ist.psu.edu/viewdoc/download?doi=10.1.1.648.7044&rep=rep1&type=pdf.

Morris, B. J. (n.d.). *History of lesbian, gay, & bisexual social movements.* Washington, DC: American Psychological Association. Retrieved from http://www.apa.org/pi/lgbt/resources/history.aspx.

National Institute on Drug Abuse. (2015). *Drugs and the brain.* Retrieved from https://www.drugabuse.gov/related-topics/drugs-brain.

Scully, J. L. (2004). What is disease? *EMBO Reports, 5*(7), 650–653.

World Health Organization. (1946). Preamble to the Constitution of the World Health Organization as adopted by the International Health Conference, New York; Official Records of the World Health Organization. Retrieved from http://apps.who.int/gb/bd/PDF/bd47/EN/constitution-en.pdf?ua=1.

World Health Organization. (1994). *Assessment of fracture risk and its application to screening for postmenopausal osteoporosis.* WHO Technical Report Series 843. Geneva: Author.

DIX, DOROTHEA LYNDE (1804–1887)

Dorothea Lynde Dix was a social reformer who observed and reported the living conditions of the mentally ill in order to create mental hospitals. "Dolly" Dix was born on April 4, 1802. Her father, Joseph, was the son of Dorothea and Elijah Dix. Elijah was a wealthy physician and merchant who donated his time to many community service projects in Worcester, Massachusetts. In 1795, Elijah moved his family to a community in Boston with other wealthy merchants. The neighbors made their fortunes by the triangular trade of shipping rum and slaves from the West Indies to America, exporting the rum to Africa in exchange for other slaves, and shipping the African slaves to the West Indies to work on sugar cane plantations.

Dorothea's father rebelled against his privileged upbringing. He dropped out of Harvard College, married a commoner, Mary Biglow, and worked as manager of several of his father's properties.

Named after her grandmother, Dorothea was a favorite grandchild. When Elijah died, he left enough money for Dorothea to support herself until she would be married. However, other heirs contested the will, and Dorothea ultimately inherited nothing. Joseph and Mary exchanged their inheritance for books, moved to a small frontier town in Vermont, and lived as religious zealots. Joseph sold religious books. Young Dorothea was responsible for collating the religious tracts and binding them into books. She was also the primary caregiver of her two younger brothers. She was miserable. At the age of 12, she ran away and found her way to her grandmother's mansion. The grandmother and granddaughter clashed. Dorothea did not measure up to Madame Dix's image of a high society young lady. She sent Dorothea to live with Sarah Fiske, a niece in Worcester.

The Fiske family offered culture and sophistication. Many young, educated women of the time opened schools on the family property and taught until they got married. Dorothea opened a school at the Fiske residence. She worked hard to dress and act the part of a young lady and schoolteacher. In 1824, she returned to her grandmother's house and opened another school. Her curriculum was haphazard. Dorothea had never had a formal education herself. She offered lessons in botany and moral development because those are the topics she was interested in. She also gathered information by reading or attending public lectures. Her independent study led to the publication of her first book, *Conversations on Common Things*. The book provided a small, steady income.

Despite her efforts, Dorothea did not fit in socially. While other young ladies were interested in getting married, Dorothea joined the Unitarian church and embraced the values of personal restraint and social activism. In 1826, Dorothea moved to a boardinghouse, proclaiming independence from her family. She worked as teacher, coedited the first children's magazine, and wrote religious meditations, poems, and children's stories. Her subsequent publications were not as successful, and her employment as a teacher was sporadic. She frequently suffered from bouts of illness during which time she stayed with friends.

In 1841, a Harvard Divinity student asked Ms. Dix to teach his Sunday school class at Middlesex County House of Correction in East Cambridge. The Industrial Revolution was pulling rural youth into the cities to work in factories. Isolated from family and friends, some developed mental illness and were destined to almshouses or jails where the mentally ill were easy victims for physical, verbal, sexual, and financial abuse. Dorothea was appalled by what she saw, frail men and women, unkempt and shivering in cold cells. She asked the jailer to light a fire in the stove, and he responded that lunatics did not feel the cold. With the help of two influential friends, Simon Gridley Howe and Charles Sumner, Dorothea went to the courts to ask for help, and the jailer agreed to improve the conditions in the cell. This experience prompted Dorothea to learn as much as she could about the mentally

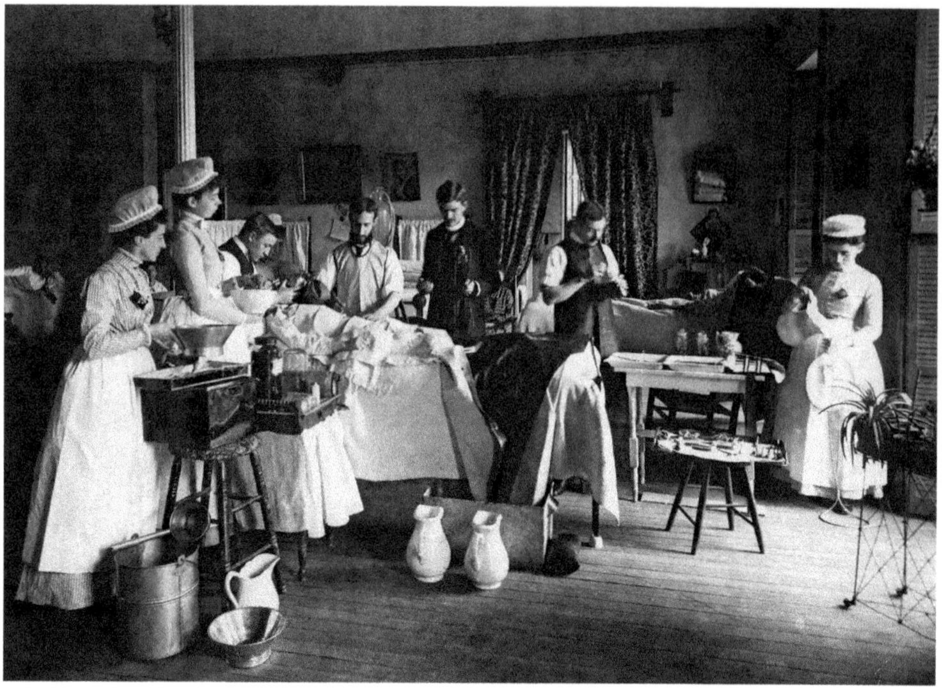

Doctors and nurses operate on a patient at Bellevue Hospital, ca. 1870. After founding specialized hospitals for mentally ill patients, Dorothea Dix studied best practices in care. Although the practices were barbaric by today's standards, philosophy of care shifted from punitive morality-based practices to biological treatments. (Bettmann/Getty Images)

ill. Little was known about mental illness, and treatment followed two streams of thought, *heroic* versus *moral*. Heroic treatment used emetics, laxatives, or narcotics to remove the evil spirits. Moral treatment used a controlled environment with scheduled activities, a nutritious diet, and restricted visiting hours. Moral treatment was consistent with Dorothea's Unitarian values. Howe, Sumner, and Horace Mann encouraged Dorothea to investigate further.

Dorothea visited every jail and almshouse in Massachusetts, recording the number of detainees, their physical, mental, and spiritual status, and naming the institution and managing official. The findings were compiled into the *Memorial to the Legislature of Massachusetts*. Howe presented the report to the Massachusetts legislature. In comparison to other areas of the country, Massachusetts had better conditions. However, Dix's descriptions were moving, "The present state of insane persons confined within this Commonwealth, in *cages, closets, cellars, stalls, pens! Chained, naked, beaten with rods,* and *lashed* into obedience!" (Dix, 1843, p. 2). According to the social norms of the day, it would have been very unladylike to visit or describe such deplorable conditions. Dix used her femininity to her advantage by claiming that female empathy forced her to use plain words, clear descriptions, and to advocate for improved conditions. She implored politicians to:

> Become the benefactors of your race, the guardians of the solemn rights you hold in trust. Raise up the fallen, succor the desolate, restore the outcast, defend the helpless, and for your eternal and great reward receive the benediction. 'Well done, good and faithful servants, become rulers over many things.' (Dix, 1843, p. 25)

Thus, Dorothea played on the men's sense of power and righteousness. The report enraged the public. Opponents wanted this woman to mind her own business. Some officials claimed she was lying. Supporters defended her by noting that since women could not run for political office, Dorothea had nothing to gain from lying. Howe, Sumner, and Mann defended Dix and convinced the legislature to increase the number of beds for the mentally ill.

Dix set off traveling across New England and Eastern Canada, documenting the conditions of prisons and almshouses and calling on state legislators to provide beds for the mentally ill. In the fall of 1843, she went to New York. The New York State Lunatic Asylum of Utica had just opened with enough beds for 225 patients. The problem was that the 1840 census had registered 2,300 mentally ill persons, and the hospital would only accommodate treatable cases. Dorothea argued for the intractable cases because mental illness is a consequence of social policies and should be addressed through social policy. Dr. Amariah Brigham, the medical superintendent of the New York hospital, opposed Dix on the argument that patients with intractable mental illness were unmanageable and would ruin the system. Dorothea headed to Pennsylvania and New Jersey. This time she met with the superintendents of mental hospitals and asked for their support. Her reports evolved. She praised modern medicine, advocated for early treatment, and cautiously suggested public policy. Dix was moving away from her focus on moral care to a medical model.

By August 1845, Dix had visited 500 almshouses, 300 jails, and several hospitals. She grew distant from friends. As a famous lobbyist and social reformer, she spent more time with politicians and wealthy patrons and less time with the mentally ill patients, whom she had so strongly advocated for. In the summer of 1845, she turned her focus to prison inmates. Prison reformers were debating keeping prisoners separated or together. In 1845, Dix published *Remarks on Prisons and Prison Discipline in the United States*. The document used the same ethnographic and epidemiological techniques, which Dix had used in previous efforts. To determine best practices in prison management, Dix interviewed prison wardens and collected data on corporal punishment. She noted:

> While we diminish the stimulant of *fear*, we must increase to prisoners the incitement of *hope*: . . . we should awaken and strengthen the *control* of the *conscience*. . . . Man is not made better by being degraded; he is seldom restrained from crime by harsh measures, except the principle of fear predominates in his character; and then he is never made radically better for its influence. (Dix, 1845, p. 25)

Dix proposed that prison guards could serve as models for prisoners, providing moral guidance. By this time, Dix had helped to establish 32 state mental institutions across the United States. After unsuccessfully trying to convince Congress to grant federal land for mental institutions, Dix traveled to Europe. She continued her crusade of educating policy makers and advocating for mental institutions until 1856 when she returned to the states.

The mental hospitals that Dix had established were becoming overcrowded. Medical superintendents were resorting to the same harsh strategies that Dix had opposed. She blamed the overcrowding on the influx of Irish immigrants escaping the Irish Potato Famine. Reflecting the bigotry of the time, Dix believed that the Irish were morally inferior and uneducable. To add to the dysfunction, the Civil War was breaking out. Hoping to work on social reforms in the North and the South, Dix stayed silent on the issue of slavery. This allowed her to travel throughout the Southern states advocating for mental institutions.

Once the Civil War started, Dix volunteered to recruit nurses to care for the Union soldiers. She wanted to replicate Florence Nightingale's efforts in the United States, and she believed her experience establishing mental hospitals provided the necessary qualifications. On June 10, 1861, Dix was commissioned as the Superintendent of Women War Nurses by Secretary of War Simon Cameron, making her the first female to earn a federal appointment. The idea of females as nurses and Dix's moral stance clashed with the military doctors. The doctors preferred untrained male assistants. Dix insisted that the doctors abstain from alcohol and that nurses dress modestly. Jewelry or other frills were banned. Any applicant under the age of 30 or who appeared to be looking for a husband was rejected. Dix was a one-person show. She did not take a salary and used her own money to buy gowns and supplies. Unfortunately, she was not trained to deal with infections, the leading cause of death in Civil War hospitals. The final straw came with the battle of Wilson's Creek, Missouri. One thousand injured men were transported 110 miles to the nearest military hospital. Moving at her own pace, Dix had not set up the hospital. Without beds or nurses, the local residents stepped in. When Dix arrived, she neglected to notify the Sanitary Commission. The Sanitary Commission was furious and Secretary of War Edwin Stanton restricted Dix's authority.

As the war escalated, both armies struggled to care for prisoners of war. In Elmira, New York, officials estimated that 8,000 Confederate prisoners would die within a year. Hoping to force the South to exchange prisoners, officials asked Dix to inspect the prison and record conditions. To their disappointment, Dix stayed faithful to her Northern allegiance and reported that the Confederate soldiers were receiving adequate care. When the war ended, Dix resigned. Despite the problems, Dix is recognized for advancing opportunities for women in nursing. Because of the power struggles during the Civil War, Dix lost her political influence, and questions were being raised about mental hospitals. Elizabeth Parsons Ware Packard (1816–1897) spent three years falsely imprisoned at the Jasonville Insane Asylum in Illinois for publicly disagreeing with her husband. She published several books on her experiences and advocated for the rights of mentally ill patients and women. Packard's case revealed weaknesses in Dix's ideas.

In 1870, Dix was diagnosed with malaria. She spent three years recuperating, staying at her favorite mental institution in New Jersey. In 1881, she moved into an apartment at the state mental hospital in Trenton and gradually grew weaker. Dorothea Lynde Dix died in her sleep on July 18, 1887.

The techniques Dorothea Dix used are now known as ethnography or shoe leather epidemiology. By investigating, reporting, and disseminating the living conditions of the mentally ill, Dix was able to confront the stigma of mental illness and founded 32 mental institutions, 15 schools, and numerous training facilities.

Sally Kuykendall

See also: Beers, Clifford Whittingham; Blackwell, Elizabeth; Mental Health; Mental Illness; *Controversies in Public Health:* Controversy 2

Further Reading

Dix, D. L. (1843). *Memorial to the Legislature of Massachusetts.* U.S. National Library of Medicine. Retrieved from https://collections.nlm.nih.gov/catalog/nlm:nlmuid-7703963-bk.

Dix, D. L. (1845). *Remarks on prisons and prison discipline in the United States.* Philadelphia: Joseph Kite. Retrieved from https://collections.nlm.nih.gov/bookviewer?PID=nlm:nlmuid-60540680R-bk.

Morin, I. V. (1995). 1: Dorothea Dix Superintendent of Army Nurses. *Women Chosen for Public Office*, 10–23.

Muckenhoupt, M. (2003). *Dorothea Dix: Advocate for mental health care.* New York: Oxford University Press.

DREW, CHARLES RICHARD (1904–1950)

Charles Richard Drew was an African American surgeon and physiologist who developed techniques of preserving blood products for life-saving transfusions. "Charlie" was born on June 3, 1904, in Washington, DC, the eldest of five children of Nora Rosella Burrell and Richard Thomas Drew. Richard worked as a carpet layer and was the financial officer of the predominantly white local trade union. Nora was a graduate of Miner Normal School, a teacher training school for young women of color. Nora was remembered as a graceful woman of great faith and culture. Charlie loved sports. Swimming in the harbor at Foggy Bottom and at the 12th Street YMCA, he won his first athletic award. As a teenager, he attended Paul Lawrence Dunbar High School, a segregated school for academically gifted minority youth. In high school, Charles ran track and played football, basketball, and baseball. He earned the James E. Walker Memorial Trophy for best all-around athlete in his junior and senior years and at graduation was recognized as the most popular student and the student who accomplished the most for Dunbar High School. By adolescence, Charles had successfully embodied his mother's graciousness and his father's ability to organize and lead.

Charles was awarded a partial college scholarship to Amherst College in Massachusetts. To cover his expenses, he worked, ran track, and played football. Despite winning the football team's most valuable player in his junior year, Drew was passed over to become football captain for a white player. His time in football was marred by racial prejudice. Opposing players frequently hurled racial slurs at him, and restaurants denied him service. He stayed silent, did not fight back, but instead turned a deep shade of red, earning the nickname "Big Red." Drew graduated in 1926 with a bachelor of arts degree and was recognized with the Howard Hill Mossman Trophy, awarded to the person who brought the most to Amherst athletics.

An injury from college football, the death of his younger sister, Elsie from tuberculosis complicated by influenza, and encouragement from his biology professor influenced Charles to go into medicine. To save money for medical school, Charles worked for two years at Morgan State University in Baltimore as a biology instructor and athletic director. Howard University Medical School, his dream college, rejected him because he did not have enough English credits. Harvard University Medical School offered a deferred admission to start the following year. McGill University offered unconditional acceptance, and Charles flourished in Montréal. He won many athletic and academic awards and was admitted to the Alpha Omega Alpha honor society. After graduating with honors, he completed his internship and residency. Working with Dr. John Beattie at Montréal General Hospital, Drew started studying the use of fluids and blood products as a treatment for shock.

Drew wanted to continue his surgical training at a major medical institution in the United States. However, large medical institutions rarely accepted African American residents because white patients refused treatment by people of color. In 1935, he accepted a position as instructor of pathology at Howard University and soon earned promotion to assistant instructor in surgery/assistant surgeon at Freedman's Hospital. To advance further in academia, Drew needed an academic doctoral degree as opposed to a clinical doctoral degree. In 1938, Drew commenced graduate studies at Columbia University. He also worked as surgical resident at Presbyterian Hospital. The combination of graduate student and surgical resident afforded Drew the opportunity to work with Dr. John Scudder studying the fluid and electrolyte balance of surgical patients. For his doctoral dissertation, Drew studied blood storage. At the time, blood donations were stored as whole blood. Since red blood cells undergo hemolysis within two days, whole blood has a short shelf life. To extend shelf life, Drew separated the plasma and red blood cells. Separately, each product could be stored up to one week. Furthermore, plasma is a protein-electrolyte solution, which means there is no need for cross-matching blood type. The plasma could be used to treat critically ill patients who were difficult to cross-match.

In 1939, Drew traveled to Atlanta for a conference. On his way, he attended a dinner party where he met Minnie Lenore Robbins, a teacher at Spelman College. Not one to waste time, Drew continued to the conference and stopped at Spelman on his return trip. Arriving after midnight, he awoke the dormitory matron, insisted that the matron ask Ms. Robbins to meet him outside, where he proposed on the spot. The couple married six months later. Knowing that her husband worked long hours, Lenore took a job as laboratory assistant at Columbia University. The following year, Dr. Drew became the first African American to receive a doctor of medical science degree from Columbia University.

The late 1930s were marred by ethnocentricity, hyper-nationality, and oppression of minority populations. Worldwide economic depression forced people to move across the globe in search of job opportunities and survival. Anti-Asian sentiment was growing across North America. Anti-Semitism was taking hold in Germany. In the Soviet Union, Stalin organized the deportation, exile, or genocide of Volga Germans, Soviet Koreans, Crimean Tatars, Chechens, Poles, Meskhetians, Ukrainians, and Russian Jews. Racism was a key factor in World War II (1939–1945). Each ethnic group believed that they were superior to others. In America, white superiority was part of everyday life. Medical ideology supporting racial oppression originated from 1907 when scientists hypothesized that people of color were closer to primitive man and apes than white people. African Americans were seen as inferior. As a surgical resident at Columbia, Drew witnessed persistent racism in patient care. And despite working long hours to develop superior medical and surgical skills, Dr. Drew was denied acceptance into the American Medical Association and the American College of Surgeons.

In June 1940, Drew returned to Howard University School of Medicine as assistant professor of surgery. By September, he was asked to assist with the Blood for Britain program. World War II was raging in Europe. Germany routinely flew bombing raids over England's cities creating a severe blood shortage. Drew's expertise was needed to organize the Blood for Britain program. Through the Blood Transfusion Betterment Association, Drew refined techniques to preserve plasma and suggested the use of bloodmobiles, refrigerated vans to transport blood. In February 1941, he was named the first director of the American Red Cross Blood Bank and organized a blood drive of more than 100,000 donors. Yet, Drew found himself frustrated by blood procurement and transfusion methods mandated by the U.S. Army and Navy. The military insisted that the Red Cross segregate blood by race. Per transfusion protocol, Caucasian blood recipients could only receive blood from white donors. The idea had no scientific merit and falsely promoted the idea that whites were superior to people of color. Drew denounced the policy, resigned from the project, and returned to Howard University where he was appointed full professor and chair of surgery and chief surgeon at Freedman's Hospital.

In 1941, the American Board of Surgery acknowledged Drew with the appointment of surgical examiner. Three years later, Drew was awarded the prestigious Spingarn Medal from the National Association for the Advancement of Colored People (NAACP). He was a model of professionalism, perseverance, and graciousness. Drew's philosophy toward racism is best described in a letter to Mrs. J. F. Bates (January 27, 1947), a Fort Worth, Texas, schoolteacher:

> So much of our energy is spent in overcoming the constricting environment in which we live that little energy is left for creating new ideas or things. Whenever, however, one breaks out of this rather high-walled prison of the "Negro problem" by virtue of some worthwhile contribution, not only is he himself allowed more freedom, but part of the wall crumbles. And so it should be the aim of every student in science to knock down at least one or two bricks of that wall by virtue of his own accomplishment. (U.S. National Library of Medicine, n.d.)

Through science, knowledge, and creativity, Charles R. Drew knocked more than a few bricks out of the wall.

On April 1, 1950, Dr. Drew was driving with three other surgeons to a conference at Tuskegee Institute. Exhausted after performing lengthy surgery the day before, he fell asleep at the wheel. The car veered off the road. Drew was ejected from the car and suffered a spinal cord injury and traumatic brain injury. Surgeons at the hospital recognized the famous colleague and worked diligently to save his life. Unfortunately, the injuries were too serious and at the age of 45, Dr. Charles Richard Drew passed away. After his death, the American College of Surgeons elected him as a fellow. The Charles R. Drew University of Medicine and Science in Los Angeles is named in his honor.

Dr. Charles Richard Drew was an African American surgeon who overcame enormous prejudice and discrimination to advance the use of blood products as a way to treat victims of traumatic injury and blood dyscrasia. Dr. Drew offered his secret to success as, "Excellence in performance will transcend artificial barriers created by man" (Dedication: Charles Richard Drew, 2006). Sadly, the world will never know what successes may have been realized if the barriers had never existed in the first place.

Sally Kuykendall

See also: Health Care Disparities; Health Disparities; Infectious Diseases; Social Determinants of Health

Further Reading

[Dedication: Charles Richard Drew]. (2006). *Journal of Blacks in Higher Education,* (52), 1. Retrieved from http://www.jstor.org/stable/25073456.

Drew, C. R. (1942). *Dr. C.R. Drew wins 29th Springarn medal.* New York: NAACP Press Service, 28, March 1944, 1–3.

Drew, L. R. (1978). Unforgettable Charlie Drew. *Reader's Digest, 112,* 135–140.

Ford, J. R., & Drew, C. R. (1950). Appendicitis in the American Negro. *American Journal of Surgery*, *80*(3), 341–344.

Gordon, R. C. (2005). Charles R. Drew: Surgeon, scientist, and educator. *Journal of Investigative Surgery*, *18*(5), 223–225. doi:10.1080/08941930500350601

Pearson, P. A. (2001). Charles R. Drew. *Black heroes* (pp. 192–196). Ipswich, MA: History Reference Center.

U.S. National Library of Medicine. (n.d.). *The Charles R. Drew papers.* Profiles in science. Bethesda, MD: National Institute of Health. Retrieved from https://profiles.nlm.nih.gov/ps/retrieve/Narrative/BG/p-nid/336.

Wynes, C. E. (1988). *Charles Richard Drew: The man and the myth.* Urbana: University of Illinois Press.

DRITZ, SELMA KADERMAN (1917–2008)

Selma Kaderman Dritz was a physician and epidemiologist who investigated unusual cases of amoebic dysentery, *pneumocystis carinii* pneumonia, and Kaposi's sarcoma among young gay men in San Francisco. The early investigation of acquired immune deficiency syndrome (AIDS) is a good example of how public health epidemiologists must navigate and collaborate with disenfranchised people in order to prevent and treat disease. With little support from the federal government and few resources, San Francisco public health staff worked long hours tracking cases, interviewing patients, and characterizing symptoms. Dritz would often say, "We can't let those kids die" (Perlman, 2008). Her analytical approach and knowledge of the victims allowed San Francisco's health department to identify the mechanism of transmission of human immunodeficiency virus (HIV) and to start programs to reduce the spread of AIDS. Dritz's shoe leather epidemiology and dedication to the cause earned the respect of scientists, health professionals, and most importantly, young men who had been discarded and dismissed by society.

Selma Kaderman was born on June 29, 1917, in Chicago. In 1941, she graduated from medical school at the University of Illinois and completed an internship and residency at Cook County Contagious Disease Hospital. After residency, Selma moved into private practice specializing in pediatrics. This was prior to the discovery of the polio vaccine, and many young patients suffered from the long-term effects of polio or other infectious diseases. From 1946 to 1947, Selma worked as a consultant to Illinois State Health Department. She married H. Fred Dritz during her pediatric residency. Soon after the union, her husband shipped overseas to serve in the navy. When he returned from World War II, the couple moved to San Francisco. Rather than starting with a new practice, Selma decided to take a break from her career and raise her children. When her children became teenagers, Selma decided to return to work. However, medicine had changed. Vaccines had been invented, and Selma noticed greater focus on problems of premature birth and mental health. Also, Dritz preferred working with groups of people rather than individual patients. She had enjoyed her work with the state health department and decided to pursue a career in public health. In 1967, she earned her master's degree in public health at the University of California at Berkeley and went to work with the San Francisco Public Health Department.

In the role of assistant director of the Disease Control department, Dritz was responsible for investigating outbreaks of measles, mumps, and whooping cough and some incidents of occupational illnesses. In 1974, the Board of Supervisors passed a bill that decriminalized private sexual acts between consenting adults. Escaping homophobia across the United States, gay men flocked to San Francisco. The population movement tripled the number of homosexual men in the city. Bars, bookshops, and bathhouses developed as places where gay men could meet. The massive population movement and sexual freedom converged to create an epidemic of syphilis and gonorrhea. The San Francisco health department had a specific division to investigate sexually transmitted diseases (STDs) and tuberculosis. The Disease Control department was responsible for investigating *other* communicable diseases, which included an epidemic of enteric infections and hepatitis A and B. Dritz quickly learned about the sexual practices of young gay men and began working with local community groups to educate men on safe sex. Her no nonsense approach and clear concern earned the trust and respect of the gay community and physicians. She was able to influence men who were suspicious of those in positions of power.

In June 1981, the Centers for Disease Control (CDC) reported five cases of *pneumocystis carinii* pneumonia (PCP) in Los Angeles. PCP is a deadly lung infection, typically seen among cancer patients with severe immune suppression resulting from chemotherapy. In late July, the San Francisco Department of Public Health received the first report of Kaposi's sarcoma, a rare, slow-growing cancer. Within a month, 20 cases of Kaposi's sarcoma were reported and two victims had already died. Cases of PCP had also started to appear in San Francisco. Health professionals were bewildered. PCP was a very rare disease as was Kaposi's sarcoma. Kaposi's sarcoma was typically limited to older men living in the Mediterranean or North Africa, and the men died of other causes, not Kaposi's sarcoma. Dritz started meeting weekly with gay and lesbian health services to review the number of cases and deaths.

By this point, public health professionals in major cities across the country were reporting similar cases of unusual communicable diseases. In an attempt to identify the cause, the CDC developed a 24-page questionnaire. Dritz administered the questionnaire to approximately 100 patients. The data were not analyzed for another two years because the CDC could not get funding for a statistician. In the meantime, epidemiologists and physicians interviewed patients and worked every lead that they could. Dritz employed techniques used by Dr. John Snow to investigate London's cholera epidemic of 1854. She confiscated an old blackboard, listed and mapped cases. She connected 44 cases that could have been transmitted through sexual or blood contact. Her hypothesis that the problem was blood borne was confirmed when a baby developed AIDS-like symptoms. The baby suffered from Rh factor disease and had received multiple blood transfusions. Dritz recognized the name of one of the 13 donors as a name on her blackboard. Evidence of blood borne transmission meant that health officials could start prevention programs. However, the federal government refused to fund research, treatment, or prevention. Dritz developed partnerships with journalists, nonprofit organizations, and community groups. Working together, they established health education for the gay community and services for people with AIDS. Dritz became recognized as the go-to person within the health department. She worked tirelessly, giving seminars. She taught men to recognize the symptoms of opportunistic infections. She trained bartenders to refer patrons with health concerns to the health department. She encouraged men to reduce the number of sexual contacts. She met with personnel departments of large businesses to allay concerns that AIDS could be transmitted in the workplace. She was instrumental in the health department's biggest challenge, closure of the city's bath houses. Bath houses were large, crowded venues where gay men enjoyed multiple anonymous sexual partners. Dritz knew that men with AIDS were still attending the bath houses and possibly transmitting disease. Under the law, health officials could close the bath houses as a potential health hazard. However, members of the gay community fought closure. The men were not going to voluntarily give up their newfound sexual freedom. Public health officials also knew that closing the bath houses could force high-risk sexual behaviors underground. Dritz was instrumental in negotiating the bath house closures because the gay community realized that her chief motive was public health, not condemnation of their lifestyle. Dritz retired from the health department on April 24, 1984, after HIV was discovered.

Dr. Jonathan Mann, founder of the World Health Organization's Global Programme on AIDS, described the contributions of early public health professionals and researchers, "Our responsibility is historic. For when the history of AIDS and the global response is written, our most precious contribution may well be that, at the time of plague, we did not flee, we did not hide, we did not separate ourselves" (Mann, 1998). Selma Dritz serves as a role model for other public health professionals. Her thorough analysis of medical reports, carefully detailed interviews with patients, and nonjudgmental interactions helped to identify an unknown disease. Dritz worked around social stigmas and limited support to focus on stopping AIDS.

Sally Kuykendall

See also: Blackwell, Elizabeth; Community Health Centers; Community Organizing; Epidemiology; Hepatitis; Human Immunodeficiency Virus and Acquired Immune Deficiency Syndrome; Infectious Diseases; Lesbian, Gay, Bisexual, and Transgender Health; Snow, John

Further Reading

Bacchetti, P., Osmond, D., Chaisson, R. E., Dritz, S., Rutherford, G. W., Swig, L., & Moss, A. R. (1988). Survival patterns of the first 500 patients with AIDS in San Francisco. *Journal of Infectious Diseases*, *157*(5), 1044–1047.

Curran, J. W., & Jaffe, H. W. (2011). AIDS: The early years and CDC's response. *Morbidity and Mortality Weekly Report Supplements*, *60*(4), 64–69.

Dritz, S. K. (1995). *Charting the epidemiological course of AIDS, 1981–1984, an oral history conducted in 1992 by Sally Smith Hughes in the AIDS epidemic in San Francisco: The medical response, 1981–1984*. Volume I. Regional Oral History Office, Bancroft Library, University of California, Berkeley. Retrieved from https://archive.org/stream/aidsepidemicinsf01chinrich/aidsepidemicinsf01chinrich_djvu.txt.

Mann, J. M. (1998, June 28–July 3). Presentation at XII International Conference on AIDS, Geneva.

Perlman, D. (2008). Selma Dritz, tracked early AIDS cases, dies. *SFGate*. Retrieved from http://www.sfgate.com/bayarea/article/Selma-Dritz-tracked-early-AIDS-cases-dies-3270092.php.

Roehr, B. (2008). Selma Dritz, obituary. *British Medical Journal*, *337*(7676), 997.

DUNHAM, ETHEL COLLINS (1883–1969)

Ethel Collins Dunham was a pediatrician who developed clinical standards for the medical care of premature infants. Ethel was born on March 12, 1883, in Hartford, Connecticut, the eldest of six children of Alice Collins and utility executive Samuel Gurley Dunham. As wealthy aristocrats, the Collins children and their 14 cousins were encouraged to support charitable organizations. After graduating from high school, Dunham spent two years at Miss Porter's School in Farmington, Connecticut. From 1903 to 1909, she played golf, traveled around Europe, and volunteered. She found the life of leisure unfulfilling and decided to go to medical school. After completing prerequisite courses in physics, she enrolled at Bryn Mawr College. At Bryn Mawr, Ethel met Martha May Eliot. Martha and Ethel decided to attend medical school together. They enrolled and were accepted at Johns Hopkins University. This was unusual because few medical schools accepted female students. At Hopkins, the two women studied and attended public lectures on the suffrage movement and philanthropy.

After graduation, Dr. Eliot and Dr. Dunham applied for internships in pediatrics at Johns Hopkins. With limited spaces for female students, they had to separate. Dunham completed her internship in pediatrics at Johns Hopkins, working under Dr. John Howland at Harriet Lane Home while Eliot interned in Boston. In 1919, Dunham moved to Connecticut where she became the first female house officer at New Haven Hospital and professor at Yale University. Dunham's ability to recognize and solve problems garnered the respect of her male colleagues. At Yale, she purchased a car so that interns could make house calls to new mothers and infants. At New Haven's outpatient clinic, she implemented an appointment system to reduce overcrowding and improve patient care. In the hospital nursery, Dunham convinced the chief obstetrician to allow pediatricians to care for infants. Consistent with her philanthropic roots, Dunham would forgo salary in order to obtain resources that might improve patient care.

Dunham's interest and expertise in the medical care of infants gained recognition. In 1927, she joined the U.S. Children's Bureau as medical officer in charge of neonatal studies. This position allowed her to stay in New Haven where she researched, developed, and piloted best practices in the care of newborns. In 1935, she left her position at Yale so that she could focus exclusively on developing national standards for the care of newborns. Within a year, she published her first study, a statistical analysis of infant mortality. Infant mortality rates were horrifying. In 1934, 1 out of 18 infants died within the first year of life and 1 out of 11 infants of color died (Department of Commerce, 1938). Prematurity was the leading cause of death in the first year of life. Dunham organized nurses and social workers from the Children's Bureau to perform home visits. The nurses monitored infant development and nutrition while the social workers supported first-time mothers in the transition to motherhood. In 1943, Dunham published the *Standards and Recommendations for the Hospital Care of Newborn Infants, Full Term and Premature*. The nation was immersed in World War II. Qualified doctors and nurses were called to army field hospitals, tending to the wounded. The health care needs of infants and mothers at home were overlooked. Dunham recommended regular medical rounds, coordination of obstetrical and pediatric services, trained pediatric nurses, nurse-to-patient ratios of 1 to 8 for full-term infants and 1 to 4 for premature infants. The standards also recommended infection control measures, ventilation and control of temperature in nurseries, equipment, infant care, and preparation for discharge (Dunham, 1943). The hospital standards were followed by a handbook for physicians. From 1949 to 1951, Dunham worked with the World Health Organization developing international recommendations in the prevention of premature births. After retiring in 1952, she continued to advocate for the specialized care of premature infants. Dunham's efforts were recognized by the American Pediatric Society when she became the first female to receive the John Howland Medal for her contributions as a teacher, researcher, and public servant. In 1957, lifelong partners Ethel and Martha moved to Cambridge to enjoy time together. Ethel died of bronchial pneumonia in 1969.

Dr. Ethel Collins Dunham laid the foundation for the fields of neonatology and perinatology. Her efforts to promote child and maternal health led to one of the greatest achievements in public health today. Hospitals have specialized nurseries and trained staff to care for premature infants, and health professionals support young mothers before, during, and after pregnancy. Dunham's ability to see a problem and identify solutions benefited millions of women and children around the world.

Sally Kuykendall

See also: Children's Health; Eliot, Martha May; Infant Mortality; Maternal Health; World Health Organization

Further Reading

Centers for Disease Control and Prevention. (2016). *Maternal and infant health*. Retrieved from http://www.cdc.gov/reproductivehealth/maternalinfanthealth/.

Department of Commerce. (1938). *Birth, stillbirth, and infant mortality statistics: 1936*. Washington, DC: U.S. Government Printing Office. Retrieved from https://www.cdc.gov/nchs/data/vsushistorical/birthstat_1936.pdf.

Dunham, E. C. (1943). *Standards and recommendations for the hospital care of newborn infants, full term and premature*. Washington, DC: U.S. Government Printing Office. Retrieved from https://archive.org/stream/standardsrecomme00dunh#page/n5/mode/2up.

Dunham, E. C. (1945). Progress in the care of premature infants. *American Journal of Nursing, 45*, 515–518.

E

EATING DISORDERS

Eating disorders are serious but treatable mental disorders that threaten nutritional status, physical, and emotional health. Mental health professionals recognize three main types of eating disorders: anorexia nervosa, bulimia nervosa, and binge-eating disorder (American Psychiatric Association [APA], 2013). Although each disorder is characterized by different behaviors, common symptoms include obsessions with food, body weight, and body shape (National Institute of Mental Health [NIMH], 2016). Eating disorders affect males, females, children, and adults and are most common during adolescence. Underlying causes are thought to be a combination of genetic, biological, behavioral, psychological, and social factors (NIMH, 2016). Treatment occurs through a team approach consisting of a primary care provider for medical care, psychologist and/or psychiatrist for psychotherapy and medication, and a registered dietitian for nutritional counseling (APA, 2013). Treatment plans are tailored to the individual's unique needs.

Individuals with anorexia nervosa are severely underweight yet see themselves as being overweight. The diagnostic criteria for anorexia nervosa are "[1] persistent energy intake restriction; [2] intense fear of gaining weight or of becoming fat, or persistent behavior that interferes with weight gain; and [3] a disturbance in self-perceived weight or shape" (APA, 2013). There are two types of anorexia nervosa behaviors. One is the restricting type where one's weight loss is accomplished by dieting, fasting, and/or excessive exercise for the last three months (APA, 2013). The second type, binge-eating/purging type, is accomplished by self-induced vomiting or the misuse of laxative, diuretics, or enemas for the last three months. Anorexia nervosa can be fatal (NIMH, 2016). Hospitalization is necessary to restore fluids and electrolytes and ensure adequate nutrition for basic body functions.

Individuals with bulimia nervosa may be hard to detect because they usually maintain a normal weight. The diagnostic criteria for bulimia nervosa are "[1] recurrent episodes of binge eating, [2] recurrent inappropriate compensatory behaviors to prevent weight gain, and [3] self-evaluation that is unduly influenced by body shape and weight" (APA, 2013). Individuals with bulimia nervosa binge eat and then force themselves to vomit, exercise, fast, and/or use laxatives or diuretics (NIH, 2016). The level of disease severity is defined by the APA (2013): mild, average of 1–3 episodes per week; moderate, average of 4–7 episodes per week; severe, average of 8–13 episodes per week; and extreme, average of 14 or more episodes per week. As the level of severity increases, so does the degree of functional disability.

The most common eating disorder in the United States is binge-eating disorder. The diagnostic criteria for binge-eating disorder are: "[1] recurrent episodes of binge eating; [2] binge-eating episodes are associated with three (or more) [criteria set by the APA]; [3] marked distress regarding binge eating is present, [4] the binge eating occurs, on average, at least once a week for 3 months; and [5] the binge eating is not associated with the recurrent use of inappropriate compensatory behavior as in bulimia nervosa and does not occur exclusively during the course of bulimia nervosa or anorexia nervosa" (APA, 2013). Shame and the attempt to conceal one's symptoms may lead an individual to hide their binge-eating behaviors. The following are triggers: "interpersonal stressors; dietary restraints; negative feelings related to body weight; body shape and food; and boredom" (APA, 2013). The level of severity for binge-eating disorder is defined by the APA (2013): mild, 1–3 episodes per week; moderate, 4–7 episodes per week; severe, 8–13 episodes per week; and extreme, 14 or more episodes per week. As the level of severity increases, so does the degree of functional disability.

There is another category of eating disorders called the "other specified feeding or eating disorder." In order for an individual to qualify for a diagnosis of anorexia nervosa, bulimia nervosa, and/or binge-eating disorder, the "behaviors must occur, on average, at least once per week for 3 months" (APA, 2013). However, if an individual has symptoms characteristic of an eating disorder that do not meet the full criteria of anorexia nervosa, bulimia nervosa, and/or binge-eating disorder, the individual would fit into this category.

Individual treatment of eating disorders consists of fluid and electrolyte replacement, nutritional counseling, and psychotherapy and medication, as needed. Public health works to prevent eating disorders through universal and indicated prevention programs and comprehensive school health education. Examples of evidence-based programs to prevent eating disorders are *The Weight to Eat* (Neumark-Sztainer & Butler, 1995), *Planet Health* (Austin et al., 2005), *Student Bodies* (Taylor et al., 2006), *The Body Project* (Stice et al., 2006), *New Moves* (Neumark-Sztainer et al., 2010) and *Eating, Aesthetic Feminine Models and the Media* (González et al., 2011). A review of nine evidence-based programs discovered common characteristics among evidence-based eating disorder prevention programs (Ciao, Loth, & Neumark-Sztainer, 2014). All programs were based on health theory, addressed one or more risk factors, were implemented through multiple sessions over a period of time, and provided hands-on activities. There is a need to continue assessing and evaluating programs to determine which are most effective and to expand programs to reach a wider range of audiences.

Susana Leong

See also: Body Mass Index; Mental Health; Nutrition; Women's Health; *Controversies in Public Health:* Controversy 2

Further Reading

American Psychiatric Association. (2013). Feeding and eating disorders. In *Diagnostic and Statistical Manual of Mental Disorders* (5th ed.). Arlington, VA: Author. doi:10.1176/appi.books.9780890425596.dsm10

Austin, S. B., Field, A. E., Wiecha, J., Peterson, K. E., & Gortmaker, S. L. (2005). The impact of a school-based obesity prevention trial on disordered weight-control behaviors in early adolescent girls. *Archives of Pediatrics & Adolescent Medicine*, *159*(3), 225–230.

Ciao, A. C., Loth, K., & Neumark-Sztainer, D. (2014). Preventing eating disorder pathology: Common and unique features of successful eating disorders prevention programs. *Current Psychiatry Reports*, *16*(7), 453. doi:10.1007/s11920-014-0453-0

González, M., Penelo, E., Gutiérrez, T., & Raich, R. M. (2011). Disordered eating prevention programme in schools: A 30-month follow-up. *European Eating Disorders Review*, *19*(4), 349–356. doi:10.1002/erv.1102

National Institute of Mental Health. (2016). *Eating disorders*. Retrieved from https://www.nimh.nih.gov/health/topics/eating-disorders/index.shtml.

Neumark-Sztainer, D., & Butler, R. (1995). Eating disturbances among adolescent girls: Evaluation of a school-based primary prevention program. *Journal of Nutrition Education*, *27*(1), 24.

Neumark-Sztainer, D. R., Friend, S. E., Flattum, C. F., Hannan, P. J., Story, M. T., Bauer, K. W., & . . . Petrich, C. A. (2010). New moves-preventing weight-related problems in adolescent girls a group-randomized study. *American Journal of Preventive Medicine*, *39*(5), 421–432. doi:10.1016/j.amepre.2010.07.017

Stice, E., Shaw, H., Burton, E., & Wade, E. (2006). Dissonance and healthy weight eating disorder prevention programs: A randomized efficacy trial. *Journal of Consulting and Clinical Psychology*, *74*(2), 263–275. doi:10.1037/0022-006X.74.2.263

Taylor, C. B., Bryson, S., Luce, K. H., Cunning, D., Doyle, A. C., Abascal, L. B., & . . . Wilfley, D. E. (2006). Prevention of eating disorders in at-risk college-age women. *Archives of General Psychiatry*, *63*(8), 881–888.

ELDER MALTREATMENT

Elder maltreatment involves any form of abuse that leads to harm or loss for a vulnerable person who is older than 60 to 65 years old. The damage could be physical, sexual, emotional, financial, or neglect, which includes failure to provide adequate care or supervision. Elder maltreatment is on the rise. Since 1986, a 150 percent increase in elder abuse occurred. Around 2 million elders experience abuse or neglect every year (Snyder, 2014, p. 132). Elder maltreatment can occur within personal relationships, as well as abuse and neglect of the aged within institutions. Cases are rarely resolved through the criminal justice system, and serious cases that occur in long-term care facilities and are reported typically end up in civil courts.

A variety of theories attempt to explain elder maltreatment. *Social learning theory* proposes that violence is learned. An abused child is more likely to grow up and abuse his or her own children. Extended to elder abuse, some adults caring for aged loved ones were socialized to believe that violence is an appropriate form of interaction and will act violently toward elders. Perpetrators normalize violence, sometimes as a legitimate response to stress, without being aware of it. Abuse also occurs when adult children consciously engage in violence toward vulnerable elders as a form of retribution. Old conflicts can reemerge or are aggravated by contradictory ideas on religion, politics, child rearing, or work. *Stressed caregiver theory* describes caretakers who are suffering from the strains associated with the responsibility of providing constant care. When the caregiver experiences peak stress levels, maltreatment is more likely. Not all caregivers respond to stress the same, so the psychopathology of caretakers is relevant. *Isolation theory* holds that the elderly experience a drop in social bonds, and this facilitates abuse. Diminished social networks help abusers avoid detection, increase dependence of the elder person, and amplifies the maltreatment. *Dependency theory* relies on traditional models in the field of victimology. It argues that anyone with fewer physical or mental resources is more susceptible to abuse and neglect. With that in mind, women, people over the age of 80, and those suffering from dementia suffer from highest rates of elder maltreatment.

Elder maltreatment is all too prevalent and the most common perpetrators are, sadly, those who are closest to the elder person. Ninety percent of abusers are family members (NCEA, 2015). In intrafamilial cases, abusers have higher unemployment rates, drug and alcohol problems, a higher rate of previous incidents with the criminal justice system, and are more likely to have a history of hospitalization for mental health issues. Situations involving one adult child as the exclusive caregiver are more likely to exhibit elder maltreatment. Adult sons are perpetrators in 64 percent of cases, and in 30 percent of cases perpetrators contend the elder previously abused them (Ulsperger, 2007, p. 291). In personal care situations, abusers fall into three categories—hostiles, authoritarians, and dependents. Hostile abusers tend to blame the elder parent for limiting their potential and dominating their personal resources. Authoritarian abusers tend to be married, have aged parents living with them, and are more likely to infantilize an elderly parent. Dependent abusers are financially reliant on the elder. In 77 percent of cases, the caretaker is somewhat or fully financially dependent on the person cared for, and in 65 percent of cases, the perpetrator is somewhat or completely dependent on the cared for with housing (Ulsperger, 2007, p. 292). Although the majority of family perpetrators are adult children, in a small number of cases the intimate partner may perpetrate maltreatment. The statistics on elder maltreatment and relatives are believed to be inaccurate. The sensitive nature of family relationship dynamics means that many cases go unreported.

Institutionalized maltreatment, which includes long-term care facilities, has developed into an important issue. In the 1970s, reports of residents receiving inedible food, staff leaving residents unattended lying in their own excrement, and physically assaulting the elderly made headlines. Reform movements led to the Omnibus Budget Reconciliation Act (OBRA) of 1987. OBRA implemented provisions on privacy rights, physical restraint use, and new requirements related to managing personal funds. It tightened the survey and certification requirements for nursing homes, but also made nursing homes one of the most highly regulated industries in the United States. Intentional elder maltreatment takes place in elder care environments due to a variety of reasons, such as racial tension, class conflict, and individual psychopathologies. However, research shows that elevated levels of bureaucracy, promoted by legislation such as OBRA, unintentionally facilitates abuse and neglect. Inundated with rules and demands for efficiency, staff focus on quality resident care diminishes. Residents turn into objects of labor. Victimology theory reasons that when perpetrators view other people as objects, the likelihood of maltreatment increases. Currently, more than 3 million people live in nursing homes in the United States. Around 44 percent report experiencing abuse, and 95 percent report either experiencing neglect or witnessing another resident neglected. More than 80 percent of staff report witnessing emotional abuse and 36 percent physical abuse (Snyder, 2014, p. 136).

The U.S. government currently provides little funding to protect against elder maltreatment. Organizations dedicated to addressing and reducing elder maltreatment often operate through state and local health agencies. Adult Protective Services (APS) is one organization dedicated to the issue. APS educates and encourages individuals to report maltreatment, provides a hotline to report suspected abuse and neglect, and provides legal services to individuals who experience maltreatment. As the baby-boomer generation ages, awareness of maltreatment issues is essential to reversing rates of abuse. This includes becoming familiar with specific laws within your jurisdiction, developing the ability to recognize signs of mistreatment, and having the capacity to assess relationships in order to understand motives for family involvement.

Jason S. Ulsperger

See also: Aging; Alzheimer's Disease; Behavioral Health; Care, Access to; Mental Health; Violence

Further Reading

Gibbs, L., & Mosqueda, L. A. (2014). *Medical implications of elder abuse and neglect.* Philadelphia: Elsevier.

National Center on Elder Abuse. (2015). *Statistics/data.* United States Department of Heath and Human Services. Retrieved from http://www.ncea.aoa.gov/Library/Data/index.aspx.

Payne, B. (2011). *Crime and elder abuse: An integrated perspective.* Springfield, IL: Charles C. Thomas.

Snyder, D. R. (2014). *Elder crimes, elder justice.* Burlington, MA: Jones & Bartlett.

Ulsperger, J. (2007). Elder abuse perpetrated by adult children. In A. Jackson (Ed.), *Encyclopedia of domestic violence* (pp. 290–296). New York: Routledge.

Ulsperger, J. S., & Knottnerus, J. D. (2011). *Elder care catastrophe: Rituals of abuse in nursing homes and what you can do about it.* Boulder, CO: Paradigm.

ELDERS, JOYCELYN (1933–)

Joycelyn Elders is a famous physician and health administrator who served as the first African American and second woman surgeon general of the United States, serving in Bill Clinton's presidential administration. She was trained as a pediatrician and was a faculty member for many years at the University of Arkansas Medical Center, beginning in 1967. As surgeon general, she was best known for her discussions of sensitive issues such as drug legalization, teenage sexuality, and distribution of contraception in schools.

She was born as Minnie Lee Jones in Schaal, Arkansas, and later changed her name to Minnie Joycelyn Lee. She grew up in a poor family, with her father working as a sharecropper. She received her BS degree in biology from Philander Smith College in Little Rock, Arkansas, in 1952. She then worked as a nurse's aide in a veteran's administration hospital in Milwaukee, before joining the U.S. Army in May 1953. While in the army, she trained as a physical therapist. After leaving the army, she attended the University of Arkansas Medical School and obtained her medical degree in 1960. She completed an internship at the University of Minnesota Hospital, followed by a residency in pediatrics at the University of Arkansas Medical Center. She also earned an MS degree in biochemistry. As a faculty member at the University of Arkansas Medical Center, she advanced from assistant professor to professor by 1976. She received a National Institutes of Health career development award while there, and certification as a pediatric endocrinologist in 1978.

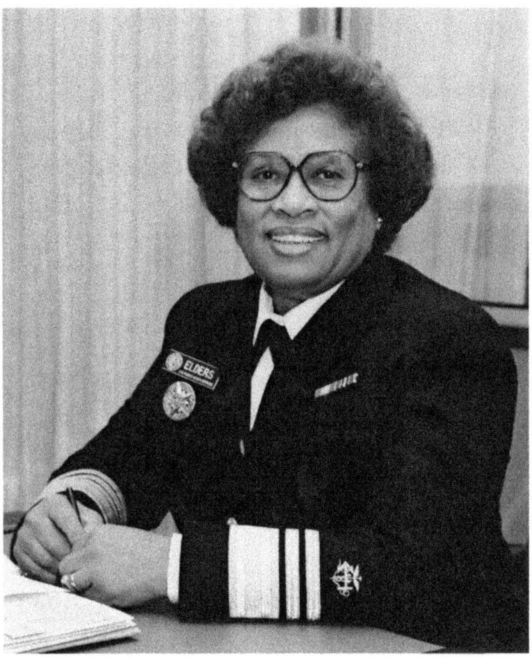

The daughter of a poor Southern sharecropper, Surgeon General Joycelyn Elders gives voice to the struggles of poor, young minority females. Controversies over birth control and sex education led to her forced resignation as the nation's top doctor. (National Institutes of Health)

Her political and administrative career, rather than her career as a medical school faculty member, began in 1987 when then Governor Bill Clinton appointed her as the director of the Arkansas Department of Health. Among her proudest achievements in that position were a tenfold increase in the number of early childhood screenings annually and almost a doubling of the immunization rates of two-year-old children in Arkansas. Elders pushed aggressive campaigns to reduce teen pregnancy by making birth control and sex education more readily available to teenagers. She also endorsed HIV testing and counseling in the state. She was elected the president of the Association of State and Territorial Health Officers in 1992.

President Bill Clinton appointed her the U.S. surgeon general in January 1993. She was a strong supporter of his health plan and became a controversial nominee whose appointment was not confirmed until September 7, 1993. She was a strong, outspoken advocate for health-related causes, such as the distribution of contraceptives in school, the exploration of drug legalization, and abortion rights. In 1994, at a speech at the United Nations, she said schools should consider teaching masturbation to students as a means to prevent sexually transmitted diseases. This statement was attacked by right wing activists, and the ensuing controversy led to her being removed from this position by President Clinton in December 1994. She returned to the University of Arkansas Medical Center and to public lecturing on issues related to AIDS and teen pregnancy. She continues to live in Little Rock, Arkansas, as a semiretired professor emerita.

Jennie Jacobs Kronenfeld

See also: Children's Health; Human Immunodeficiency Virus and Acquired Immune Deficiency Syndrome; Men's Health; Nation's Health, The; School Health; Surgeon General; Women's Health

Further Reading

Elliott, J. C. (2001). Joycelyn Elders. *Black heroes* (pp. 216–221). Ipswich, MA: History Reference Center.

Kronenfeld, J. J. (2011). Elders, Joycelyn. In M. Z. Stange, C. K. Oyster, & J. G. Golson (Eds.), *Multimedia encyclopedia of women in today's world* (pp. 470–471). Thousand Oaks, CA: Sage.

ELIOT, MARTHA MAY (1891–1978)

Martha May Eliot was a public health pediatrician who advocated for federal policies to support disadvantaged mothers and children. Martha was born on April 7, 1891, in Dorchester, Massachusetts, the second of three children of Christopher Rhodes and Mary Jackson May Eliot. The Eliot family was a member of a society referred to as the Boston Brahmins. This powerful and elite group dominated art, drama, education, politics, and philanthropy on the East Coast. Martha's grandfather was the first chancellor of Washington University in St. Louis, her father was a respected Unitarian minister, and her cousin was the Nobel Prize–winning poet, playwright, and literary critic T. S. Eliot. Martha attended Radcliffe College, majoring in classical literature. During her undergraduate studies, she spent one year at Bryn Mawr College where she met her future partner, Ethel Collins Dunham. Ethel was eight years older but one academic year behind Martha. In order that they could attend medical school together, Martha spent a gap year working in the Social Service Department at Massachusetts General Hospital. This experience gave her direct experience with poor women and children and introduced her to the concept of social medicine.

Martha's first choice of medical school was Harvard School of Medicine. However, Harvard rejected her because she was female. Johns Hopkins University School of Medicine accepted both Ethel and Martha. During their time at Hopkins, they attended lectures on the suffragette movement and philanthropy. Dr. Eliot graduated with honors and was offered an internship at Johns Hopkins. She turned the internship down because she wanted to stay near Dunham who was denied a position. However, as males were being called to war, Hopkins was forced to expand their pool and subsequently offered an internship to Dunham. Thus, Dunham stayed in Baltimore while Eliot interned at Peter Bent Brigham Hospital in Boston. After an additional year in pediatrics residency at Saint Louis Children's Hospital, Dr. Eliot joined Dr. Edwards A. Parks, teaching and researching at Yale Medical School's new Department of Pediatrics.

In 1923, the U.S. Children's Bureau reached out to the Yale researchers requesting collaboration in a study of rickets. Rickets is a disease caused by vitamin D deficiency. Descriptions of the disease are recorded as early as the first and second centuries CE by the Greek physician Sorano of Ephesus. In places with less sunlight or dietary sources of vitamin D, children's bones do not develop normally. The bones are soft and weak, causing structural deformities. In 1890, zookeepers in London successfully treated ricketed monkeys with cod liver oil and ultraviolet light. The U.S. Children's Bureau decided to test similar treatments among young children in Boston. Within the first year of the study, pediatricians observed remarkable success. In the two untreated control groups, 23 percent and 34 percent of children developed moderate to severe rickets. In the treatment group, 4 percent of the children developed moderate rickets, and none developed severe rickets (Eliot, 2004). Parks and Eliot presented their results to the American Medical Association, recommending widespread use of cod liver oil and sunlight to treat and prevent rickets. Because of these simple treatments, rickets is now considered an extremely rare disease.

In 1924, Eliot was named director of the Division of Child and Maternal Health within the U.S. Children's Bureau. Led by Katharine Frederica Lenroot (1891–1982), the Children's Bureau focused on improving health outcomes for women and children. At the time that Eliot took public office, infant mortality rate was 128 deaths per 1,000 live births, maternal deaths due to sepsis were 23 deaths per 1,000 live births, and maternal deaths due to "other puerperal causes" (i.e., hemorrhage, hypertension or embolism during pregnancy, and childbirth) were 43 deaths per 1,000 live births (Department of Commerce, 1927). Qualified doctors shunned obstetrics, leaving the care of pregnant women and infants to untrained staff. Lenroot and Eliot designed and drafted federal policies to support maternal and infant nutrition, prenatal services, postnatal home visits by trained nurses, parent education, and formal medical training in obstetrics and pediatrics. Title IV, the Aid to Dependent Children, Title V, and Title VII of the Social Security Act of 1935, and later, the child labor laws of the Fair Labor Standards Act of 1938 were critical in advancing maternal and child health and continue to support the health and well-being of women and children today. Over the next 80 years, child welfare policies and advancements in science and clinical care reduced infant mortality rate to 7.2 per 1,000 live births and reduced maternal mortality rate to less than 0.1 per 1,000 live births (Centers for Disease Control and Prevention, 2016).

In 1934, Eliot was appointed assistant chief of the Children's Bureau. The following year, Dunham joined the Children's Bureau as director of child development. Eliot's responsibilities included managing the Emergency Maternity and Infant Care Program. The program provided medical, nursing, and hospital care for the wives and children of men enlisted in World War II. The program was designed to alleviate servicemen's concerns for their wives and children at home so that they could focus on war efforts. Eliot traveled to England to investigate the impact of war on children. The British government was evacuating children, mothers, and disabled people from areas heavily bombed by Germany to the safety of rural villages. Eliot studied the British system and children's ability to cope with the trauma of war. Her interviews and field study published as *Civil Defense Measures for the Protection of Children* advocated for more social workers to support children displaced by war. After the war, Eliot moved into global advocacy, working with the United Nations Children's Fund (UNICEF) and helping to establish the World Health Organization (WHO). Eliot was the only female to sign the founding documents of the WHO. In 1949, she served as assistant director general of the WHO and in 1957, became chair of the Department of Child and Maternal Health at the Harvard School of Public Health (the school that had rejected her for medical school). Eliot retired in 1960 but continued her work with UNICEF and the WHO, advancing care for women around the world.

Eliot's public health advocacy was well recognized within her lifetime. In 1947, she was elected the first female president of the American Public Health Association (APHA). In 1948, she was awarded the prestigious Lasker Award for her work with the Emergency Maternal and Infant Care Program and was also elected president of the National Conference on Social Welfare. In 1958, the APHA awarded Eliot the Sedgwick Memorial Medal for distinguished service and advancement of public health knowledge and practice. In 1964, the APHA established the Martha May Eliot award recognizing outstanding service in maternal and child health. Despite numerous professional awards and acknowledgments, Eliot was often the target of gender and heterosexual biases. Critics questioned how an unmarried woman without children could know how to care for pregnant women and children. Politicians referred to her as "Godmother to the Nation's Youngsters." Despite criticism, Eliot stayed focused on her mission. In personal notes to family members, she relates how her relationship with Dunham provided personal and professional support as well as reprieve from her work. In 1957, Ethel and Martha moved to Cambridge, Massachusetts. Ethel died of bronchial pneumonia in 1969. Martha died on Valentine's Day in 1978.

Martha May Eliot was a member of the far-reaching, liberal Eliot clan, a family that masterminded the culture, education, and social welfare of a developing nation. Unmarried, without children of her own, and openly lesbian, Eliot was a woman of enormous influence and resilience dedicated to the physical and emotional development of children. Her efforts in maternal and child health research, advocacy, and policy proved to be enormously successful, creating a downward trend in infant and maternal mortality rates that continued into the next century.

Sally Kuykendall

See also: Blackwell, Elizabeth; Dunham, Ethel Collins; Infant Mortality; Maternal Health; World Health Organization

Further Reading

Barclay, D. (1952, April 6). Godmother to the nation's youngsters. *New York Times Magazine*, 17.

Centers for Disease Control and Prevention. (2016). *Maternal and infant health.* Retrieved from http://www.cdc.gov/reproductivehealth/maternalinfanthealth/.

Department of Commerce. (1927). *Mortality statistics: 1924.* Washington, DC: U.S. Government Printing Office. Retrieved from https://www.cdc.gov/nchs/data/vsushistorical/mortstatsh_1924.pdf.

Eliot, M. (2004). The control of rickets. *American Journal of Public Health, 94*(8), 1321–1323. Retrieved from https://www.ncbi.nlm.nih.gov/pmc/articles/PMC1448445/.

Eliot, M. M. (1942). Effect of war and civil defense on children: The British experience. *Social Service Review, 16,* 1–36.

Hansen, B. (2002). Public careers and private sexuality: Some gay and lesbian lives in the history of medicine and public health. *American Journal of Public Health, 92*(1), 36–44.

Lasker awards for 1948. (1948). *American Journal of Public Health, 38,* 1717.

Parry, M. S., & Tedeschi, S. K. (2004). Martha May Eliot: "Spinster in steel specs adviser on maternity." *American Journal of Public Health, 94*(8), 1322.

Schmidt, W. M. (1979). Some kind of a social doctor: Martha May Eliot, 1891–1978. *Pediatrics, 63*(1), 146.

U.S. National Library of Medicine. (2015). *Martha May Eliot.* Retrieved from https://cfmedicine.nlm.nih.gov/physicians/biography_99.html.

ELLERTSON, CHARLOTTE EHRENGARD (1966–2004)

Charlotte Ehrengard Ellertson advocated for women's right to self-determination in reproductive health. Maternal mortality increases among women who have four or more children (WHO, 2017). The use of birth control to space pregnancy provides multiple health and social benefits. Birth control improves maternal health and well-being, reduces the need for abortion, allows parents to focus resources and attention on a fewer number of children, and empowers women to pursue further education, employment, or community service. Male and female condoms have the added advantage of protecting against human immunodeficiency virus (HIV) and other sexually transmitted diseases (STDs). Nationally and internationally, birth control slows population growth, supporting the earth's resources and the health of nations. Ellertson was instrumental in identifying the most effective methods of birth control when regular methods fail or sex is forced.

Charlotte was born in 1966 in Johannesburg, South Africa, to Gabrielle and Reverend Carroll Ellertson. Gabrielle was an artist. Carroll was a Lutheran minister based in Minnesota. The Lutheran ministry worked against apartheid in South Africa, providing education to black men and women and advocating for women's rights and racial equality. The family lived in the ZwaZulu-Natal province. Charlotte learned to speak several languages and developed a passion for exotic animals. Gabrielle and Carroll were active supporters of the Rorke's Drift Art and Crafts Centre. Established in 1962, the arts center was designed to train local women in the traditional African arts of weaving and pottery. The hope was that the women would work as art therapists at Ceza Mission Hospital in Zululand. The center provided a rigorous education to aspiring artists and is now world renowned for advancing African arts and crafts. In addition to his work at the mission, Reverend Ellertson directed a radio show, the Radio Voice of the Gospel. In 1979, the Ellertsons moved to Minnesota. Gabrielle went back to school for her bachelor's degree in fine arts, and Reverend Ellertson continued his work with the Lutheran church.

In 1987, Charlotte graduated from Harvard University with a degree in biological anthropology. Her roommates recalled her love of practical jokes and her pet python, "Precious." During her undergraduate studies, Charlotte worked as a contraceptive counselor. She continued her education at Princeton University, earning a master's in public affairs (1992) and a PhD in demography and public affairs (1993). After graduation, Dr. Ellertson moved to Africa, working on reproductive rights with the U.S. Agency for International Development and as a health educator providing family planning information to a radio broadcasted soap opera.

In 1995, Ellertson joined the Population Council, an international organization, which works to empower adolescent girls, support family planning, prevent STDs, and eliminate sexual and gender violence. The Population Council supported research into emergency contraception, medical and surgical abortions, unintended pregnancy, the point of pelvic examinations prior to contraceptive prescription, intimate partner violence, adolescent pregnancy, and STDs. The intention was to develop evidence-based programs and practices in family planning. Ellertson developed expertise in emergency contraception (EC), an oral formula of estrogen and progestin used by women to prevent pregnancy when the woman is mid-cycle and other birth control methods either failed or were not used. EC was discovered in the 1920s when researchers noticed that estrogenic extracts interrupted pregnancy. Soon after discovery, veterinarians used EC to avert pregnancy in dogs and horses. If an animal mated too early, before the female was physically mature enough to carry a pregnancy or while she was still recovering from a previous birth, the veterinarians could stop the pregnancy. In the 1960s, Dutch doctors successfully used EC on a 13-year-old who had been raped during the middle of her menstrual cycle (Haspels, 1994). Women began to use EC with some harmful side effects. In the 1970s Dr. Albert Yuzpe developed a regimen that featured four doses of easily accessible hormones and had fewer side effects (Ellertson, 1996). Independent researchers found Yuzpe's method to be safe and effective. In 1994, the International Conference on Population and Development officially supported women's right to use EC. During her research, Ellertson often found that women were reluctant to report intimate sexual behaviors and concerns to their health care providers, and some health care providers refused to provide services, referrals, or information to women seeking EC. In 2002, she founded the organization Ibis Reproductive Health. The purpose of Ibis was to bridge research and women's health practices. In 2004, at the age of 38, Ellertson died of breast cancer. In her short lifetime, she published more than 100 journal articles, book chapters, and technical reports. Her research continues to raise questions of whether women need a pelvic examination in order to use birth control and whether prescriptions are truly needed for birth control (Grossman, Ellertson, Abuabara, Blanchard, & Rivas, 2006).

Charlotte E. Ellertson performed multiple research studies comparing effectiveness and cost of birth control and emergency contraception. From her research, public health organizations were able to develop programs and guidelines to promote women's health and reduce maternal and infant mortality. Ellertson believed in demedicalization of family planning. She believed that women are capable of identifying their own needs for birth control, are capable of attaining birth control pills from a local pharmacy, and are capable of following the instructions on the package. She was instrumental in improving women's health by advocating for FDA approval of RU-486 and emergency contraception. Today, many women enjoy a better quality of life, free from the fear of unintended pregnancy, due to the efforts of Charlotte Ellertson.

Sally Kuykendall

See also: Elders, Joycelyn; Family Planning; Maternal Health; Planned Parenthood; Sanger, Margaret Louise Higgins; Women's Health

Further Reading

Ellertson, C. (1996). History and efficacy of emergency contraception: Beyond Coca-Cola. *Family Planning Perspectives*, *28*(2), 44–48.

Grossman, D., Ellertson, C., Abuabara, K., Blanchard, K., & Rivas, F. T. (2006). Barriers to contraceptive use in product labeling and practice guidelines. *American Journal of Public Health*, *96*(5), 791–799.

Haspels, A. A. (1994). Emergency contraception: A review. *Contraception*, *50*, 101–108. doi:10.1016/0010-7824(94)90046-9

Population Council. (2017). Available at http://www.popcouncil.org/.

Princeton Alumni Weekly. (2016). *Charlotte E. Ellertson *93*. Retrieved from https://paw.princeton.edu/memorial/charlotte-e-ellertson-93.

Trussell, J., Stewart, F., Potts, M., Guest, F., & Ellertson, C. (1993). Should oral contraceptives be available without prescription? *American Journal of Public Health*, *83*(8), 1094–1099.

World Health Organization. (2017). *Family planning/contraception*. Retrieved from http://www.who.int/mediacentre/factsheets/fs351/en/.

EMERGENCY MEDICAL TREATMENT AND LABOR ACT (EMTALA)

Congress enacted the Emergency Medical Treatment and Labor Act (EMTALA) in response to patient dumping, a practice where private hospitals would discharge or transfer medically indigent patients even when the patient was not stable. The maneuver was primarily motivated by finances, an effort by hospitals to avoid treating patients on Medicare. Physicians at Cook County Hospital in Chicago were concerned for the patients and shed light on the practice through published research studies. The research indicated that 87 percent of patient transfers to other hospitals were due to lack of insurance, 24 percent of the transferred patients were unstable at the time of transfer, and transferred patients were twice as likely to die in comparison to other patients in the receiving hospital (Ansell & Schiff, 1987; Schiff, Ansell, Schlosser, Idris, Morrison, & Whitman, 1986). The doctors concluded that dumping jeopardized patient safety and that minority and unemployed individuals were disproportionately targeted. Under EMTALA, emergency departments must screen and stabilize patients before transfer or discharge. Anyone with a medical emergency who seeks treatment at an emergency room, regardless of ability to pay, has the right to medical screening and stabilization. The law applies to all facilities that accept Medicare, approximately 98 percent of all U.S. hospitals (Zibulewsky, 2001). Transfers are permitted under certain conditions. Facilities are responsible for posting notices advising patients of their rights to treatment. Although EMTALA was originally designed for emergency departments, the regulations have expanded to all aspects of patient care in hospitals. The law is one of the most comprehensive laws prohibiting discrimination against individuals based on ability to pay. EMTALA supports public health by ensuring that people receive the emergency care that they need, when they need it.

There are four key parts to EMTALA: (1) the patient, (2) an emergency medical condition, (3) right to medical screening, and (4) right to stabilization or medically indicated transfer. EMTALA states that anyone who comes to the emergency department with a medical condition cannot be turned away. The statute does not simply mean patients who are formally admitted. Someone who collapses on the street outside of the emergency department or has a heart attack in the ambulance on the way to the emergency department is covered by the law. The person does not have to be physically in the hospital building. The emergency medical condition includes acute illnesses as well as labor and delivery when the woman is having contractions or there is not enough time for transfer to a maternity hospital. Medical screening is defined as the type of screening exam provided to insured patients. Medical screening goes beyond history and physical exam to include blood tests, X-rays, or consults by specialists (Zibulewsky, 2001). The obligation of medical screening is fulfilled when possible diagnoses are ruled out or stabilized. Stabilization varies by disease or injury. Stabilization may mean medication, immobilization, fluid replacement, or mechanical ventilation. For the purposes of the law, stabilization means that the patient is not reasonably expected to deteriorate due to transfer or during transfer. Patients may be transferred if the patient requests transfer or the physician advises transfer for medical reasons and the benefits of transfer outweigh the risks. As part of the regulations, hospitals that specialize in certain diseases or treatments must accept medically indicated transfers. As with any law, penalties are imposed for violation. Fines range from $25,000 (for hospitals fewer than 100 beds) to $50,000 per patient. The fines are paid out of pocket and are not covered by malpractice insurance. Physicians and hospitals found in violation may be denied future participation in the Medicare program, which essentially means they are out of business.

EMTALA, also known as the patient antidumping law, was passed as part of the Consolidated Omnibus Reconciliation Act (COBRA) of 1986. EMTALA requires hospitals to provide adequate care to uninsured or underinsured individuals. The law has become a significant factor in ensuring that patients who are supported through public funds have access to the emergency care that they need.

Leapolda Figueroa and Sally Kuykendall

See also: Administration, Health; Centers for Medicare and Medicaid Services; Public Health Law

Further Reading

Ansell, D. A., & Schiff, R. L. (1987). Patient dumping. Status, implications, and policy recommendations. *Journal of the American Medical Association*, 257(11), 1500–1502.

Centers for Medicare and Medicaid Services. (2016). *Emergency Medical Treatment & Labor Act (EMTALA)*. Retrieved from https://www.cms.gov/Regulations-and-Guidance/Legislation/EMTALA/.

Schiff, R. L., Ansell, D. A., Schlosser, J. E., Idris, A. H., Morrison, A., & Whitman, S. (1986). Transfers to a public hospital: A prospective study of 467 patients. *The New England Journal of Medicine, 314*(9), 552–557.

Zibulewsky, J. (2001). The Emergency Medical Treatment and Active Labor Act (EMTALA): What it is and what it means for physicians. *Proceedings (Baylor University. Medical Center), 14*(4), 339–346. Retrieved from http://www.ncbi.nlm.nih.gov/pmc/articles/PMC1305897/.

EMERGENCY PREPAREDNESS AND RESPONSE

Emergency preparedness and response is a specialized field of public health that plans for, prepares, and practices responses to public health emergencies resulting from natural disasters, infectious diseases, bioterrorism, chemical, or radiation and nuclear threats. Although different incidents require different interventions, there are common actions individuals and organizations may take to minimize the impact of a disaster. Public health organizations play critical roles in identifying threats, mobilizing resources, aiding victims, and supporting communities.

The need for a specialized field in public health emergency preparedness and response was first realized with the 2001 World Trade Center terrorist attacks. On 9/11, 2,996 people died and more than 6,000 were injured. Emergency responders pulled victims from the wreckages, sacrificing their own lives to help others. Critically ill survivors were taken to the nearest hospitals. In New York City, non-critically injured survivors were ferried to waiting ambulances in Jersey City. Physicians, nurses, and medical technicians treated thousands of victims through the organized chaos. Dust, rubble, and smoke filled the air. Confused and shocked residents walked for miles to safety. Teachers carried wheelchair-dependent students by piggyback. People with respiratory conditions covered their faces with wet towels to filter the air. Before the nation had time to recover, a second bioterrorist attack occurred, deadly anthrax delivered via the U.S. Postal Service to media outlets and senate offices. The horrific events exposed the need for an organized public health response to disasters.

In public health, the first line of defense is the 250,000 public health workers, 760,000 doctors, 2.7 million nurses, and other medical staff who screen, diagnose, and treat patients every day. Medical professionals are trained to detect unusual diseases, patient complaints, or symptoms that may signal a threat to public health. The Centers for Disease Control and Prevention (CDC) Emergency Operations Center (EOC) fields calls from health professionals, government officials, and members of the general public. A team of experts reviews all reports to identify possible patterns of disease and at-risk groups and to recommend a plan of action. Public health laboratories are on call 24 hours a day. Located throughout the nation, public health laboratories are equipped to handle and test potentially biohazardous specimens. When an urgent threat is identified, the CDC deploys scientists to the area to provide expert advice. The threat is communicated to the Division of Strategic National Stockpile, a stockpile of over seven billion dollars' worth of drugs and medical supplies, which may be needed for catastrophic events.

During a natural or man-made disaster, the general public needs clear, concise, and accurate information in order to make smart decisions to either move to safety or shelter in place. Scare tactics do not work. Fright paralyzes people. Health communications is a specialized field of public health. The Health Alert Network (HAN) is a communication network that disseminates clear and accurate information during public health emergencies. Messages are classified as health alerts (high priority), health advisories (warnings), health updates, and general information. Health alerts provide background information on the specific causal mechanism, identify at-risk groups, and provide recommendations for intervention, treatment, and prevention. The information is disseminated directly to federal, state, territorial, and local health officers, public health practitioners, health organizations, and the media. The Crisis & Emergency Risk Communication (CERC) uses evidence-based practices to communicate with the general public. CERC provides training, resources, and materials on how to communicate in ways that empower people to make life-saving decisions. The CDC supports health communications in a disaster by maintaining an online database of fact sheets for use by the public in an emergency.

Individuals play a critical role in emergency situations. Failure to act or to respond wisely threatens the life of the person, family members, and first responders who may need to deploy search and rescue. Individuals can prepare for emergencies by knowing potential natural disasters or weather emergencies that occur within their geographic region. Planning for severe earthquakes, floods, hurricanes, landslides, tornadoes, tsunamis, volcanoes, wildfires or extreme heat or cold can save precious minutes. The CDC recommends gathering a three-day supply of food and water, personal care items, safety supplies, electronics, important documents, and cash. Depending on individual and family circumstances, it may also be necessary to pack prescription medicine, medical supplies, infant formula, or baby or pet supplies. The supplies should be stored in portable waterproof containers. Homeowners and renters can control damage by knowing where and how to turn off residential gas, electric, and water supplies. It is important for friends and family members to have a plan to communicate during an emergency. Children should be taught to dial 911 and how to respond to an emergency. It is helpful to memorize important telephone numbers or keep a contact card with telephone numbers in a wallet, purse, or book bag. Beyond communicating with family members, individuals should listen to credible sources of information to determine what is going on in the area, safe places to go, and how to access shelter resources.

The CDC is prepared to respond to numerous anticipated and unanticipated emergencies, for example, an anthrax attack. Anthrax is a deadly bacterium that lives in the soil, easily grown in a laboratory and manipulated as a weapon of bioterrorism. Anthrax is tasteless and odorless. It could be released in the air, water, or food without immediate detection. To prevent unintentional transmission, the federal government and international agreements regulate the possession and use of hazardous biological materials. To control intentional transmission, the CDC educates local, state, territorial, and tribal health departments on ways to detect and respond to threats. Initially, a patient may appear at a clinic, doctor's office, or hospital with signs of anthrax. The health care provider would contact the EOC. Specimens would be sent to public health laboratories through the Laboratory Response Network (LRN), and the patient would start treatment with antibiotics. Federal agencies would deploy field staff to complete an epidemiological investigation, identifying the source of contamination. And doctors would treat symptomatic patients using best practices clinical guidelines published by the CDC. If the event is a mass-casualty incident, beyond the scope and ability of local health care services, the CDC would deploy medical professionals and stockpiled medical countermeasures (MCMs) to Points of Dispensing (PODs). PODs are schools, community centers, or areas familiar and easily accessible to local residents. Residents would be directed by the media and local officials to report to the PODs, where symptoms would be assessed and possibly exposed people would be treated with antibiotics or antitoxins. After the threat is contained, the CDC assesses what worked and what did not work in order to improve future responses.

People respond to traumatic events in different ways. It is normal to feel sorrow, anxiety, or grief after a life-challenging event. Many people can become overwhelmed by shock, fright, sorrow, or anger. Public health assists in recovery after natural and man-made disasters. Experts recommend that survivors stay informed, take care of themselves, rest, and connect with others. Volunteering, creative expression, stress management, and advocacy can help survivors to create their own story out of disaster. To assist individuals and families, the Substance Abuse and Mental Health Services Administration (SAMHSA) offers the Disaster Distress Helpline (1-800-985-5990 or TTY for the hearing impaired, 1-800-846-8517).

Responding to disasters and assisting in control and recovery are part of the mission of public health of preventing infectious diseases, controlling injuries, protecting against environmental hazards, facilitating access to quality health services, and promoting overall well-being. The public health system detects and responds to disasters by maintaining a formal surveillance system for sudden and urgent health events. In the event of an emergency, the Department of Homeland Security, CERC, the Office of Public Health Preparedness and Response, and the Centers for Disease Control and Prevention work with state, local and other federal agencies to coordinate effective responses. The main goal of public health preparedness and response is to empower individuals in order to contain the event, minimize loss, and restore health and well-being.

Sally Kuykendall

See also: Antibiotic Resistance; Association of Public Health Laboratories; Bioterrorism; Centers for Disease Control and Prevention; Environmental Health; Environmental Protection Agency; Epidemiology; Infectious Diseases; Substance Abuse and Mental Health Services Administration; Violence; Zombie Preparedness

Further Reading

Centers for Disease Control and Prevention. (2007). *Emergency preparedness and response.* Retrieved from https://emergency.cdc.gov/.

Centers for Disease Control and Prevention. (2016). *Coping with a disaster or traumatic event.* Retrieved from https://emergency.cdc.gov/coping/index.asp.

Substance Abuse and Mental Health Services Administration. (n.d.). *Disaster distress helpline.* Retrieved from http://www.samhsa.gov/find-help/disaster-distress-helpline.

U.S. Department of Health and Human Services, Centers for Disease Control and Prevention. (2001). *The public health response to biological and chemical terrorism: Interim planning guidance for state public health officials.* Retrieved from https://emergency.cdc.gov/Documents/Planning/PlanningGuidance.PDF.

U.S. Department of Homeland Security. (2017). Retrieved from https://www.ready.gov/.

ENVIRONMENTAL HEALTH

A recent report published by the World Health Organization (WHO) estimated that 12.6 million people die each year due to unhealthy living or working environments (WHO, 2016). The National Environmental Health Association Committee (NEHA, 2013) defines environmental health as a component of public health that prevents injury and illness, promotes wellness, reduces the impact of hazardous agents in the environment, and improves the safety of air, food, water, and soil. Hazards develop as a result of interaction between human beings and their environment. Environmental health focuses on assessing, evaluating, and controlling environmental contaminants that pose threat to human health, and seeking ways to prevent against diseases and injury caused by pollutants. The most critical environmental toxins are those that affect the quality of the outside air, surface, or ground water supply. The presence of such contaminants adversely affects body systems and quality of life detracting from years of healthy life.

The average adult breathes more than 24 kilograms of air daily (Moeller, 2005). Disposal of airborne waste in the form of gases, droplets, or particulates pollutes the air and impairs the ability to breathe. Environmental health researchers study air quality. The most common air pollutants come from emissions by automobiles, airplanes, or industrial sites; dust raised during agricultural processes; and smoke from forest fires or wood burning. Pollution is created when engine and fuel gases interact with the air under direct sunlight. The pollution contributes to poor air quality. Secondhand smoke is another serious air pollutant. The World Health Organization (WHO, 2016) reports an estimated 8.2 million people die annually due to secondhand inhalation of cigarette smoke. Direct and indirect smoking irritates the eyes, respiratory tract, and lungs, resulting in coughing, sneezing, asthma, tightness of the chest, or death due to severe acute respiratory syndrome (SARS), lung cancer, or cardiovascular disease. Air pollution also occurs within homes. Household pollutants occur from cooking and heating homes with stoves, wood, or other nonventilated fires. Household air pollution contributes to pneumonia, stroke, ischemic heart disease, chronic obstructive pulmonary disease (COPD), lung cancer, and premature death (WHO, 2016). Environmental health focuses on improving the quality of air, both outside and inside the home, as a way to minimize health issues and promote quality of life.

Global warming is a specific environmental health problem evidenced by rising average temperature across the globe. Higher temperatures are caused by large amounts of carbon dioxide and greenhouse gases in the atmosphere. Human activities, such as burning fossil fuels, forest fires, industrial processes, and agricultural practices, create global warming with subsequent climate change. Climate change affects the environment in a variety of ways, including persistent rising ocean tides and sea levels, heavy rains, floods, storms, winds, and severe heat waves. Changes result in reduced air quality, promotion of communicable pathogens, and potential for more frequent national disasters. All of these factors affect human health and promote human suffering. The role of the U.S. Environmental Protection Agency (EPA) is to control and monitor greenhouse gas (GHG) emissions, to protect human life, and to minimize human suffering. The EPA works through partnership with private sectors and local government to promote voluntary energy and climate programs. To reduce GHG, the EPA initiated several regulatory initiatives, including vehicle greenhouse gas rules. These rules are expected to eliminate 6 billion metric tons of GHG pollution and save $1.7 trillion at the pump by 2025 (EPA, 2016).

Ground and surface water are the main sources of drinking water for many families. In many areas of the country, ground water can be accessed from rain, snow, well, or bore hole. Using ground or surface water provides an inexpensive and convenient source of water. However, such sources can be easily contaminated by human activities. Lakes, rivers, and streams may become polluted with inorganic contaminants, volatile organic chemicals, pesticides, radioactive materials, or minerals (Moeller, 2005). Environmental health focuses on providing safe, clean water for drinking and sewage.

Another component of environmental health is monitoring and promoting a healthy environment by reducing exposure to harmful waste products. Hazardous wastes are solid wastes produced from manufacturing and industrial processes that have been identified by the Environmental Protection Agency (EPA) to cause serious disease or illness. Nonhazardous wastes are often called municipal wastes, and they include refuse, garbage, sludge, plastics, and municipal trash. Experts estimate that the United States produces about 6 billion tons of hazardous waste and 160 million tons of municipal waste each year (Moeller, 2005). Government and local environmental health officials take the disposal of toxic and hazardous waste seriously. Whereas municipal waste, which has minimal health risks to humans, is buried under the ground, hazardous waste is carefully disposed through sanitary landfill. Toxic substances and hazardous wastes are classified as solid waste by Congress in the Resource Conservation and Recovery Act (RCRA) of 1976. The EPA has the jurisdiction to enforce the mandate of the RCRA.

An environmental health professional or specialist is a university graduate with a bachelor's degree and certification from an approved environmental health program. Additional specialization is available to those individuals who want to pursue advanced degrees in environmental health, environmental epidemiology, toxicology, or public health. Environmental health specialists are trained to investigate and assess air, water, soil, and the living and working environments in order to determine compliance with government regulations. Responsibilities include handling complaints, collecting data, interpreting evidence, resolving concerns, and providing health education to the public. Positions are available in government and private sectors, as well as in academic, research, and consulting firms. According to the Bureau of Labor Statistics, the salary for an environmental health specialist ranges from $36,300 to $102,610 per year.

The field of environmental health continues to expand and embrace emerging issues that affect human health. In the United States, as well as in other parts of the world, climate change and global warming, disaster preparedness, exposure to unknown hazards, and bioterrorism are becoming great challenges to the field of environmental health, especially as they relate to human safety. Furthermore, global warming is changing the nature of public health to include greater focus on natural disasters due to floods, hurricanes, and drought. Although current efforts focus on disaster readiness to protect human health and safety, future efforts must include structural designs for solid roads, bridges, water banks, and a transportation system that can withstand strong storms, wind, and tornados. Emerging issues, such as clean energy, disposal of electronic devices, and overuse of plastic, should be part of the national agenda. Achievement of these goals begins with creating and supporting strong alliances with environmental shareholders, policy makers, government, and community leaders.

Victor Okparaeke

See also: Air Pollution; Bioterrorism; Environmental Protection Agency; Global Health; Modern Era, Public Health in the; Population Health; Prevention; U.S. Public Health Service; World Health Organization; *Controversies in Public Health:* Controversy 4

Further Reading

Environmental Protection Agency (EPA). (2016). *Climate change indicators in the United States* (4th ed.).

Moeller, D. W. (2005). *Environmental health* (3rd ed.). Cambridge, MA: Harvard University Press.

National Environmental Health Association. (2013). New perspective on environmental health: The approval of new definition. *Journal of Environmental Health, 76*(3), 72–73. Retrieved from http://neha.org/sites/default/files/about/JEH-Oct-2013-Definition-Environmental-Health.pdf.

World Health Organization (WHO). (2016). *Preventing disease through healthy environments* (2nd ed.). Geneva: Author.

ENVIRONMENTAL PROTECTION AGENCY (EPA)

Life on earth depends on water, nutrients from the soil, energy from the sun, and oxygen from the atmosphere. Environmental degradation causes disease. Water pollution causes hepatitis, cholera, typhus, yellow fever, and West Nile virus. Water pollution disrupts the food chain and destroys the ecosystem, increasing infectious diseases. Land pollution causes cancer and respiratory problems and breeds rats and other vectors that transmit disease. Air pollution causes asthma, birth defects, cancer, developmental disabilities, heart disease, and reproductive problems. Global warming increases the frequency and severity of heat waves, floods, and other extreme weather events, which expands the regions of disease-carrying vectors (mosquitos and ticks) and lengthens the seasons for mold, plant allergen, and pollen growth. Rising sea levels contaminate water and food supplies. The Environmental Protection Agency (EPA) is the federal agency responsible for supporting public health by protecting the air, water, and land.

The social and political movement of conservation and environmentalism started with environmental degradation. During colonial times, drinking water was drawn from a centralized spring or well or a nearby river. Boston was the first city to build waterworks to provide a plentiful source of clean water (Kempe, 2006). Boston's *Conduit* was not so much for drinking, bathing, or cleaning as it was for fighting fires. The thatched rooves of the city spread fires quickly. The system of wooden pipes was intended to fight fires. As city populations grew, so did refuse, waste, noise, and odors. People disposed of garbage and trash wherever they could, attracting rats and other vermin. In urban communities, neighbors shared an outhouse. Animals wandered through the streets, dropping refuse and spreading germs. Industries discharged waste and chemicals into rivers, streams, and lakes. Cemeteries sprung up near lakes and streams, contaminating drinking water during rainy seasons. Not surprisingly, deadly epidemics of cholera, typhoid, smallpox, and yellow fever occurred regularly. The industrial movement of the 1800s further compounded overcrowding, lack of sanitation, and deadly diseases. Attitudes and practices started to change with John Snow's study of cholera and Robert Koch's four postulates of infectious disease. Although germ theory created awareness, the problems of bacterial contamination were limited by the lack of tests for contamination. It was not until Julius Richard Petri's discovery of Apgar in 1887 that state boards of health could test public drinking water for bacterial contamination. Even with available testing, boards did not have the authority to close public wells or waterworks. Boards could only recommend that a community stop using a contaminated source. In 1893, the Quarantine Act gave boards of health the authority and responsibility to prevent the transmission of communicable diseases, which included ensuring the safety of public sources of drinking water.

As humans invaded forests, fields, and mountains, interest in conservationism grew. The literature of Herman Melville, Henry David Thoreau, John Burroughs, and John Muir presented people with the beauty and spirituality of nature (EPA,

1992). Preservation of natural resources became a priority under President Theodore Roosevelt. In 1916, President Woodrow Wilson founded the National Park Service. In 1933, President Franklin Roosevelt founded the Civilian Conservation Corps, a work relief program aimed at protecting natural resources. After World War II, economic growth and the baby boom pushed families into the suburbs, replacing farms and fields with housing developments. Confronted directly by nature, interest in land preservation and ecology increased along with fears of radioactive fallout and air and water pollution. When marine biologist Rachel Carson published *Silent Spring* (1962), the nation took notice. Carson's book warned of the harmful effects of indiscriminate pesticide use. The landmark event that led to the creation of the EPA occurred in 1969. Oil, trash, and debris floating on the Cuyahoga River in Ohio caught fire (Rotman, 2016). The river had actually caught fire several times. The largest and most destructive fire was in 1952 and caused more than $1 million in damage. Ohio's factories and towns had dumped waste, sewage, and trash into the river for decades. When industries closed, Cleveland residents were left with the most polluted river in America. After the 1969 fire, *Time* magazine published a photograph from the 1952 fire, the image of a small tugboat fighting multistory flames with thick, black, oil-fueled smoke.

A combination of events, the publication of *Silent Spring,* the Cuyahoga River fire, and public concern launched the environmental movement and demand for action by federal and state authorities. Wisconsin senator Gaylord Nelson brought the environmental movement to Washington, DC. The founder of Earth Day, Nelson believed, "Environment is all of America and its problems. It is rats in the ghetto. It is a hungry child in a land of affluence. It is housing not worthy of the name; neighborhoods not fit to inhabit" (Nelson Institute for Environmental Studies, n.d.). Presidents Kennedy, Johnson, and Nixon used the popularity of the environmental movement to campaign for and win their presidencies. Under public and political pressure, Nixon created the EPA in 1970. The regulatory agency provided an umbrella for what were previously piecemeal efforts in pesticide research and control, air pollution, water quality, solid waste management, and radiation control. The EPA assumed responsibilities from the Department of Agriculture, Department of Health, Education and Welfare, Department of the Interior, Food and Drug Administration, and the Bureaus of Solid Waste Management, Water Hygiene and Radiological Health. Nixon named William D. Ruckelshaus as the first EPA administrator.

Today, the EPA's purpose is to (1) protect all Americans from significant environmental health risks, (2) ensure that efforts to reduce environmental health risks are based on accurate science, (3) provide fair and effective enforcement of federal laws designed to protect the environment, (4) integrate environmental protection practices into new federal policies, (5) ensure access to accurate environmental information by all members of society, and (6) support and lead international efforts in protecting the global environment (EPA, 2017). As history has shown, not everyone

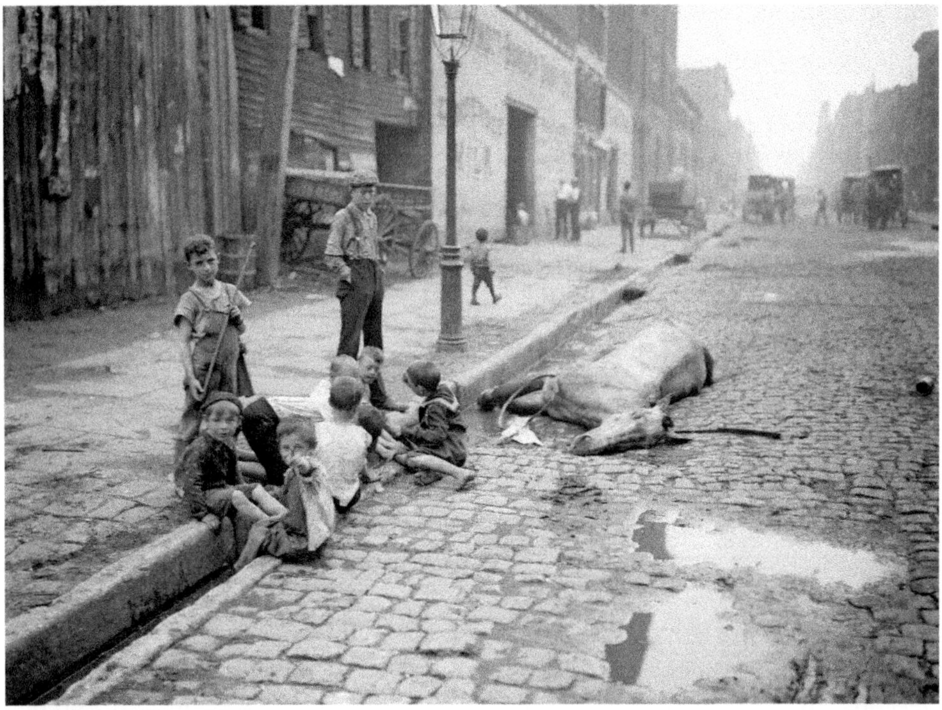

Children playing near a dead horse in New York City, ca. 1905. As city populations grew, so did refuse, waste, noise, odors, and pollution. Deadly epidemics of cholera, typhoid, smallpox, and yellow fever occurred regularly and local health officers held little authority. In 1970, President Richard Nixon created the Environmental Protection Agency (EPA) to protect Americans from environmental hazards. (Library of Congress)

voluntarily supports environmental protections. The EPA fulfills its mission through regulations and enforcement, grant funding, research, partnerships with businesses, nonprofit agencies, state and local governments, and health and environmental education. Some of the many public health concerns covered by the EPA are acid rain, air quality, bed bugs, climate change, drinking water, hazardous waste cleanups, lead poisoning, mold, pesticides, radon, and recycling. The agency is critical in ensuring that businesses, communities, and nations respect the earth and do not cause harm to human life.

Sally Kuykendall

See also: Air Pollution; Association of Public Health Laboratories; Centers for Disease Control and Prevention; Children's Health; Disease; Environmental Health; Food Safety; Grants; Quarantine; Waterborne Diseases

Further Reading

Environmental Protection Agency (EPA). (1992). *The guardian: Origins of the EPA*. Retrieved from https://archive.epa.gov/epa/aboutepa/guardian-origins-epa.html.

Environmental Protection Agency (EPA). (2017). Retrieved from https://www.epa.gov/.

Kempe, M. (2006). New England water supplies: A brief history. *Journal of the New England Water Works Association, 120*(3), 1–158. Retrieved from http://www.mwra.com/04water/html/historypaper/historypaper-mwra-kempe.html.

Nelson Institute for Environmental Studies. (n.d.). *Gaylord Nelson and Earth Day: The making of the modern environmental movement*. Madison: University of Wisconsin. Retrieved from http://www.nelsonearthday.net/nelson/.

Rotman, M. (2016). Cuyahoga River fire. *Cleveland historical*. Retrieved from https://clevelandhistorical.org/items/show/63.

EPIDEMIC

Epidemic is defined as an unexpected outbreak or spread of disease(s) within a group of people at a specific period of time. The word *epidemic* is a combination of two Greek words *epi*, meaning "upon, among, toward," and *demos*, meaning "common people." The term may apply to both infectious and noninfectious diseases. Noninfectious disease epidemics are health events, occurrences, conditions, or cases affecting a particular population. Examples of noninfectious epidemics are lead poisoning among children living on former Superfund sites, mesothelioma related to asbestos exposure among shipyard workers, or post-traumatic stress disorder (PTSD) among veterans. In comparison to sporadic cases of disease, epidemics are statistically significant increases in cases. For example, in 2013, there were 2,372 cases of pertussis (whooping cough) in California. In 2014, cases increased to 10,831, and by 2015 the number of cases decreased to 4,683 (California Department of Public Health, 2016; Winter, Glaser, Watt, Harriman, & CDC, 2014). The 2014 incidence rates were in excess of expected. When an epidemic spreads beyond the initial, immediate region or across continents, the spread is upgraded to a *pandemic*. Cardiovascular disease, obesity, and HIV/AIDS are pandemic health issues. When a disease is contained within a population and becomes a natural part of life, the problem is classified as *endemic*. Rocky Mountain spotted fever is endemic to certain areas on North, Central, and South America. Travelers to and residents of endemic regions are warned to take precautions to avoid tick bites. An epidemic with an alarmingly high rate of mortality is referred to as a *plague*. The Justinian plague (541–542) is estimated to have killed more than 25 million people throughout the Mediterranean region. Understanding the history and science of epidemics offers insight into public health prevention and control of future epidemics and significant loss of life.

Since epidemics are an emerging health threat, as opposed to an existing problem, several commonalities exist in when or how epidemics occur. Epidemics develop when the virulence of the pathogen or strength of the causal mechanism increases, the pathogen develops new portals of entry or modes of transmission, or the host becomes more susceptible to the causal agent. In 2000, the bacteria *Clostridium difficile* mutated to a stronger strain and over the next seven years, deaths increased 400 percent (CDC, 2013). Multiple environmental, socioeconomic, cultural, and geographic conditions influence susceptibility of potential hosts. Cases of mosquito borne diseases are higher in years with a mild winter, early and warm spring, dry spring and summer, or wet autumn. Geography can either facilitate or inhibit the spread of infections. Mountain ranges, deserts, and dense forests limit human interaction, stopping the spread. Waterways and transportation routes enhance opportunities for communicable disease transmission. Scientists note that the genomes of Zika have not changed in more than 70 years (Maron, 2016). What did change was geography. Zika was traditionally contained within remote areas of Uganda, Nigeria, Senegal, Malaysia, and South Africa, and health professionals were unaware of the health consequences. When the virus spread to other areas of the globe, public health professionals noted severe birth defects among infants of mothers who contracted the virus. Cultural practices may also facilitate disease transmission. In some cultures, funeral goers kiss the body of the departed loved one. This tradition can spread highly contagious microorganisms, such as Ebola. Therefore, at a time when people need the comfort of cultural traditions, public health professionals must intervene to stop practices. Although epidemic diseases may appear to be new and unexpected health threats, in reality, there are common characteristics that can be used as warning signs of impending problems.

Epidemics are classified based on the source of outbreak. The two main classifications are *common source outbreak* and *multiple source outbreak*. With common source outbreak, there is one reservoir. The pathogen is transmitted from this reservoir to potential victims from this one common source. Exposure from common source outbreaks may be either *point*, *continuous*, or *intermittent*. Point source outbreak refers to one source that infects people over a short period of time and within a limited geographic area. Food poisoning or cholera in the water supply are examples of point source outbreaks. It is easier to identify point sources because the victims will all report the same common exposure, eating at the same restaurant, living in the same area, or using water from the same well. In a continuous common source outbreak or intermittent outbreak, the individuals are exposed to the source of disease over an extended period. This is critical because prolonged exposure can lengthen time of recovery and may make it difficult to identify the source. Some people exposed to the source may not get ill, depending on how virulent the source is at the time of exposure.

Multiple source outbreak means that there are multiple sources transmitting the pathogen. Multiple source outbreaks are classified as *propagated*, *vector borne*, *vehicle borne*, and *seasonal*. Propagated refers to when one infected person transmits the disease to a second, uninfected person. Pertussis is an example of propagated transmission. *Bordetella pertussis* is passed from person to person through infected respiratory secretions. Vectors are insects (mosquitos, fleas, or lice) or arachnids (mites or ticks) that carry a parasite from area to area. The Zika virus is carried and transmitted by mosquitos. Vehicle borne transmission is transmission of the infection through inanimate objects. Meningitis may be spread by sharing drinking straws, toothbrushes, lipstick, or cigarettes. Seasonal outbreaks are influenced by climatic factors, such as seasons, prevailing wind conditions, and excess rainfall. For example, cold breezy weather during the winter season helps in the spread and transmission of influenza (flu). In the United States, seasonal flu epidemics occur from October to May, peaking in the winter. Regional air streams and local and seasonal prevailing wind conditions are a medium of transmission. Prevailing winds may help in arthropod transmission and migration of vectors. Heavy rainfall and flooding are associated with sewage overflow leading to widespread food and drinking water contamination with diseases such as dysentery, cholera, viral gastroenteritis (stomach flu), *cryptosporidiosis* (water diarrhea), *Escherichia coli*, and norovirus.

Numerous biological, behavioral, environmental, and socioeconomic factors influence the spread of diseases and resulting epidemics. Factors that create opportunities for an epidemic are deforestation, population movement, globalization, and overcrowding. Deforestation displaces animals from their natural habitat, which forces the migration and spread of vector borne illnesses. When people move from one area to another, they are at risk for new diseases and also carry pathogens that are endemic to their homeland. In the summer of 1837, the steamboat SS *St. Peter's* sailed from St. Louis to the fur trading post of Fort Union, delivering supplies along the Missouri River. Several of the deckhands and passengers were suffering from smallpox. Native Americans had struggled with smallpox epidemics since Spanish exploration in the 1500s. Inoculation practices, common throughout Europe and the East were unheard of among Native Americans. As the *St. Peter's* sailed along the route, it spread smallpox at each stop. More than 15,000 Native Americans died and several tribes were wiped out by the 1837 Great Plains smallpox epidemic. Socioeconomic factors can compound the threat of an epidemic. Overcrowding puts a strain on public amenities, resulting in poor living conditions, environmental health, hygiene, and unsafe food and drinking water. Areas with high population density suffering from unemployment, poverty, lack of education, and access to medical care are the most vulnerable.

Public health management of epidemics involves forecasting, investigation, control, and prevention. Through forecasting, public health professionals recognize the potential for an epidemic and take measures to prepare for the threat. Infectious disease scientists monitor the virulence and modes of transmission of various pathogens in order to categorize threats as urgent, serious, or concerning (CDC, 2013). State and local public health departments monitor immunization rates to ensure that an adequate number of people within the population receive vaccination and therefore cannot transmit the communicable disease. High immunization rates function similar to geographic obstacles. When 92 to 94 percent of the population are immunized against pertussis, it is harder for the bacterium to move from host to host. The probability of an infected host coming in contact with another susceptible person is low, a concept known as herd immunity. Events of man-made disasters (war or nuclear explosion) or natural disasters (famine, flooding, mud slides, tropical storms, hurricanes, earthquakes, or drought) are the perfect storm for potential epidemics. Forecasting can prevent or control the potential damage of an epidemic by ensuring that communities and health systems are prepared and the public is warned of impending threat and necessary precautions. During investigation, experts seek to identify the impact of the outbreak, time trend, affected population, and geographic location. Through such investigation, epidemiologists can identify causes, sources, and patterns in order to suggest ways to control epidemics. Controlling an epidemic involves identification of the source and mode of transmission. The goal of control is to eliminate the source, treat affected people, and prevent further spread. Affected individuals are treated through isolation, quarantine, vaccination, use of personal protection equipment, and education in personal hygiene. Fighting an epidemic requires the coordinated efforts of many individuals and groups from inside and outside of the affected community.

Epidemics of communicable diseases have plagued mankind since early civilization. As people, animals, and insects moved from one area to another, they carried tiny microorganisms capable of reaping immense havoc. Advances in microbiology, immunizations, and surveillance systems improved public health responses to these potential threats. Currently, public health professionals monitor epidemics around the world in order to forecast and prevent future outbreaks. As systems are developed to control the spread of infectious diseases, the nature of epidemics seems to change to the noninfectious communicable diseases of obesity, violence, and substance abuse. Future directions include applying the science of infectious diseases to noninfectious diseases in order to prevent the spread of imminent health threats.

Godyson Orji

See also: Cholera; Epidemiology; Global Health; Immigrant Health; Infectious Diseases; Influenza; Mallon, Mary; Measles; Middle Ages, Public Health in the; Modern Era, Public Health in the; Obesity; Pandemic; Polio; Quarantine; State, Local, and Territorial Health Departments; World Health Organization; *Controversies in Public Health:* Controversy 3; Controversy 5

Further Reading

California Department of Public Health. (2016). *Pertussis summary report.* Retrieved from http://www.cdph.ca.gov/programs/immunize/pages/pertussissummaryreports.aspx.

Centers for Disease Control and Prevention (CDC). (2012). *Principles of epidemiology in public health practice* (3rd ed.). Atlanta: U.S. Department of Health and Human Services. Retrieved from http://www.cdc.gov/ophss/csels/dsepd/ss1978/.

Centers for Disease Control and Prevention (CDC). (2013). *Antibiotic resistance threats in the United States, 2013.* U.S. Department of Health and Human Services. Retrieved from http://www.cdc.gov/drugresistance/threat-report-2013.

Centers for Disease Control and Prevention (CDC). (2016). *Zika virus*. Retrieved from http://www.cdc.gov/zika/index.html.

Maron, D. F. (2016). The Zika virus has changed little over 70 years—So why is it a problem now? *Scientific America*. Retrieved from http://www.scientificamerican.com/article/the-zika-virus-has-changed-little-over-70-years-so-why-is-it-a-problem-now/.

Winter, K., Glaser, C., Watt, J., Harriman, K., & Centers for Disease Control and Prevention (CDC). (2014). Pertussis epidemic—California, 2014. *Morbidity and Mortality Weekly Report, 63*(48), 1129–1132. Retrieved from http://www.cdc.gov/mmwr/preview/mmwrhtml/mm6348a2.htm?hc_location=ufi.

EPIDEMIOLOGY

The word *epidemiology* is a combination of three Greek words *epi*, meaning "upon, among," *demos*, meaning "people, district," and *logos*, meaning "study, word, discourse." From the three Greek words, epidemiology literally means the study of what is upon the people or what befalls the population. Epidemiology investigates health-related issues in a particular place at a specific time. By studying and mapping events and health outcomes, such as cases of infections, disabilities, birth defects, suicides, or injuries, health professionals can identify who gets the disease and possibly why. This information can spur ideas for cure and prevention. Epidemiology maps *disease* of a specific *population* at a particular *place* and *time*. For example, 7,840 men (population) were diagnosed with prostate cancer (disease) in New Jersey (place) in 2011 (time), which calculates to a prostate cancer incidence of 16 per 100 men, or 16 percent. *Population* might be an individual, group, community, or persons with defined characteristics, such as a specific age group, gender, ethnicity, profession, or socioeconomic status. *Time* could be measured in seconds, minutes, hours, days, weeks, duration, season, frequency of occurrence, or as a set period in time (one year after childbirth). *Place* focuses on the geographic locations of community, neighborhood, town, city, state, country, continent, or other location affected by the problem. Epidemiology is an interdisciplinary science, using scientific practices from public health, life sciences, biomedical, mathematical, behavioral, and social sciences. Through systematic inquiries and investigations, epidemiologists collect and analyze data in order to interpret and understand disease occurrences or other health-related events.

Outbreaks of disease follow logical patterns. Historically, infectious diseases were spread by people moving along heavily traveled ports and roads. AIDS transmission in Europe can be traced along trade routes in West-Central Africa. By mapping cases, epidemiologists estimate how a disease is spread and suggest ways to interrupt transmission. Similar to other disciplines, epidemiological studies are undertaken through systematic scientific methods. The process of studying a disease consists of (1) reviewing previous studies of similar health topics to identify best approaches, (2) developing research questions or hypotheses, (3) planning the study design and procedures, (4) collecting and analyzing data, and (5) drawing logical conclusions, based on the study results. The aims and objectives for epidemiological studies vary based on needs and our current understanding of the disease of interest. With emerging diseases, where the mode of transmission is unknown, epidemiologists might be interested in investigating etiology, transmission, risk factors, and how the disease is distributed within a population. This information allows public health to predict at-risk populations and to implement selective prevention programs. With reemerging diseases or health problems where the etiology is known, epidemiologists might study treatment and policy interventions as ways to mitigate or eradicate the problem. Epidemiological studies also look at the number of people affected by a specific disease or health status within a population of interest. One example might be investigating overweight and obesity among children and adolescents. Epidemiologists would want to study how many youth are affected overall and differences by gender, geographic region, or age.

Health data can be collected directly through interviews, observation, or survey of the affected population or indirectly through school records, public health records, census reports, medical records, registries (birth, death, cancer, immunization, or reportable diseases), insurance claims, or previous surveys. Collecting data directly from the affected population is referred to as primary data collection, whereas collecting data through intermediate sources is secondary data collection. Once the numbers of cases are tallied, results are analyzed by mathematical formula, standardizing the number of cases per 100, 1,000, 10,000, or 100,000 people in the population of interest. Incidence rates, prevalence rates, morbidity rates, and mortality rates allow statisticians to make comparisons between groups to determine which groups are at lowest, moderate, or highest risk. In Philadelphia, Pennsylvania, 13.7 per 100 (13.7 percent) of female high school students drink one soda two to three times per day. In comparison, 3.5 per 100 (3.5 percent) of female high school students in San Diego, California, drink one soda two to three times per day (Kann et al., 2016). Identifying risk allows professionals to focus limited public health resources or policy on those who are most affected by the problem. In an effort to counteract advertising by the beverage industry, Philadelphia became one of the first major cities in the United States to implement a soda tax. Identifying low-risk groups informs public health professionals of ways to build resistance against the health problem. By investigating why youth in San Diego drink less soda or pop than youth in other areas of the country, program planners can suggest other ways to reduce sugary beverage consumption and ultimately childhood obesity.

There are two major branches of epidemiology: *descriptive epidemiology* and *analytic epidemiology*. Descriptive epidemiology *describes* the pattern, distribution, and occurrences of a disease within a population in relation to the characteristics of the people (gender, race, or age), geographic location, and time (duration, season, or year). In addition to using numbers, descriptive epidemiologic studies also use qualitative methods. Interviewing people affected by the disease can provide insight into prevention and management. Analytic epidemiology measures cause-effect relationships and risk factors of disease, seeking to answer the why and how a disease affects specific populations. John Snow used descriptive epidemiology to map cholera cases in London in 1854. His map directed him to the cholera source, a contaminated water pump in Soho. Officials removed the pump handle, limiting further transmission and saving numerous lives. Analytic epidemiology is used to compare groups. Analytical epidemiologists analyze data through specialized mathematics, known as biostatistics. Complex mathematical calculations allow epidemiologists to control for differences between groups in order to draw inferences about the data.

Epidemiologic study designs are categorized as experimental or observational. Experimental designs manipulate a variable in order to test a research hypothesis. Clinical trials, cluster randomized trials, and field and community trials are used to test treatments or confirm causal relationships. These study designs provide strong evidence, linking exposure to outcomes. Observational studies measure the natural degree of exposure and status of disease within populations through cohort, case-control, and cross-sectional study methods. *Cohort studies* are used to estimate disease incidence over time or in comparison to other populations with varying levels of exposure. A cohort study may be both analytic and descriptive and may study present disease conditions (concurrent or prospective) or past disease (retrospective). Investigators do not manipulate variables or provide interventions in cohort studies. The Nurses' Health Study, the Framingham Heart Study, and the Black Women's Health Study are examples of large cohort studies. The Nurses' Health Study started in 1972 when Dr. Frank Speizer wanted to study long-term effects of oral contraceptive use. Dr. Speizer chose to study nurses because of their health knowledge and ability to report health information accurately and thoroughly. Since data collection started in 1976, more than 280,000 nurses have participated. Large cohort studies provide a wealth of information. *Case control studies* are used to compare people with disease (cases) to people without disease (controls). Data may be collected directly from the patient or indirectly from medical, laboratory, employment, or pharmacy records. Comparing cases to controls provides insights into potential risk or protective factors. Prospective study designs look forward in time, tracking people without the disease to learn who becomes affected by the disease and who does not. Retrospective studies investigate people with the disease and people without the disease to determine what exposures may have caused the disease. Prospective study designs are scientifically stronger because prospective studies collect data as events occur whereas retrospective studies rely on the individual's memory. People with disease will often reflect on past experiences and exposures, wondering why or how they got the disease. Thus, people with disease are more likely to recall exposures that those without disease may have forgotten. This time or reason to reflect creates a limitation known as recall bias. Cross-sectional studies provide a snapshot in time, examining rates of exposure and rates of disease at the same point in time. Cross-sectional studies are used to collect information about health and risk factors. Although cross-sectional studies are useful for preliminary investigation, planning and allocation of health resources and prevention programs, cross-sectional studies also have limitations. Cross-sectional studies only tell us whether two variables existed together in higher numbers than expected. The designs do not tell us whether one variable caused the other. For example, a cross-sectional survey of student athletes may reveal that football players report higher rates of traumatic brain injury (TBI) than track and field athletes. Because cross-sectional surveys only measure variables at one point in time, we don't know whether football increases risk of TBI or whether athletes with TBI are more attracted to football, or if a third, moderating variable influences the relationship. Only prospective studies can tell us which came first, football or TBI.

Epidemiological studies are embedded in scientific research using carefully planned methods, data collection, and statistical analysis to identify trends in disease and to find solutions to cure, treat, prevent, and control diseases. Descriptive and analytic studies analyze patterns of disease to identify who is affected, where, and when. Results provide information on risk factors, effects, causes, prevention, and control. Epidemiology provides a backbone to public health planning and action, exploring the causes of disease, and suggesting ways to advance prevention, treatment, and cure.

Godyson Orji

See also: Cholera; Epidemic; Food Safety; Global Health; Infectious Diseases; Modern Era, Public Health in the; Pandemic; Research; Snow, John

Further Reading

American College of Epidemiology. (2017). Retrieved from http://acepidemiology.org/.

Aschengrau, A., & Seage, G. R. (2013). *Essentials of epidemiology in public health*. Burlington, MA: Jones & Bartlett.

Epimonitor. (2017). *The epidemiology monitor.* Retrieved from http://www.epimonitor.net/.

Friis, R. H., & Sellers, T. (2013). *Epidemiology for public health practice*. Burlington, MA: Jones & Bartlett.

Kann, L., McManus, T., Harris, W. A., Shanklin, S. L., Flint, K. H., Hawkins, J., & Zaza, S. (2016). Youth risk behavior surveillance—United States, 2015. *Morbidity and Mortality Weekly Report. Surveillance Summaries (Washington, DC: 2002)*, *65*(6), 1–174. doi:10.15585/mmwr.ss6506a1. Retrieved from http://www.cdc.gov/healthyyouth/data/yrbs/pdf/2015/ss6506_updated.pdf.

Nurses' Health Study. (2017). Retrieved from http://www.nurseshealthstudy.org/.

Rothman, K. J., Greenland, S., & Lash, T. L. (1998). Types of epidemiologic studies. *Modern Epidemiology*, 3, 95–97. Retrieved from http://www.medicine.mcgill.ca/epidemiology/hanley/bios601/Comparativegeneral/..%5CRothmanGreenland98/RothmanGreenland05TypesEpiStudies.pdf.

ETHICS IN PUBLIC HEALTH AND POPULATION HEALTH

Public health ethics is an interdisciplinary field where ethical issues and possible interventions are investigated and analyzed in order to develop ethically sound health promotion policies and practices. Public health refers to the network of health promotion and disease prevention systems designed to meet the needs of the general population and at-risk populations. Population health refers to the health outcomes of a population or the general population's health status in reference to the existing health care systems. Improving population health means reducing health disparities, enhancing overall quality of the health care system, and promoting a health-conscious culture. The fundamental ethical principles that guide public health practice and research are respect for persons, beneficence, and justice. These ethical principles define professional boundaries and norms of conduct that differentiate acceptable from unacceptable behavior. Problems arise when two or more ethical principles come in conflict with each other. For example, consider the idea that laws requiring people to eat healthily would be a quick and highly effective way of reducing heart disease, diabetes, high blood pressure, and other obesity-related diseases. However, public health is guided by ethical principles, one of which requires practitioners and policy makers to respect the autonomy (free will) of individuals. Public health ethics present a systematic process of identifying, prioritizing, and justifying a course of action based on ethical principles.

The principle of respect for persons demands that each person has the right to be treated with dignity and respect. The principle of beneficence dictates a responsibility to promote and enhance the good of others. Beneficence complements nonmaleficence, which prohibits the infliction of harm, injury, or death. Nonmaleficence originates from the Hippocratic Oath. In ancient Roman medicine, beneficence is presented in the negative form. The agent is cautioned not to inflict harm, injury, or death on others. Justice refers to the fair distribution of burdens and benefits where vulnerable populations, groups lacking political or social power, do not have a greater burden of illness or responsibility than others in society. Ethical issues in population health research and policy often revolve around the concept of distributive justice. The issue of distributive justice begins with designating a particular population group. The group typically already exists and has agreed to basic sociopolitical systems through formal or informal social contract. Attempts toward just distribution of health (and health care) resources are determined by or within the social system.

The traditional sense of distributive justice (henceforth "justice") is justice as desert, that is, everyone should get what they deserve. However, this view is too simple to employ for our complex capitalist system. Also, it has apparent difficulty locating the meaning of what kind of health resource in what quality is deserved, who deserves it, and how much one deserves; thus, it lacks practical import to become our ethical justification. Needs-based theory of justice states that goods must be distributed based on everyone's needs. However, this is fundamentally the Marxist/Communist ideology, which does not fit in with the current health care system in the United States. The U.S. capitalist health and health care economy is run by a free market economy where better quality of care or "luxury care" is available for those who can pay. The ethical justification we are looking for is a type of market distributive justice. Contribution-based theory argues that goods should be distributed to match an individual's overall contribution to the society. However, the theory justifies the system that the vulnerable in society continuously suffers because, according to the theory, it is ethically just to let the poor and the handicapped access poor quality of or less health care because they contribute to the society less than other members. However, the theory is fragile because it is exposed to a practical contraction. For example, the capitalist society allows, say, a handicapped person to be treated with great health care when the patient's rich family members who contribute greatly to the society pay for the patient. Then, the same act will be considered just and unjust at the same time. Another popular theory of justice, utilitarianism, says that just distribution will be allocating goods in the way of producing the best consequences for the greatest number of people by taking everyone's goods impartially into account. However, this may demand sacrifice of some members for the good of others in an unrealistic, utopian fashion. Since the poor outnumber the rich, the just distribution of health for the greatest number will be to provide health resources for the poor via harsh taxation for the rich, which is against the principle of market economy.

Philosopher John Rawls's difference principle argues that social and economic inequalities are granted but to be arranged in such a way that the least privileged have the greatest benefit. Granted that population health thinking concerns, first, improving the overall quality of general health system while, second, reducing health and health care disparities, the difference principle gives the ethical direction in which the former concern should be fulfilled in reference to the latter concern. In other words, the effort to improve the overall health system should be carried out in order for the most vulnerable population to have the greatest benefit. There is difficulty coming to an agreement on the identification of the most vulnerable group and also the greatest benefit for them. However, this is not a notorious difficulty. We have a specific focus, the health system in the capitalist-liberal democratic country. Also, there exists the relatively accurate statistics that shows that racial/ethnic minorities and low-income individuals are the most vulnerable groups. There is a pretty good sense of distinguishing basic health care from luxury care. There should be other ethical concerns to deal with along the way, as particular health policies or programs develop. However, provided that we have agreed on these basic terms and data, the policies developed and refined in accordance with the difference principle can be ethically sound interventions.

Through such consideration, scholars may suggest ethical justifications and directives for particular population health research and policies in order to obtain ethical soundness. In many cases, ethical principles are what differentiate public health from other professions and businesses. Pharmaceutical companies are not held to the same level of responsibility for beneficence; otherwise they would not be earning millions of dollars per year. In all functions and all matters, public health professionals consider the ethical implications of each decision, action, and policy.

Marvin J. H. Lee

See also: Belmont Report, The; Code of Ethics; Epidemiology; Greco-Roman Era, Public Health in the; Health Care Disparities; Hippocrates; Population Health, Tuskegee Syphilis Study; *Controversies in Public Health:* Controversy 1; Controversy 3; Controversy 4; Controversy 5

Further Reading

Allingham, M. (2014). *Distributive justice*. London and New York: Routledge.

Beauchamp, T. L., & Childress, J. F. (1994). *Principles of biomedical ethics*. New York: Oxford University Press.

Department of Health, Education, and Welfare. (1979). *The Belmont report*. Retrieved from http://www.hhs.gov/ohrp/regulations-and-policy/belmont-report/.

Rawls, J. (1993). *Political liberalism*. New York: Columbia University Press.

EVALUATION

Public health professionals use a wide variety of initiatives, interventions, treatments, and programs to promote health and prevent illness. Evaluations are a type of research design used to investigate whether these activities are (1) feasible for the target audience, (2) effective in addressing the health concern of interest, and/or (3) cost effective. Ideally, evaluation results add to our existing knowledge of the topic and guide ways to improve practices, new policy, or community initiatives. Program objectives are used to guide and structure the evaluation. A program to reduce smoking among teenagers is evaluated by investigating whether the youth who attended the program actually stopped or reduced cigarette smoking. Program objectives may be short term, such as improving knowledge about the adverse effects of cigarette smoking; intermediate, changing attitudes to decrease the attraction of smoking; or long term, reducing the number of people who currently smoke. Through program evaluations, public health professionals can determine which programs work for the target population, and stakeholders can determine if program funding should continue. Limitations of program evaluations are that they often measure outcomes over a short period. If the behavior relapses or improves outside of the evaluation period, this result may not be captured by the evaluation study. Also, many different factors influence health behaviors. The smoking cessation program may successfully educate participants on the negative effects of smoking. However, if the participants are simultaneously exposed to heavy product placement, where tobacco companies embed their product into popular movies or videos, the evaluation could show increased usage. Evaluations tell us *if* a program works; they do not tell us *how* a program works. The field of evaluation research continues to develop as a science, seeking to inform communities on the best ways to allocate public health resources.

Evaluation studies range in formality and purpose. Formal evaluations are planned in advance, before the program or treatment is offered. Preplanning with an evaluation expert ensures that the evaluation is feasible, follows ethical practice guidelines, legitimately measures what it is intended to measure, and addresses the needs of funders, collaborators, and participants. Data are collected at the start and the end of the program and sometimes, throughout the program. For example, the researchers evaluating a smoking cessation program might collect urine samples from participants to measure urine cotinine levels. (Cotinine is produced when the body breaks down nicotine.) The first cotinine levels, collected before the program starts, are referred to as pretest or baseline data. Posttest data are gathered at the end of the program or at a set time point, such as six months or one year post-program. The evaluator compares posttest results with pretest to identify any changes that occurred. Although urine cotinine levels are a convenient and accurate way to measure smoking, the transtheoretical model tells us that people typically take two years to change a health behavior. An evaluation that measures cotinine immediately at the end of the program will miss participants who stop smoking within the two years after the program. Informal evaluations are less structured and may consist of asking participants or the instructor what they feel are strengths and weaknesses of the program or how the program could be improved. Formal evaluations are designed to gather credible evidence that a program is effective. Informal evaluations are designed to describe, improve, or refine a program.

Whenever possible, evaluations use existing instruments with proven validity and reliability. Instruments are the tools that researchers use to collect data. Examples of instruments are height and weight scales to measure BMI, a sphygmomanometer to measure blood pressure, or a survey to measure participant knowledge, attitudes, and behaviors. Validity and reliability assess the quality of the instrument. Validity describes how well the instrument measures what it is intended to measure. With a few exceptions, using a good quality medical scale to assess BMI is a fairly valid measure of underweight, normal weight, overweight, or obese status. Reliability describes how stable the instrument is over time. We expect a good quality medical scale to give the same results under the same circumstances. If someone weighs 135 pounds today and does not gain or lose weight, we expect the scale to measure 135 pounds the next day, and the next day, as long as the individual's weight does not change. An instrument could be invalid, measuring 5 pounds higher than the person actually weighs. However, as long as the scale is consistently 5 pounds higher, it is still reliable. On the other hand, BMI is less valid when used to assess athletes with high muscle mass, women who are pregnant, and children. The evaluator will select a quality instrument with proven validity and reliability whenever possible because using the same instrument allows researchers to compare study results. With some health topics, instruments do not exist and the evaluator must develop a new instrument.

There are different types of evaluations that target different aspects of a program. Formative evaluations, also known as process evaluations, assess the project during planning and/or implementation. Process evaluations gather information from participants, the instructor, or key stakeholders on how the program is progressing. Formative assessment of the smoking cessation program may survey participants to see if they prefer certain learning activities over others, whether they feel the instructor is qualified, or if the classroom or physical surroundings are comfortable. Summative evaluations assess the outcomes of the program. Ideally, the smoking cessation program would measure the number of participants who stop smoking. Summative evaluations allow reviewers to draw conclusions on how effective the program is by studying impact and/or outcome. Impact evaluations examine the short-term or intermediate benefits, such as changes in knowledge, attitudes, or skills. Outcome evaluations study long-term benefits, such as improving quality of life or reducing morbidity and mortality. Evaluation studies can be simple, studying only one aspect such as process, or very complex, studying process, impact, and outcome. Larger studies use the concept of triangulation, evaluating several different impact and outcome measures in order to get a bigger picture of program effects.

Although it seems that all evaluations should focus on process, impact and outcome simultaneously, in reality the type of evaluation depends on where we are in understanding the problem. In the early days of smoking research, the researchers did not have a set definition for smoking. They needed to perform a process evaluation, developing and testing a definition. After experts agreed on the definition, it became important to measure program impact, whether programs changed attitudes toward smoking. Today, evaluators look at process, impact, outcome, and an additional variable, fidelity of implementation. Fidelity of implementation measures whether the instructors are presenting the program as it was intended by the original program author. Evaluation studies are like relay races. The first evaluator completes a process evaluation, passing the results to the next evaluator who confirms or refutes the initial results, and enhances ideas for the next study, which are passed to the next evaluator. Results and ideas for improving evaluations are communicated through technical reports, conferences, professional journals, and books. This process ensures that the field of research continues to move forward, improving techniques and understanding of the issue. When enough evidence is gathered to suggest that a program works, the evaluation studies are reviewed by groups of independent experts. This review determines whether the program meets the criteria necessary to be granted the status of evidence-based program. Examples of evidence-based programs in smoking cessation are Adolescent Smoking Cessation: Escaping Nicotine and Tobacco Program (ASCENT), Good Behavior Game, Not On Tobacco (N-O-T), and Project EX.

Evaluations are an unusual form of research known as translational research. In some disciplines, the scholar depends primarily on books or existing documents for ideas and information. This ivory tower research remains disconnected from the real world, providing few practical benefits. The evaluation researcher must take complex models and theories from the ivory tower and translate the concepts into real-world practices. This is particularly important where people want a quick fix or have ill-conceived ideas as to how to fix a problem. For example, many schools like bringing the local police in for smoking and drug prevention education. In theory, using the local police as health educators seems like a great idea. Police-sponsored programs are usually free, officers are readily available, and this seems like a great way to build community connections. In practice, police are not trained as health educators, often lack knowledge of the unique traits of adolescent brain development and how this applies to health promotion programs, or have severely alienated at-risk populations. What message is conveyed to the victim of bullying when a police officer walks into the classroom with a gun and suddenly commands immediate respect? A well-planned and insightful evaluation is like a finger on the pulse of the community, constantly assessing and evaluating whether the program works the way that it was intended to work. Translational research not only tells us what happened within the program but also what needs to be done next.

The real-life nature of program evaluations presents limitations. It may be hard to measure the variable of interest or new technology may come out that changes behavior. Smoking cigarettes is being replaced by e-cigarettes, which can also be harmful to health. New forms of social media provide tobacco companies with never-ending ways to sell their product. Program planners may be wary of the evaluator or the evaluation instrument, resulting in reluctance to share data or access participants. A major issue with program evaluations is that typically when a program is implemented, participant awareness increases. Individuals who previously considered themselves nonsmokers because they only smoked one to two cigarettes a week may now realize that they are, in fact, smokers.

People might have a wonderful idea of how to address a health issue. However, if the idea does not work in the real world or makes the problem worse, we've wasted precious funding and resources, while allowing the problem to continue. Evaluations are a unique part of program implementation that studies whether public health initiatives, techniques, treatments, or programs work to enhance health and prevent disease. Through evaluation studies, we are able to move forward and develop better ways to handle health issues.

Sally Kuykendall

See also: Body Mass Index; Causality; Evidence-Based Programs and Practices; Goals and Objectives; Health Education; PRECEDE-PROCEED Planning Model; Public Health Department Accreditation; RE-AIM (Reach, Effectiveness, Adoption, Implementation, and Maintenance); Research; Syringe Service Programs; Transtheoretical Model; Truth Campaign, The

Further Reading

Craig, P., & Campbell, M. (2015). Evaluability assessment: A systematic approach to deciding whether and how to evaluate programmes and policies. *What works Scotland.* Retrieved from https://edge.sagepub.com/system/files/Evaluability%20Assessment.pdf.

Newcomer, K. E., Hatry, H. P., & Wholey, J. S. (2015). *Handbook of practical program evaluation* (4th ed.). San Francisco: Jossey-Bass.

Smith, M. F. (2015). Evaluability assessment. In S. Mathison (Eds.), *Encyclopedia of evaluation.* Thousand Oaks, CA: Sage. Retrieved from https://edge.sagepub.com/system/files/Evaluability%20Assessment.pdf.

EVIDENCE-BASED PROGRAMS AND PRACTICES

Evidence-based programs and practices are health promotion or disease prevention activities that have been tested and proven to work. Evidence-based medicine has been around since ancient healers first recorded which herbs successfully treated diseases. The same logic and science is applied to social and behavioral programs. Teams of researchers, experts, and practitioners review evidence from program evaluations to determine which programs are effective. Organizations, such as the Campbell Collaboration, the Center for the Study and Prevention of Violence of the University of Colorado at Boulder, Cochrane Collaboration, Office of Juvenile Justice and Delinquency Prevention (OJJDP), and the Substance Abuse and Mental Health Services Administration's National Registry of Evidence-Based Programs and Practices (NREPP) list and report effectiveness of programs. Several groups provide searchable databases for community members to assist in deciding on which program is best for a particular school or community. The databases allow users to search by gender, age of the target population (middle school or high school), demographic location (urban, suburban, or rural), and purpose (bullying prevention, substance abuse prevention, or other behavior). The main advantage to evidence-based programs is that the curriculum or activities are already developed, refined, and tested, saving a great deal of time, resources, and effort. Unfortunately, some people have strong views on how to fix social problems and are either unable or unwilling to use the available science. There is still a misconception that the flashy, expensive program advertised by a popular talk show host is preferable to a scientifically developed and tested program.

In 2001, public health experts produced *Youth Violence: Report of the Surgeon General*. The report reviewed existing violence programs and concluded that some of the most popular and well-recognized programs did not work. The problem with using ineffective programs is that they distract attention and resources from programs that do work. Community leaders, school officials, and parents are not likely to use an evidence-based program if they believe (incorrectly) that the current program will prevent violence or substance abuse. The surgeon general's report was followed up with work by researchers at the Center for the Study and Prevention of Violence (CSPV) at the University of Colorado at Boulder. After reviewing more than 600 programs, the researchers found that only 20 percent actually reduced youth violence. Some of the most popular programs were either ineffective or caused greater harm. For example, group therapy for young offenders can increase risk of offending because the group provides informal training in antisocial behavior. Lower offending youth learn worse behaviors.

When experts assess program effectiveness, they look at how the program was implemented and evaluated, the quality of evaluation measures, and evaluation results. They carefully review the evidence supporting the program. Effective public health programs are carefully planned integrating models and theories of how people learn and how people change health behaviors. Program outcomes should match program objectives. A program designed to prevent smoking should, in fact, prevent smoking. Quality evaluations compare data before and after the program and to a similar control group. Results are expected to show statistical significance. This means that the smoking prevention program does not simply lower the number of smokers, but the differences are large enough that they did not occur by chance. After review of the evidence, the program is categorized as harmful, unsupported, promising, supported, or well supported. Communities are advised not to use harmful programs. Unsupported programs or promising programs may be used within particular contexts. Ideally, the program designers need to gather further evidence and resubmit the program for review. When available, supported and well-supported programs are preferred.

Implementing evidence-based practices can be challenging. In schools, teachers may need to change practices and learn new ways to address behavioral problems. In communities, adults in positions of power may need to give up power in order to work with public health educators. The benefits of using evidence-based programs are substantial. Researchers estimate using evidence-based bullying programs in 125,000 public and private schools would cost $625 million per year. With school violence costing $14.4 billion to $40.3 billion per year, evidence-based programs would save up to $39.7 billion per year (Pereznieto, Harper, Clench, & Coarasa, 2010). Even after a program has achieved model status, program authors will continue to evaluate, review, and update program materials to proactively address health problems. For example, early evidence-based bullying prevention programs did not include cyberbullying because at the time they were created most children did not have regular access to technology. With the growth in social networking, programs were updated to include cyberbullying.

In the past, social programs were controversial because many did not work, and stakeholders felt that the resources used toward such programs were wasteful. Efforts by the federal government, academics, researchers, and public health practitioners identified effective and ineffective programs, developing databases for use by communities. In using evidence-based programs, communities can effectively reduce issues of substance abuse and youth violence. The next steps are to educate politicians, educators, and parents on the science and benefits of evidence-based programs.

Sally Kuykendall

See also: Addictions; Behavioral Health; Causality; Evaluation; Goals and Objectives; Health Education; Intervention; Research; Substance Abuse and Mental Health Services Administration; Violence

Further Reading

Campbell Collaboration. (2016). *What helps? What harms? Based on what evidence?* Retrieved from http://www.campbellcollaboration.org/.

Injury Prevention and Control, Division of Violence Prevention, Centers for Disease Control and Prevention. (2017). *Violence education tools online.* Retrieved from Centers for Disease Control and Prevention, http://vetoviolence.cdc.gov/.

Institute of Behavioral Science, University of Colorado Boulder. (2016). *Blueprints for healthy youth development.* Retrieved from http://www.blueprintsprograms.com/.

Office of Juvenile Justice and Delinquency Prevention. (2016). *Model programs guide.* Retrieved from http://www.ojjdp.gov/mpg/.

Pereznieto, P., Harper, C., Clench, B., & Coarasa, J. (2010). *The economic impact of school violence: A report for plan international.* London: Overseas Development Institute. Retrieved from http://www.odi.org/sites/odi.org.uk/files/odi-assets/publications-opinion-files/6289.pdf.

Substance Abuse and Mental Health Services Administration. (2016). *NREPP: SAMHSA's National Registry of Evidence-Based Programs and Practices.* Retrieved from http://www.samhsa.gov/nrepp.

U.S. Department of Health and Human Services. (2001). *Youth violence: A report of the surgeon general.* Rockville, MD: U.S. Department of Health and Human Services, Centers for Disease Control and Prevention, National Center for Injury Prevention and Control; Substance Abuse and Mental Health Services Administration, Center for Mental Health Services; and National Institutes of Health, National Institute of Mental Health.

F

FALSE CLAIMS ACT (FCA)

The False Claims Act (FCA) was not originally intended for the health care industry. Started during the Civil War, the FCA was established to combat merchants who tried to defraud the federal government by selling rancid food, poor quality shoes and clothing, broken down horses and mules, and faulty rifles to the Union and Confederate Armies. Also referred to as the "Lincoln Law," the law contained a provision compensating whistleblowers who reported fraud that resulted in recovery for the government. *Qui tam* is a legal term that means "who as well for the king [government] as for himself sues in this matter." The term refers to a civil suit where the person is suing on behalf of the government. By World War II, people had found ways to manipulate the system. When the Department of Justice filed criminal charges, lawyers would file civil suits claiming a *qui tam* reward. Congress was going to eliminate the FCA and instead ruled to reduce the amounts paid to whistleblowers. In 1986, the law was extended to make it a crime for any individual to defraud the federal government, including making a false medical record or payment claim. False Medicare and Medicaid claims were a growing concern. Under the FCA, providers cannot knowingly make a false claim, submit a false record, misrepresent goods, or buy government property from other than authorized sellers. In 2010, the FCA was further refined by the Affordable Care Act. Under the ACA, only the original source of a fraud disclosure may file for *qui tam* reward. If the fraud has already been disclosed through public sources, *qui tam* suits are automatically dismissed. Under the FCA, health providers and those who do business with local departments of public health must have a strong compliance plan. Penalties range from $5,000 to $11,000 per claim as well as additional penalties three times the initial claim. Between 1996 and 2005, the government recovered $9.3 billion of fraudulent Medicare and Medicaid claims (Kesselheim & Studdert, 2008). Of the 379 cases, only 13 cases were against pharmaceutical companies, yet those cases totaled $3.6 billion. Whistleblowers were primarily physicians or business executives motivated by a sense of integrity and ethics. As health care systems continue to grow and become more complex, health care fraud will most likely continue to be a problem. Given the temptations of some, it is the responsibility of the individual employee to report suspected abuse. Unfortunately, many employees fear retaliation by those in positions of power within the company. Finding ways to protect and support whistleblowers can reduce fraud and increase available health care resources.

Sally Kuykendall and Leapolda Figueroa

See also: Administration, Health; Affordable Care Act; Public Health Law; Stark Law

Further Reading

Kesselheim, A. S., & Studdert, D. M. (2008). Whistleblower-initiated enforcement actions against health care fraud and abuse in the United States, 1996 to 2005. *Annals of Internal Medicine*, *149*(5), 342–371.

Stubbs, J. D. (2013). The 2009 Amendment expands the types of fraud subject to the federal false claims act. *Florida Bar Journal*, *87*(2), 16–23.

Total Healthcare. (2016). *False claims act overview.* Retrieved from https://thcmi.com/PDF/common/False%20Claims%20Act%20Policy.pdf.

FAMILY PLANNING

Family planning refers to health and medical services that empower women to control the timing, spacing, and number of pregnancies. The services include access to contraception, pregnancy testing, counseling, preconception health screening and treatment, infertility care, and screening and treatment for sexually transmitted diseases (STDs). The ability to control reproduction promotes maternal, infant, family, and community health. Reproductive health services reduced maternal death rate from 608 women per 100,000 live births to 12 women per 100,000 live births (Hoyert, 2007). Contraceptives prevent 1.9 million pregnancies per year, reducing the demand for elective abortions (Guttmacher Institute, 2016). Family planning builds healthier communities with less poverty and better quality of life. Women are free to work or volunteer and can focus their time and resources on fewer children. Every tax dollar spent on family planning services saves $7 in Medicaid and other expenditures (Guttmacher, 2016). Contraceptive and infertility services also provide an opportunity for health care providers to screen for breast or cervical cancer, hypertension, lipid disorders, skin cancer, osteoporosis, and intimate partner violence. Early screening, referral, and treatment improve health and reduce premature mortality. The major obstacles to family planning are a lack of education, limited access to services, and lack of support by partners or society.

In the United States the birth control movement was started by a public health nurse. Working with poor, immigrant women in New York City, Margaret Sanger witnessed a frighteningly high number of infant and maternal deaths. For every 1,000 live births, 102 to 181 infants died and 6 to 11 women (Lindner & Grove, 1947, tables 26 and 36). (The lower numbers report "white" death rates, and the higher numbers report death rates of "other races," i.e., African American, Italian American, Greek American, and Jewish American, the community that Sanger served.) The medical causes of infant death, infectious diseases, diarrhea, premature birth, congenital malformations, pneumonia, and injury were primarily due to social problems of poor nutrition, poverty, and neglect. Without the benefit of unlimited resources, mothers struggled to care for their children. Sanger witnessed how botched abortions, too many pregnancies, and family violence claimed the physical and emotional lives of women. She started teaching her patients about birth control, reproduction, and women's health. The information was considered radical and immoral, a threat to puritan values. Sanger was charged and indicted with violating federal obscenity laws. She fled to England. However, as she left U.S. territory, she signaled a publisher to print and distribute 100,000 copies of *Family Limitation,* a 16-page booklet describing different methods of birth control. Sanger returned from England the following year and opened the first birth control clinic in the United States. Women stood in line for care until the New York police closed the clinic. Sanger's case stimulated public discourse, and physicians were given permission to counsel patients on birth control. In 1952, Sanger founded International Planned Parenthood and a decade later, the United States legalized birth control for married couples. As concerns for population growth increased, the federal government established the Family Planning Services and Population Act (1970) and created Title X of the Public Health Service Act. Title X is the health program of the Office of Population Affairs designed to provide family planning and related health services.

As the cost of raising children increased and opportunities for females expanded, the image of the ideal family size dropped from four children to two children (Gao, 2015). The American Academy of Pediatrics describes many benefits to smaller family size. Parents can focus attention, resources, and educational opportunities on a fewer number of children, which means higher self-esteem for the child, lower household costs, fewer families in poverty, better life-career balance, less stress, and greater financial security. This means that many women spend the majority of their reproductive lives *trying to avoid pregnancy*. Too often, the 30-year effort results in at least one error. By the age of 45, 49 percent of women report an unintended pregnancy and 3 out of 10 women report having an abortion (Guttmacher, 2016). Highest risk groups for unintended pregnancy are adolescents, minority women, and women with incomes below the federal poverty line. The United States has one of the highest teen pregnancy rates (40 pregnancies per 1,000 females aged 15 to 17) (Office of Disease Prevention and Health Promotion, 2017). *Healthy People 2020* lists 16 family-planning objectives. The objectives focus on increasing the number of females and males who use reproductive health services and contraception; increasing the proportion of intended pregnancies; increasing the number of teenagers who receive formal instruction on reproductive health; increasing the number of teenagers who talk with a parent or guardian about reproductive health; reducing teen sexual activity and pregnancies; reducing pregnancies that occur as a result of contraceptive failure; reducing the number of pregnancies that occur within 18 months of previous childbirth; and increasing publicly funded family planning clinics and health insurance plans that offer access to FDA-approved contraception (Office of Disease Prevention and Health Promotion, 2017).

Healthy People 2020 objectives show how family planning extends beyond contraception to include comprehensive sex education, STD prevention, preconception health, infertility treatment, pregnancy testing and counseling, and postpartum care.

Since the publication of *Family Limitation*, contraceptive options have significantly increased and improved. Although abstinence is the most effective method of preventing pregnancy and STDs, sexually active women and men can choose from a wide variety of birth control methods. Choice varies based on individual preferences, safety, efficacy, reversibility, accessibility, and need for protection from STDs. National and local organizations, such as Planned Parenthood, offer free family planning services. Preconception care can significantly reduce infant mortality. An estimated 23,000 infants die each year, and more than half of these deaths are caused by birth defects, preterm birth, maternal complications due to pregnancy, sudden infant death syndrome (SIDS), and injuries (Centers for Disease Control and Prevention, 2017). Pregnancy planning and counseling gives health care professionals time to screen for and detect preventable diseases, improving the health of the mother and improving pregnancy outcomes. Unfortunately, the quality of services can vary. The key features of quality health services are the provision of safe, effective, client-centered, timely, efficient, accessible, and equitable value-based care. Public health clinics use these features to assess the quality and value of their services.

Family planning is one of the greatest public health achievements of all time. Comprehensive sex education, contraception, and pregnancy counseling empower women to control the number and spacing of pregnancies, thus promoting maternal and child health. Despite successes, restrictive policies and laws often limit funding. Public health efforts to reduce unintended pregnancies and provide an array of reproductive health services are challenged by personal values and misconceptions that limit funding and service provision. As populations grow and demands on natural resources exceed supply, the need for family planning services will continue to grow.

Sally Kuykendall

See also: Children's Health; Dunham, Ethel Collins; Ellertson, Charlotte Ehrengard; *Healthy People 2020*; Infant Mortality; Maternal Health; Planned Parenthood; Sanger, Margaret Louise Higgins; Women's Health; World Health Organization

Further Reading

American Academy of Pediatrics. (2017). *Small families.* Retrieved from https://www.healthychildren.org/English/family-life/family-dynamics/types-of-families/Pages/Small-Families.aspx.

Centers for Disease Control and Prevention. (1999). Achievements in public health, 1900–1999: Family planning. *Morbidity and Mortality Weekly Report, 48*(47), 1073–1080. Retrieved from https://www.cdc.gov/mmwr/preview/mmwrhtml/mm4847a1.htm.

Centers for Disease Control and Prevention. (2017). *Maternal and infant health.* Retrieved from https://www.cdc.gov/reproductivehealth/maternalinfanthealth/.

Gao, G. (2015). *Americans' ideal family size is smaller than it used to be.* Pew Research Center. Retrieved from http://www.pewresearch.org/fact-tank/2015/05/08/ideal-size-of-the-american-family/.

Gavin, L. Moskosky, S., Carter, M., et al. (2014). Providing quality family planning services: Recommendations of CDC and the U.S. Office of Population Affairs. *MMWR Recommendations and Reports, 63*(4).

Guttmacher Institute. (2016). *Publicly funded family planning services in the United States.* Retrieved from https://www.guttmacher.org/fact-sheet/publicly-funded-family-planning-services-united-states.

Henshaw, S. K. (1998). Unintended pregnancy in the United States. *Family Planning Perspectives, 30,* 24.

Hoyert, D. L. (2007). Maternal mortality and related concepts. National Center for Health Statistics. *Vital Health Statistics, 3*(33). Retrieved from http://www.cdc.gov/nchs/data/series/sr_03/sr03_033.pdf.

Lindner, F. E., & Grove, R. D. (1947). *Vital statistics rates in the United States 1900–1940.* Washington, DC: U.S. Government Printing Office. Retrieved from http://www.nber.org/vital-stats-books/vsrates1900_40.CV.pdf.

Office of Disease Prevention and Health Promotion. (2017). *Healthy People 2020.* Retrieved from https://www.healthypeople.gov/.

World Health Organization (WHO). (2017). *Family planning/contraception.* Retrieved from http://www.who.int/mediacentre/factsheets/fs351/en/.

FLUORIDATION

Fluoridation is the process of adding therapeutic doses of fluoride to public drinking water in order to promote oral health. The history of fluoridation is a classic example of public health in action (CDC, 1999). Initially, dentists from the western and midwestern United States and Argentina, Japan, and England reported cases of brown stained and pitted tooth enamel. Dental experts assumed that the irregular teeth were susceptible to decay. In 1931, the National Institutes of Health hired public health dentist Henry Trendley Dean to investigate. Dean's team traced the problem to high levels of fluoride in local water sources. To their surprise, they found that children with mottled teeth had fewer cavities. Dean suggested adding low doses of fluoride to public water sources and today, millions of people benefit fluoridation with better oral health and fewer cavities. Despite numerous studies supporting the safety and efficacy of fluoridation, the practice remains a controversial issue. Opponents question the government's right to add chemicals to public water supplies while advocates argue that public benefit outweighs individual rights.

The story of fluoridation started in 1901 when Dr. Frederick S. McKay graduated from University of Pennsylvania dental school and moved to Colorado Springs. He noticed a permanent brown stain on the teeth of long-term residents and named the condition *Colorado brown stain*. McKay was curious and wanted to learn more about the condition. However, other local dentists and colleagues on the East Coast were uninterested. He started his own local field study, tracking the source to Pike's Peak watershed. In 1909, McKay presented clinical cases of Colorado brown stain to the Colorado Springs Dental Society. His presentation attracted the attention of preeminent dental expert Dr. Green Vardiman Black. McKay convinced Black to visit Colorado Springs and collaborate in his research. Black recalled his first visit to the area:

> I spent considerable time walking on the streets, noticing children in their play, attracting attention and talking to them about their games, etc., for studying the general effect of the deformity. I found it prominent in every group of children. One does not have to search for it, for it is continually forcing itself on the attention of the stranger by its persistent prominence. (National Institute of Dental and Craniofacial Research, 2014)

Black renamed the problem *mottled enamel.* By 1915, McKay and Black had discovered that mottled enamel was more severe among long-term residents and especially children. Children who lived in the region when they were developing their secondary teeth appeared to have the most obvious discoloration. McKay believed that the cause of the problem was trace elements in drinking water. But water analyses revealed nothing unusual. In 1920, 78 children in Oakley, Idaho, developed similar characteristics of brown, pitted teeth. Townspeople dug a well to a different spring, and within eight years the children had normal teeth. In Arkansas, Dr. F. L. Robertson also noticed mottled enamel among children living in nearby Bauxite. Suspecting the town's water source, local officials dug a new well. Bauxite was owned by the Aluminum Company of America (ALCOA). ALCOA's chief chemist H. V. Churchill was worried ALCOA might be blamed for water contamination. He instructed an assistant to test the town's water supply using the company's sophisticated photospectrometer. Analysis revealed high levels of fluoride. Churchill contacted McKay and offered to test samples from other affected areas. Tests revealed similar results, high levels of fluoride in the water supply. The U.S. Public Health Service sent health alerts to 300 areas warning that minute amounts of fluorine could cause pitted teeth.

Robertson, McKay, and others were frustrated by the lack of support and interest from government officials. They spoke out publicly, pushing public health officials to act. In 1931, the National Institutes of Health engaged the services of Dr. Henry Trendley Dean. Dean was a public health dentist who served in World War I providing oral care to soldiers suffering from trench mouth. He was very analytical and methodical. Colleagues described his innate ability to look at clinical cases and epidemiological data and to develop workable solutions. Dean read reports from around the world and designed a large-scale epidemiological study. Dental researchers studied children's teeth while chemists analyzed water samples. The NIH's investigation revealed high levels of fluoride in the water where mottling existed along with significantly lower levels of caries. Dean designed a second study comparing levels of fluoride in the local water supply to degree of dental fluorosis in children. This correlational study identified levels of fluoride that were ineffective, safe, or harmful. With this new information, Dean designed a third study to evaluate the impact of titrated fluoridation of public drinking water. Grand Rapids, Michigan, agreed to serve as a pilot site, adding the recommended level of fluoride, one part per million to the public water system. Over the next 15 years, public health dentists and researchers monitored the oral health of around 30,000 children. The pilot was a success. Caries rates decreased 60 percent (Arnold Jr., Dean, Jay, & Kuntson, 1953). Other large cities soon adopted fluoridation methods. In 1999, the Centers for Disease Control and Prevention estimated that fluoridation improves oral health by 68 percent.

Fluoride works in several ways. When we eat, bacteria in the mouth produce acid that initiate the breakdown of carbohydrates. The acid does not differentiate between food and teeth. The acid will attack and demineralize enamel, the hard, protective, outer layer of teeth. Fluoride protects tooth enamel by adhering to the surface and attracting calcium ions. The calcium ions bond with phosphate ions forming an acid-resistant protective layer. Fluoride in the mouth enters the bacterial cell and interrupts acid production. Reducing the amount of acid in the mouth minimizes tooth decay. In children who are developing their second set of teeth, fluoride strengthens tooth structure by replacing the mineral hydroxyapatite ($Ca_5(PO_4)_3OH$) with the harder, more durable fluorapatite ($Ca_5(PO_4)_3F$. Water fluoridation benefits people of *all* ages, socioeconomic status, or dental practices. This means that community members who are least able to afford dental care also benefit, which ultimately reduces health disparities. The American Dental Association (2016) estimates that each dollar spent on fluoridation saves $38 in dental treatment.

Fluoridation is one of the greatest public health achievements of the 20th century. Unfortunately, fluoridation occurred during the Cold War (1947–1991) and was quickly overshadowed by the fear-mongering and conspiracy theories of the time. Some conspiracy theorists believed that ALCOA was intentionally dumping toxic chemicals into the local water system. Others believed fluoridation was a communist plot to control the minds of American citizens. Antifluoridationist groups continue today with claims that fluoridation causes AIDS, Alzheimer's, low IQ, cancer, and gastrointestinal diseases. Seventy years of research have shown that, at the correct levels, fluoride is safe and effective in improving dental health.

Ethicists point out that fluoridation creates an ethical dilemma pitting the common good against individual rights. With respect to the common good, federal, state, local, and territorial governments have the power and responsibility to develop policies and procedures that benefit all or most members of society. This is why Oakley and Bauxite dug new wells. Authorities had a responsibility to protect children's teeth. Individuals also have rights. Those advocating for individual rights point out that fluoridation is a medical treatment, and thus local governments are medicating people without their consent. Fluoride is not a necessary ingredient of water purification, and individuals should have the right to refuse unnecessary water additives. The dilemma was created by science and, like other dilemmas, it may end with science. Fluoride is now readily available in bottled water, toothpastes, mouthwashes, and tablets. Starting in the 1970s, West Germany, Sweden, Japan, and the Netherlands stopped fluoridating public water supplies. England allows local health authorities to determine if fluoridation is necessary based on local data. As new techniques emerge, the necessity for public water fluoridation may diminish.

Fluoridation, adding fluoride to the water supply, protects teeth, making them resistant to decay. Prior to fluoridation, most people lost their teeth by the age of 40. Today, many Americans enjoy nutritious foods, clear speech, and attractive smiles because of the efforts and perseverance of a few dedicated public health dentists. From a public health perspective, fluoridation is ideal because it helps those who can least afford dental care. Fluoridation benefits everyone, the young and old, healthy or ill, and rich and poor.

Sally Kuykendall

See also: Community Health; Dean, Henry Trendley; National Institutes of Health; Nutrition; Oral Health; U.S. Public Health Service

Further Reading

American Dental Association. (2016). *5 Reasons why fluoride in water is good for communities.* Retrieved from http://www.ada.org/en/public-programs/advocating-for-the-public/fluoride-and-fluoridation/5-reasons-why-fluoride-in-water-is-good-for-communities.

Arnold, F.A., Jr., Dean, H., & Knutson, J. (1953). Effect of fluoridated public water supplies on dental caries prevalence: Seventh year of Grand Rapids-Muskegon study. *Public Health Reports, 68*(2), 141–148.

Centers for Disease Control and Prevention (CDC). (1999). Achievements in public health, 1900–1999: Fluoridation of drinking water to prevent dental caries. *Morbidity and Mortality Weekly Report, 48*(41), 933–940. Retrieved from https://www.cdc.gov/mmwr/preview/mmwrhtml/mm4841a1.htm.

Centers for Disease Control and Prevention (CDC). (1999). H. Trendley Dean, D.D.S. *Morbidity and Mortality Weekly Report, 48*(41), 935. Retrieved from https://www.cdc.gov/mmwr/preview/mmwrhtml/mm4841bx.htm.

Dean, H. T. (1938). Endemic fluorosis and its relation to dental caries. *Public Health Reports, 53*(33), 1443–1452.

Dean, H. T., & McKay, F. S. (1939). Production of mottled enamel halted by a change in common water supply. *American Journal of Public Health, 29*, 590–596.

Mottled teeth. (1940). *Time, 35*, 40.

National Institute of Dental and Craniofacial Research. (2014). *The story of fluoridation.* Retrieved from https://www.nidcr.nih.gov/OralHealth/Topics/Fluoride/TheStoryofFluoridation.htm.

FOOD AND DRUG ADMINISTRATION (FDA)

The Food and Drug Administration (FDA) is the oldest comprehensive consumer protection agency in the United States. It has been known as the FDA since 1930, but it has earlier origins. It is an agency of the U.S. Department of Health and Human Services. Major responsibilities include protecting and promoting public health through the regulation and supervision of a variety of types of food and drug products. This includes tobacco products, dietary supplements, prescription and over-the-counter drugs, vaccines, biopharmaceuticals, blood transfusions, medical devices, and electromagnetic drugs. The FDA also enforces other laws, some of which are not directly related to food or drugs, such as sanitation requirements on interstate travel and control of disease on products for pets. A commissioner of Food and Drugs heads the FDA and reports to the secretary of Health and Human Services.

Although perhaps the best-known and most-important parts of the FDA are its regulation of drugs and approval of new drugs, these responsibilities are only a small part of the overall agency scope. The FDA regulates more than $1 trillion worth of consumer goods, about 25 percent of consumer expenditures in the United States, including food sales, drugs, cosmetics, and vitamin supplements. It is also responsible for an array of goods imported into the United States. In terms of its costs and generated revenues, it is a large agency with a budget of more than $4 billion, about half of which is generated by user fees, most paid by pharmaceutical firms to expedite drug reviews.

The history of the agency is important to understand its current roles. Its origins date back to the appointment of Lewis Caleb Beck around 1848 in the patent office, where he was given a responsibility to carry out chemical analyses of agricultural products. This was shifted to the newly created Department of Agriculture in 1862 when chemist Charles L. Wetherill was appointed to head the Chemical Division. What we think of now as among the most essential functions of the FDA began with the passage of the 1906 Pure Food and Drug Act, a law that prohibited interstate commerce in adulterated or misbranded food and drugs. The agency responsible for FDA has been modified many times. The agency was shifted in 1940 to the newly created Federal Security Agency. It was moved to the newly created Department of Health, Education and Welfare (HEW) in 1953, becoming part of the Public Health Service within HEW in 1968. It was moved to the Department of Health and Human Services in 1980 when the education function was removed from HEW. Most federal laws concerning the FDA are part of the Food, Drug, and Cosmetic Act, first passed in 1938 and extensively amended since. This act improved the 1906 legislation by mandating that all new drugs be proved safe before marketing, by making therapeutic devices and cosmetics subject to regulation, and by requiring that standards of identity and quality be established for foods. The law also made explicit FDA's ability to conduct factory inspections.

Although most offices of the FDA are located around Washington, DC, and are part of the Headquarters Division, two important parts have field offices and a workforce spread across the United States, the Office of Regulatory Affairs (ORA) and the Office of Criminal Investigation (OCI). The ORA conducts most of the FDA's work in the field. Consumer safety officers, commonly called investigators, inspect production and warehousing facilities, investigate complaints, illnesses, or outbreaks, and review documentation in the case of medical devices, drugs, biological products, and other items where it may be difficult to conduct a physical examination or take a physical sample of the product. The ORA is divided into five regions and, within those, 13 districts. The OCI is a newer part of the FDA, established in 1991 to investigate criminal cases, such as fraudulent claims, or knowingly and willfully shipping adulterated goods in interstate commerce.

Two of the best-known activities of the FDA are food and drug regulation. For foods, the Center for Food Safety and Applied Nutrition handles most safety and labeling concerns for food products except for those with meat, which are handled by the Department of Agriculture, and alcohol-related products, which are also handled separately. The Dietary and Supplement Health and Education Act of 1994 led to the FDA regulating dietary supplements, but as foods, rather than as drugs. Thus, these products are not subject to safety and efficacy testing. Action can only occur against supplements if they are unsafe. Manufacturers of dietary supplements are permitted to make specific claims of health benefits but they may not claim to treat, diagnose, cure, or prevent disease and must include a disclaimer on the label. Bottled water is also regulated by the FDA.

For drug regulation, there are different requirements for each of three types of drugs: new drugs, generic drugs, and over-the-counter drugs. A "new" drug is a product made by a different manufacturer using different or inactive or other ingredients, and with a different purpose than the older drug. The most rigorous requirements apply to drugs not based on existing medications. These new drugs receive extensive scrutiny before FDA approval. Once approved, the sponsor must review and report to the FDA every patient adverse drug experience. If the drug event is an unexpected serious and fatal one, it must be reported within 15 days. Other events are reported quarterly. Generic drugs are chemical equivalents of name-brand drugs whose patents have expired. They are generally less expensive. Generic drug approval requires scientific evidence that the generic drug is interchangeable with or therapeutically equivalent to the originally approved drug. Over-the-counter (OTC) drugs are those that do not require a doctor's prescription. Often, they were previously approved prescription drugs but now considered safe for use without a physician's supervision.

Jennie Jacobs Kronenfeld

See also: Food Insecurity; Food Safety; Nutrition; Prescription Drugs; Prevention; Public Health in the United States, History of; Vaccines; *Controversies in Public Health:* Controversy 1

Further Reading

Food and Drug Administration, DHHS. (2012). Retrieved from http://www.fda.gov.

Healy, D. (2012). *Pharmageddon.* Berkeley: University of California Press.

Hilts, P. J. (2003). *Protecting America's health: The FDA, business, and one hundred years of regulation.* New York: Alfred E. Knopf.

FOOD INSECURITY

Food insecurity is the inability to attain an adequate or consistent supply of nutritious food in socially acceptable ways. The definition includes three main concepts:

1. quantity, quality, or variety of food is inadequate for nutritional needs;
2. limited availability of food leads to feelings of deprivation and anxiety; and
3. food can only be obtained through stealing, begging, trash-picking, or charity.

Food insecurity goes beyond hunger in that hunger is a physiological state, relieved by eating. Food insecurity is a socioemotional state of poverty, anxiety, and disordered eating. Effective, sustainable interventions work to address the lack of food, unstable household finances, and negative emotions.

The human body is amazingly resilient to food deprivation. However, over time, chronic nutrient deprivation leads to fatigue, malnutrition, muscle wasting, susceptibility to infection, and death. Infants and children are particularly vulnerable because micronutrients and macronutrients are needed for physical, social, and emotional development. With an inconsistent food supply, the body attempts to compensate. During times of plenty, the person overeats. More expensive or nutrient dense foods, milk, milk products, fruits and vegetables, are neglected in favor of inexpensive high-fat, high-calorie foods. This hunger-obesity paradox creates mental health issues of helplessness, shame, humiliation, stress, anxiety, and depression and long-term problems of obesity, diabetes, cardiovascular disease, and hypertension. The body also compensates by slowing down metabolic processes, which exacerbates the potential for obesity. One in seven U.S. households suffers from food insecurity (Coleman-Jensen, Rabbitt, Gregory, & Singh, 2016). Children and females are at highest risk. Chronic food insecurity is associated with alcohol, tobacco, and substance abuse, cravings for unhealthy comfort foods, and high-risk sexuality (trading sex for food). Children suffer from delayed development, protein-energy malnutrition (PEM), and behavioral problems. The need for food competes with other needs, such as housing or medical care. Caregivers will often forgo their own nutritional or medical needs so that their children may eat. The adverse consequences of food insecurity affect females and female-headed households more than males.

Although extreme weather events, such as droughts or floods, can destabilize local food supplies, on the broad level, food insecurity is related to political and social injustices. The inability to access nutritious food is rooted within the household economy. The inability to earn a living wage, chronic poverty, low educational achievement, limited job skills, and gender and racial inequities create social disadvantage and limit the ability to access and utilize nutritious foods. Programs designed to address food insecurity are Supplemental Nutrition Assistance Program (SNAP)/food stamps, the Women, Infants, and Children (WIC) program, National School Lunch program, food distribution programs, disaster assistance, and financial assistance to families living below the poverty line. Formerly known as food stamps, the Supplemental Nutrition Assistance Program (SNAP) is a program of the U.S. Department of Agriculture (USDA) Food and Nutrition Service. SNAP provides electronic debit cards to eligible, low-income individuals and families. The majority of SNAP recipients are children (44 percent) and/or households with at least one working adult (75 percent). The debit cards are limited to food purchases. The Women, Infants, and Children (WIC) program provides supplemental food, nutrition education, and health referrals for low-income, at-risk infants, children up to age five, and pregnant and postpartum women. WIC is offered through county and city public health departments, health centers, schools, and community centers. The National School Lunch Program (NSLP) is a federally assisted program available in public and private schools and residential child care institutions. The NSLP provides free or reduced-price lunches to school-aged children. Food distribution centers provide a safety net for people regardless of federal income guidelines on nutritional assistance. Food pantries accept donations from the community and redistribute food to people in need. Other policies and programs that work to alleviate the problems of food insecurity are laws and policies that raise families out of poverty, govern minimum wage, or provide earned income tax credit (EITC) and Temporary Assistance to Needy Families (TANF). In addition to providing a secure source of safe and nutritious foods, these programs provide opportunities for

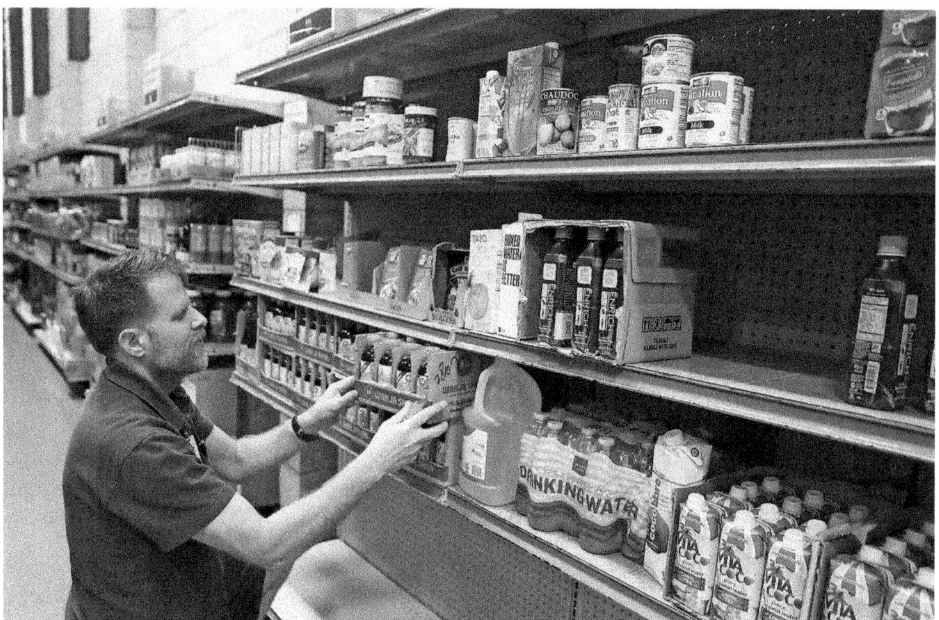

Daniel Katz sorts food at SF-Marin Food Bank in San Francisco, California. The food bank supports 225,000 people through neighborhood pantries, morning snacks for high-need students, nutrition education, and home-delivered groceries to seniors and people with disabilities. (Justin Sullivan/Getty Images)

health screening and referrals, nutrition education, and courses in literacy or English as a second language. A major obstacle to nutritional assistance programs is the stigma associated with food stamps and free school lunches. Many children and families who need and are eligible for nutritional assistance programs refuse to use the programs because they do not wish to be labeled as poor.

Food insecurity is a problem that extends beyond hunger and the need for nourishment. The inability to attain a steady source of food leads to long-term emotional and physical health problems. Government and nonprofit organizations offer a number of programs designed to address food insecurity. Policies focused on social inequity and living wages among the nation's working poor may empower households to achieve a reliable and steady source of food. For public health, challenges remain in how to identify and interrupt the cycle of disordered eating.

Sally Kuykendall

See also: Body Mass Index; Food and Drug Administration; Food Safety; Nutrition; Obesity; Rural Health; Social Determinants of Health; U.S. Department of Agriculture

Further Reading

Coleman-Jensen, A., Rabbitt, M., Gregory, C., & Singh, A. (2016). *Household food security in the United States in 2015.* Economic Research Report No. (ERR-215). Retrieved from https://www.ers.usda.gov/publications/pub-details/?pubid=79760.

Dixon, L., Winkleby, M., & Radimer, K. (2001). Dietary intakes and serum nutrients differ between adults from food-insufficient and food-sufficient families: Third National Health and Nutrition Examination Survey, 1988–1994. *Journal of Nutrition, 131*(4), 1232–1246.

Ivers, L. C. (2015). *Food insecurity and public health.* Boca Raton, FL: CRC Press.

Radimer, K. L. (2002). Measurement of household food security in the USA and other industrialised countries. *Public Health Nutrition,* 5(6A), 859–864.

United States Department of Agriculture. (2017). Retrieved from https://www.usda.gov/wps/portal/usda/usdahome.

FOOD SAFETY

Every day, people take fruits, vegetables, meat, eggs, and other products from the outside environment into their body. The potential for consumption of pesticides, bacteria, allergens, or other toxic substances is not unreasonable. Public health focuses on keeping food safe and preventing foodborne illnesses. The most common sources of foodborne illnesses are bacterial, viral, or other contamination during growing, harvesting, transporting, processing, storing, handling, or service. Food poisoning affects 48 million people each year, causing 128,000 hospitalizations and 3,000 deaths (CDC, 2016). Common pathogenic contaminants are *Salmonella, Norovirus, Campylobacter jejuni, Escherichia coli, Listeria monocytogenes,* and *Clostridium perfringens.* Although many pathogens are killed by salivary enzymes or stomach acid, some get past the body's natural defenses. Secondary lines of defense are attempts to isolate, expel, or kill the organism through nausea, vomiting, diarrhea, or high fever. Healthy individuals can recover from bouts of illness with only brief and transient incapacitation. Infants, young children, elderly, people with chronic diseases, and people with immune suppression are highly vulnerable to infections. Some strains of *Salmonella* can cause intestinal rupture, leaking contaminated gastrointestinal contents into the abdominal cavity causing sepsis and death. *Clostridium botulinum* secretes a deadly toxin, which blocks nerve transmission. The resulting paralysis can extend to facial and respiratory muscles, interfering with speaking, swallowing, or breathing. Beyond health consequences, the financial implications of foodborne illnesses are devastating to the food industry. The estimated cost of foodborne illnesses is as high as $152 billion per year (Scharff, 2012).

Methods in food safety go beyond preventing microbial contamination to include prevention of intentional or unintentional contamination by chemical residues, potential allergens, or other hazardous additives. Multiple agencies work together to ensure that the food we eat is safe for consumption. The Environmental Protection Agency (EPA) regulates the use of harmful pesticides and monitors water quality. The Food Safety and Inspection Service (FSIS) is responsible for inspecting food products for bacterial contamination, allergens, correct labeling, hazardous chemical residues, and foreign materials; promoting food safety; studying foodborne illnesses in order to identify emerging risks; and developing policies to protect the public from food borne illnesses (USDA, 2013). Environmental health specialists, formerly known as sanitarians, are employed by local and state public health departments to inspect restaurants, grocery stores, school cafeterias, nursing homes, and other food establishments to ensure food safety protocols are in place and followed. Many health departments post inspection results online for consumers to review. Health departments are also responsible for investigating and reporting cases of food borne illness. The CDC monitors cases nationwide in order to manage product recalls. The CDC also promotes food safety through health education.

Foodsafety.gov is an educational website of the Centers for Disease Control and Prevention (CDC), Food and Drug Administration (FDA), National Institutes of Health (NIH), and U.S. Department of Health and Human Services. The resource gives four primary steps to food safety: *clean*, *separate*, *cook*, and *chill*. *Cleaning* hands, food preparation surfaces, utensils, and fruits and vegetables stops the transmission of bacteria. Best practice in cleaning fruits and vegetables is to remove any damaged or bruised sections, rinse the produce under running water (scrubbing with a clean produce brush, if necessary), and dry with a paper towel or clean cloth. It is not necessary to wash eggs, meat, or poultry because eggs are washed before sale and washing raw meat can cause the juices to splash onto and contaminate food preparation areas. *Separating* aims to stop cross-contamination. Grouping food types into their own spaces while grocery shopping, transporting, storing, and preparing helps prevent contamination of bacteria from meats or seafood onto ready-to-eat foods. Using separate plastic grocery bags for meats and seafood, storing meats in a bowl in the refrigerator (or freezing) to contain leakage, and using different cutting boards, bowls, or serving plates during food preparation are a few of the recommended strategies. The site calls attention to common practices that enable cross-contamination. For example, when barbecuing outside, cooked food should go on a clean plate, not the same (unwashed) plate that was used to carry raw meat to the grill. *Cook* refers to heating and maintaining food at safe temperatures to prohibit the growth of bacteria. Temperatures between 40°F and 140°F are considered the danger zone. Microwaved meals should be heated to at least 165°F. Food waiting to be served should be kept at 140°F or above. *Chill* means using the recommended techniques to thaw frozen foods, refrigerating or freezing food promptly after serving, and throwing out food that is past the recommended use date. The safest way to thaw frozen meat, poultry, or seafood is in the refrigerator, in cold water (changing the water every 30 minutes), in the microwave, or to cook directly from frozen. Meats, such as the Thanksgiving turkey, should never be thawed on countertops as this is within the danger zone. Leftovers should be stored in the refrigerator within two hours of cooking during cooler seasons and one hour during warmer seasons. Foodsafety.gov provides several charts with recommended cooking temperatures, food storage times, and thawing times.

Public health focuses on preventing food poisoning through food safety systems, processes, inspections, training, and education. Public health allows us to safely ingest, digest, and metabolize foods. The fact that people do not experience food poisoning more often is a credit to the many systems and personnel who work to keep food safe.

Sally Kuykendall

See also: Centers for Disease Control and Prevention; Food and Drug Administration; Food Insecurity; Handwashing; Infectious Diseases; Mallon, Mary; National Institutes of Health; U.S. Department of Agriculture; U.S. Department of Health and Human Services

Further Reading

Centers for Disease Control and Prevention (CDC). (2016). *Foodborne germs and illnesses.* Retrieved from https://www.cdc.gov/foodsafety/foodborne-germs.html.

Scharff, R. (2012). Economic burden from health losses due to foodborne illness in the United States. *Journal of Food Protection*, 75(1), 123–131.

U.S. Department of Agriculture (USDA). (2013). *One team, one purpose, Food Safety Inspection Service: Protecting public health and preventing foodborne illness.* Retrieved from https://www.fsis.usda.gov/wps/wcm/connect/7a35776b-4717-43b5-b0ce-aeec64489fbd/mission-book.pdf?MOD=AJPERES.

U.S. Department of Agriculture (USDA). (2017). Retrieved from https://www.usda.gov/wps/portal/usda/usdahome.

G

GENETICS

Genetics is a field of biology that studies genes and heredity. Genetic mutations can create a spectrum of disorders ranging from minor deficiencies (color blindness) to life-threatening diseases (cystic fibrosis). Abnormalities are commonly caused by the insertion or deletion of a base pair, chromosomal abnormality, or extended length of a gene. Although some mutations cause a problem directly, others act indirectly, predisposing the individual to disease or malfunction. Examples of genetic disorders are alcoholism, Alzheimer's disease, hemochromatosis, hemophilia, Huntington's disease, Marfan syndrome, phenylketonuria, sickle cell anemia, Tay-Sachs, and breast, colon, and prostate cancers. The genetic field offers new perspectives for public health helping to understand disease, identify at-risk groups, and develop personalized treatments. Genetic science is used in newborn screening, carrier screening, pharmacogenetics, and ecogenetics. It is worth noting that such applications stretch the concept of public health. Whereas public health traditionally works at the population level, genetics functions on the individual level. As a result, public health administrators must consider whether screening, treatment, or interventions are warranted. Decisions are made based on how common a genetic disease is, whether effective treatments exist, and cost of treatment. It may be difficult to justify universal screening for rare genetic diseases that only affect few individuals or have limited, expensive treatment options. The application of genetics to medicine and public health raises ethical and legal concerns of how genetic information is used, confidentiality, DNA banking, and potential for discrimination or embryo selection.

Cystic fibrosis (CF) is one example of how genes influence health. CF is transmitted as an autosomal recessive condition. Both parents carry the mutated gene, typically without signs or symptoms. The point of mutation is the cystic fibrosis transmembrane conductance regulator (CFTR) gene, the gene that provides the body with instructions on how to make a particular protein, which allows chloride ions to move in and out of cells. Chloride ions are critical to the body's fluid and electrolyte balance. CFTR malfunction replaces normal mucus secretions with thick, sticky secretions. Body systems that are dependent on lubrication to function are affected, the respiratory, pancreatic, gastrointestinal, and reproductive systems. The person with CF struggles to clear respiratory passages and is at high risk for clogged airways, chronic lung infections, and formation of scar tissue in the lungs. Gastrointestinal (GI) problems include blockage of the GI system or pancreatic ducts, diarrhea, malnutrition, failure to thrive, weight loss, and cystic fibrosis–related diabetes mellitus. Early diagnosis is important to prevent and control adverse health consequences. Physicians make the diagnosis based on physical examination, personal and family medical history, and laboratory tests, including genetic testing. Interventions focus on keeping the airways clear with postural drainage, regular chest physiotherapy, deep breathing exercises, and medicine to thin mucus secretions. Malnutrition is prevented by high protein/high calorie diet, vitamin supplements, and pancreatic enzymes. Efforts in the home are to avoid dust, fumes, mold, or mildew, drink plenty of fluids, and exercise regularly. Pharmaceutical treatments to address the physiological problem are coming on the market. Ivacaftor (Kalydeco) works to open new channels for chloride ions, correcting the underlying deficiency. The drug costs more than $300,000 per year. The only way to prevent CF is carrier screening, genetic screening of couples prior to pregnancy. Carrier screening informs the couple of their chance of transmitting mutations to a child. For example, if both biological parents carry the mutated CFTR gene, there is a 25 percent chance that the child will have CF. Genetic counselors work with the couple to determine reproductive options based on the couple's values.

Phenylketonuria (PKU) is a good example of genetic screening in public health. All infants are screened for PKU at birth by drawing a tiny drop of blood from the heel. PKU testing is simple, and early intervention is highly effective in reducing long-term disability. Newborn screening is also used to diagnose congenital hypothyroidism, sickle cell disease, tyrosinemia, or galactosemia. Genetic screening raises ethical concerns of potential stigma, confidentiality, cost, insurability, and employment. Insurance companies or employers could use genetic information to discriminate or deny coverage. Since genes are transmitted within the family, genetic information of one individual may confer information about other family members. This raises concerns regarding confidentiality and informed consent. To overcome concerns, it is important to ensure that a community or population supports screening and does not believe they are being targeted for discrimination. Depending on the disorder, screening efforts may be cost-contained by focusing on populations at risk. For example, CF affects 1 in 2,500 Caucasian Americans, 1 in 2,270 Ashkenazi Jewish Caucasians, 1 in 13,500 Hispanic Americans, 1 in 15,100 African Americans, and 1 in 35,100 Asian American couples (Palomaki, FitzSimmons, & Haddow, 2004). If testing is expensive, it may not be necessary to screen all populations for all genetic disorders.

Two emerging fields of genetics with application to public health are behavioral genetics and precision medicine. Behavioral genetics proposes that individuals are born with certain traits that are only exhibited when *switched on* by environmental factors. Behavioral genetic theories have been applied to alcohol abuse, violence, and criminality. The premise of behavioral genetics should be used to strengthen public and policy concern for the social determinants of health. Precision medicine optimizes disease treatments and prevention by considering the individual's lifestyle, environment, and genetic makeup. For example, trastuzumab (Herceptin) is used to treat breast cancer among women with a specific genetic profile known as

HER-2 positive (The Cancer GenomeAtlas, n.d.). Precision medicine allows physicians to individualize treatments for more effective results.

The application of genetics to public health offers promise to understanding, treating, and preventing common diseases and health issues. However, like many scientific advances, the information can also be used to hurt or to harm. The eugenics movement advocated to use genetic screening to eliminate "undesirable traits" (alcoholism, criminality, feeble-mindedness, poverty, and deafness) and replace with "desirable traits" (whatever those in power determine is desirable). The horrors of Nazi Germany helped people to realize how arrogant, ridiculous, and narrow-minded such ideas were. Eliminating people with "undesirable traits" would deprive the world of the genius and contributions of Abraham Lincoln (Marfan syndrome), Frédéric Chopin (believed to have CF), Vincent van Gogh (bipolar disorder), Henri de Toulouse-Lautrec (pycnodysostosis), Miles Davis (sickle cell anemia), Niccolò Paganini (Ehlers-Danlos syndrome), John F. Kennedy (Addison's disease), King Charles II (prognathism), and Queen Victoria (hemophilia).

Sally Kuykendall

See also: Association of Public Health Laboratories; Bioterrorism; Birth Defects; Cancer; Eating Disorders; Health; Health Care Disparities; Hypertension; Maternal Health

Further Reading

The Cancer Genome Atlas. (n.d.). *Impact of cancer genomics on precision medicine for the treatment of cancer.* National Cancer Institute. Retrieved from https://cancergenome.nih.gov/cancergenomics/impact.

Cystic Fibrosis Foundation. (2017). Retrieved from https://www.cff.org/.

Ho, N. C., Park, S. S., Maragh, K. D., & Gutter, E. M. (2003). Famous people and genetic disorders: From monarchs to geniuses—A portrait of their genetic illnesses. *American Journal of Medical Genetics, Part A, 118A*(2), 187–196.

Palomaki, G. E., FitzSimmons, S. C., & Haddow, J. E. (2004). Clinical sensitivity of prenatal screening for cystic fibrosis via CFTR carrier testing in a United States panethnic population. *Genetics in Medicine: Official Journal of the American College of Medical Genetics*, 6(5), 405–414.

U.S. Department of Human Services. (2017). *Genetics home reference.* Retrieved from https://ghr.nlm.nih.gov/.

GLOBAL HEALTH

Global health is a process of international collaboration focused on addressing complex and challenging public health issues or threats. Global health issues of Zika virus, severe acute respiratory syndrome (SARS), avian influenza, and Ebola affect people directly and indirectly. These illnesses cause disability and death and strain health services, impacting regional and national economies. The issues cross geographic and regional boundaries and demand a high level of cooperation between nations. Courses in global health engage multidimensional approaches in health promotion, health equity, disease prevention, epidemiology, and health policy. As an interdisciplinary field, global health adopts information and practices from public health, medicine, biology, economics, environmental sciences, social sciences, and behavioral sciences. The United States spends about $10.2 billion annually on global health programs (Wexler & Kates, 2016). The President's Malaria Initiative (PMI), the President's Emergency plan for AIDS Relief (PEPFAR), the Global Fund, United States Agency International Development (USAID), and the Global Health Security Agenda provide services in family planning and reproductive health, maternal and child health, nutrition and treatment and prevention of AIDS, tuberculosis, and malaria. Collaborative actions draw scientific and technical assistance, human resources, and capital development from many countries to strengthen health systems in regions of need.

Historically, communicable diseases were blocked by geographic landforms. Mountains, deserts, or large bodies of water impaired face-to-face contact. Air travel and the expansion of international commerce and trade created new social and environmental conditions leading to urbanization, food borne illnesses, climate change, and microbial adaptations (De Cock, Simone, Davison, & Slutsker, 2013). Endemic and epidemic diseases are easily spread through human migration and international travel. Infectious diseases crossing transnational boundaries can create public health emergencies. In 2014, passengers returning from the West African countries of Guinea, Liberia, and Sierra Leone spread Ebola virus to the United States. Although the cases were contained and treated, the potential exists for other communicable diseases. Preventing, controlling, or extinguishing diseases at the place of origin saves lives and resources.

Infectious diseases are illnesses caused by pathogenic microorganisms, such as bacteria, viruses, parasites, or fungi. The diseases can be transmitted directly or indirectly through contact with infected bodily fluids, air, water, food, or vectors. Diseases spread through direct bodily fluid contact include HIV/AIDS, Ebola, and hepatitis C. Tuberculosis, influenza, measles, SARS, and pertussis are transmitted through the air. Malaria and Zika virus are vector borne infectious diseases transmitted by mosquitoes to humans. Cholera is transmitted through contaminated water. Infectious diseases account for 19 percent of deaths internationally (Lozano et al., 2013). HIV/AIDS, tuberculosis, and malaria are the leading causes of death. Internationally, 37 million people are infected with HIV, and more than 10.4 million people are infected with tuberculosis (WHO, 2017b). People living in developing countries, low socioeconomic status, malnourished, unemployed, with inadequate education, poor sanitation, inadequate health care, and lacking basic amenities are most affected. In Africa, infectious diseases, malnutrition, and maternal and child health problems accounted for 56 percent of deaths in 2015 (WHO, 2017a). Sub-Saharan Africa accounts for 50 percent of infectious disease deaths, globally (WHO, 2017a). Infectious diseases such as HIV/AIDS, malaria, diarrhea, and lower respiratory tract infections are the leading causes of death in Africa.

Food marketing and trade are a global health concern. Varying standards in food safety, production, and processing create the potential for food borne illnesses. Forty-eight million Americans are affected by food borne illness yearly (CDC, 2016a). Salmonella infections account for more cases of hospitalizations, illness, and death than any other food borne pathogen. To prevent food borne illnesses, Congress enacted the Food Safety Modernization Act (2010). The law empowers and mandates the Food and Drug Administration (FDA) to recall contaminated food from the United States and other countries.

Anthropogenic activities such as the emission of radioactive materials, burning of fossil fuels, use and improper disposal of industrial chemicals, water pollution, and deforestation due to urbanization threaten global health. Anthropogenic activities increase climatic temperatures, creating factors that promote communicable diseases. Global warming enhances the survival, breeding, and transmission of vector borne diseases such as malaria, dengue, and yellow fever. Rising sea levels create flooding conditions promoting waterborne illnesses of viral gastroenteritis and cholera.

Noncommunicable diseases (NCDs) are chronic and acute diseases that affect millions of people around the world. NCDs account for 80 percent of all deaths globally and include various types of cancers, chronic respiratory diseases, cardiovascular diseases, and diabetes (WHO, 2017c). These conditions are not contagious but require costly long-term management. Sufferers experience pain, disability, loss of income, disruption of family stability, and impaired quality of life. Globally, cardiovascular disease accounts for 17.7 million deaths, cancers cause 8.8 million deaths, chronic lung diseases cause 3.9 million deaths, and diabetes causes 1.6 million deaths (WHO, 2017b). In developed countries, individuals ages 60 and below account for 13 percent of NCD-related deaths, while low and middle income countries consist of 29 percent of NCD-associated deaths (Baldwin & Amato, 2012). The WHO (2011) projects a 15 percent increase in NCDs globally by 2025 and a 20 percent increase in South-East Asia, Africa, and the Eastern Mediterranean. NCDs carry substantial health care costs. For every dollar spent on health care in the United States, seventy cents goes toward treating chronic health conditions (CDC, 2016b). NCDs can be prevented by reducing common risk factors such as tobacco use, alcohol use, physical inactivity, and unhealthy diet.

Global health interventions are collaborative strategies focusing on identification, control, prevention, and treatment of disease, and overall improvement of health. Global health challenges are organized mostly through United Nations agencies, nongovernmental organizations (NGOs), charities and foundations, and private donors. These agencies coordinate funds and share information on disease outbreaks and containment. Global health agencies include the United Nations agencies such as the WHO, UNICEF, and UNIAIDS. USAID is an agency under the Department of State with responsibilities for coordinating and organizing the U.S. global health programs. The Clinton Foundation and the Bill and Melinda Gates Foundation are private organizations with initiatives on global health challenges. Global health interventions involve coordination and collaborative actions that aim at disease surveillance and mitigation, health system strengthening through scientific and technical assistance, human resource management, and capital development. Other global health interventions include vaccination and immunization programs, medical and pharmaceutical product supply, community advocacy and education programs, poverty reduction programs, and provision of medical equipment and infrastructural amenities that meet the needs of vulnerable or special populations.

The study of global health investigates international environmental and socioeconomic determinants of health. Issues include outbreak of emerging or reemerging infectious diseases, food safety, bioterrorism, global warming, vaccines and immunizations, access to health care, chronic diseases, and the proliferation of contaminated or counterfeit pharmaceutical products. Comparing data on health outcomes and living standards and infant and child mortality highlights the differences between developing and developed countries. Because infectious and chronic diseases do not recognize political boundaries, efforts to train medical personnel, share medical information, and strengthen the infrastructure of existing health systems are needed to treat and prevent global health concerns.

Godyson Orji

See also: Bioterrorism; Epidemic; Immigrant Health; Pandemic; Smallpox; World Health Organization

Further Reading

Baldwin, W., & Amato, L. (2012). *Fact sheet: Global burden of non-communicable diseases.* Retrieved from http://www.prb.org/Publications/Datasheets/2012/world-population-data-sheet/fact-sheet-ncds.aspx.

Centers for Disease Control and Prevention (CDC). (2016a). *Estimates of foodborne illness in the United States.* Retrieved from http://www.cdc.gov/foodborneburden/2011-foodborne-estimates.html#annual.

Centers for Disease Control and Prevention (CDC). (2016b). *Multiple chronic conditions.* Retrieved from http://www.cdc.gov/chronicdisease/about/multiple-chronic.htm.

De Cock, K. M., Simone, P. M., Davison, V., & Slutsker, L. (2013). The new global health. *Emerging Infectious Diseases, 19*(8), 1192–1197. doi:10.3201/eid1908.130121

Koplan, J. P., Bond, T. C., Merson, M. H., Reddy, K. S., Rodriguez, M. H., Sewankambo, N. K., & Wasserheit, J. N. (2009). Towards a common definition of global health. *The Lancet, 373*(9679), 1993–1995. doi:10.1016/S0140-6736(09)60332-9

Lozano, R., Naghavi, M., Foreman, K., Lim, S., Shibuya, K., Aboyans, V., & AlMazroa, M. A. (2013). Global and regional mortality from 235 causes of death for 20 age groups in 1990 and 2010: A systematic analysis for the global burden of disease study 2010. *The Lancet, 380*(9859), 2095–2128. doi:10.1016/S0140-6736(12)61728-0

Smith, K. F., Goldberg, M., Rosenthal, S., Carlson, L., Chen, J., Chen, C., & Ramachandran, S. (2014). Global rise in human infectious disease outbreaks. *Journal of the Royal*

Society Interface, 11(101), 20140950. doi:10.1098/rsif.2014.0950. Retrieved from http://rsif.royalsocietypublishing.org/content/11/101/20140950.

Wexler, A., & Kates, J. (2016, January 20). *The US global health budget: Analysis of appropriations for fiscal year 2016*. Retrieved from http://kff.org/global-health-policy/issue-brief/the-u-s-global-health-budget-analysis-of-appropriations-for-fiscal-year-2016/.

World Health Organization (WHO). (2011). Burden: Mortality, morbidity and risk factors. *Global status report on non-communicable diseases, 2011*. Retrieved from http://www.who.int/nmh/publications/ncd_report_full_en.pdf.

World Health Organization. (2017a). *Global health observatory (GHO) data*. Retrieved from http://www.who.int/gho/en/.

World Health Organization. (WHO). (2017b). *HIV/AIDS data and statistics*. Retrieved from: http://www.who.int/hiv/data/en/.

World Health Organization (WHO). (2017c). *Noncommunicable diseases fact sheet*. Retrieved from http://www.who.int/mediacentre/factsheets/fs355/en/.

GOALS AND OBJECTIVES

In public health, goals and objectives define the intended aim or outcome of a particular health promotion or disease prevention activity. Goals and objectives are tools used to focus the project, motivate participants, and evaluate efforts. Goals are broad statements that name the population of interest and what is expected to happen because of the planned activity. Objectives are precise statements that define the interim steps or tasks necessary to meet the intended goal. Due to this precision, health educators follow common rules in writing goals and objectives. The main advantage of goals and objectives is that they ensure that projects stay on track. A disadvantage is that even well-developed objectives are susceptible to moderating influences. Goals can only be accomplished with adequate resources, knowledge, and effort.

The idea of goals and objectives originated from business psychology. In 1897, Dr. William Lowe Bryan and Mr. Noble Hartner studied people learning the skill of telegraph code-writing. The researchers concluded that learners were more successful when given progressive tasks with specific targets for achievement. In 1911, Dr. Frederick Winslow Taylor studied time and motion in factories. He concluded that businesses could improve output (and therefore profit) by identifying specific and challenging tasks for each worker. At the time, workers were viewed as raw materials, a commodity for making money. Winslow failed to consider factors that might influence the individual worker, moderating the relationship between goals and achievement. Wyatt, Frost, and Stock (1934) studied industrial workers assigned to boring, repetitive tasks. They noted that workers paid by work output (number of widgets produced) were more productive than workers paid by the hour (time on the work clock). The researchers cautioned that while financial incentives compensated for boring tasks, the incentives did not compensate for tasks that the workers disliked or thought were meaningless. In 1935, Dr. Cecil Alec Mace further discredited the belief that employees are motivated by money.

Mace proposed the idea of goal setting. Dr. Edwin A. Locke (1968) investigated the relationship between goals, aims, and task performance and surmised that high goals are better motivators than low, easy goals and defined goals are more effective than general goals ("do your best"). Locke and Latham (1990) developed a formal theory of motivation and task performance. Goal setting theory (GST) outlines the various moderating and mediating factors that influence motivation, such as financial incentives, time constraints, competition, praise, punishment, shared knowledge of outcomes, and personal intentions (Latham & Locke, 2007). GST is applicable to business, education, psychology, sociology, and health behavioral change.

Goals describe broad, long-range states or conditions that the individual or group hopes to achieve. One example is the *Healthy People 2020* goal for adolescents (aged 10–19) and young adults (aged 20–24): "Improve the healthy development, health, safety, and well-being of adolescents and young adults" (Office of Disease Prevention and Health Promotion [ODPHP], 2016). *Improving health* encompasses multiple components for adolescents and young adults; this means reducing homicides, suicides, motor vehicle crashes, substance abuse, smoking, sexually transmitted diseases, unplanned pregnancies, and homelessness. In comparison to goals, objectives address short, intermediate, or long-term outcomes. Objectives state a specific measure of achievement and time period. Health educators and program planners use the acronym SMART (Specific, Measurable, Achievable, Relevant, and Time-bound) to write program objectives. One *Healthy People 2020* objective for adolescent and young adult mental health is: "Reduce the proportion of adolescents who engage in disordered eating behaviors in an attempt to control their weight." The defined outcome is a reduction of 10 percent. The objective is *specific*, targeting one aspect of mental health, disordered eating among adolescents (aged 10–19). Disordered eating is clearly defined as fasting in order to lose weight or prevent gaining weight; using pills, powders, or liquids without a doctor's advice in order to lose weight or prevent gaining weight; or taking laxatives to lose weight or prevent from gaining weight. This high degree of specificity sets conditions on who, what, where, or how. The adolescent who loses weight due to food insecurity is excluded from the count because weight loss is unintentional. *Measurable* defines how much of a change is desired. The objective seeks to reduce the proportion of teens affected by 10 percent, from 14.3 percent to 12.9 percent. *Achievable* means that the objective is realistic. With sufficient support for evidence-based programs, a reduction of 10 percent is not unreasonable. *Relevant* means that the objective logically relates to the overall goal. Reducing disordered eating not only improves mental health, but also improves other aspects of health, such as reducing malnutrition, osteoporosis, kidney failure, electrolyte imbalances, gastric ulceration, tooth decay, and heart disease. *Time-bound* refers to the period of time in which the outcome will be achieved. *Healthy People 2020* objectives are 10-year objectives, starting in 2010 and completing in 2020. Other programs might use a particular time point (by the end of the program), a particular time period (within one year), or an event frame (after childbirth). Since program objectives are accomplished through program activities, the objectives convey active learning. Verbs, such as recognize, describe, apply, demonstrate, construct, and evaluate, are used to define what the participants must achieve in order to meet the objective. Some grant writers, program planners, and evaluators use templates to write objectives. For example, "By [date/time], [who] will [verb] [noun] at [level/condition]" translates to "By the end of the program, adolescents will construct healthy daily menus that reflect adequate protein, carbohydrate, and fat intake."

Goals and objectives define the aims of a health program that will be accomplished through program activities. They provide program organizers with realistic and measurable targets for participants. The most effective and useful objectives are practical, well written, logical, and clearly state desired outcomes. Although goals and objectives are used in many disciplines, they serve a special purpose in public health, aiding in grant writing, program planning, evaluation, and national health planning.

Sally Kuykendall

See also: Administration, Health; Eating Disorder; Evaluation; Evidence-Based Programs and Practices; Grants; *Healthy People 2020*; Heart Truth® (Red Dress) Campaign, The; Intervention; Leading Health Indicators; Logic Model

Further Reading

Bryan, W. L., & Hartner, N. (1897). Studies in the physiology and psychology of the telegraphic language. *Psychological Review*, 4, 27–53.

Latham, G. P., & Locke, E. A. (2007). New developments in and directions for goal-setting research. *European Psychologist*, *12*(4), 290–300. doi:10.1027/1016-9040.12.4.290

Locke, E. A. (1968). Toward a theory of task motivation and incentives. *Organizational Behavior & Human Performance*, 3(2), 157–189.

Locke, E. A., & Latham, G. P. (1990). *A theory of goal setting and task performance.* Englewood Cliffs, NJ: Prentice Hall.

Mace, C. A. (1935). Incentives: Some experimental studies. *Industrial Health Research Report* (Great Britain), 72.

McKenzie, J. F., Neiger, B. L., & Thackeray, R. (2012). *Planning, implementing, & evaluating health promotion programs: A primer* (6th ed.). New York: Pearson.

Office of Disease Prevention and Health Promotion. (2016). *Healthy People 2020: Adolescent health.* Retrieved from https://www.healthypeople.gov/2020/topics-objectives/topic/Adolescent-Health.

Taylor, F. (1911). *Principles of scientific management.* New York: Harper.

Tulane University. *Tips for writing goals and objectives.* Retrieved from http://www2.tulane.edu/publichealth/mchltp/upload/Tips-for-writing-goals-and-objectives.pdf.

Wyatt, S., Frost, L., & Stock, F. G. L. (1934). *Incentives in repetitive work.* Industrial Health Research Board (Great Britain) Report, No. 69.

GRANTS

Grants are funds disbursed by government or nonprofit organizations, corporations, or foundations to support a specific research or intervention project. The grant system is designed to support public health research and prevention efforts in HIV/AIDS, suicide, health disparities, neurosciences, substance abuse, smoking, communicable diseases, and sleep disorders as well as numerous other problems. Although many public health grants are related to health goals identified by *Healthy People 2020*, grants may also support research and development in novel emerging health issues. Grant funding is competitive or noncompetitive depending on the source and the focus of the grant. Grants allow public health professionals to investigate problems, develop solutions, evaluate programs, and suggest policies to enhance health and alleviate disease.

Grant application is a very detailed process. Grant announcements are advertised in professional newsletters, government listservs, and on grants.gov. A research or community group interested in addressing a specific problem would start by identifying relevant grant opportunities. Announcements typically list the number of awards available, whether the grant requires the recipient to match the grant funds with other funding sources, start date and end date of the award, eligibility criteria, and proposed grant amount. Prior to full application, the grantor may suggest filing a letter of intent. The letter of intent allows the funder to filter applicants based on advertised criteria. For example, the letter of intent would screen community agencies from applying for a grant specifically for schools. In public health, grant applications present a brief review of the science behind the health problem; describe the purpose of the proposed project and the intended target population; methods; timeline for completion; and budget. Nonprofit organizations are required to show nonprofit status. The grant application is very specific. Failure to follow instructions may result in automatic rejection.

Once a grant is awarded, the grantor may formally announce grantees through the media. All government grants are announced to the public. The funding is allocated throughout the project based on length of the grant. The funder may check in at regular intervals to ensure that the project is progressing as planned. At the end of the grant, the recipients submit a technical report detailing the project, outcomes, successes, and next steps. Research findings or program outcomes are disseminated to other public health professionals through conference presentations and professional journals. One issue that grant recipients face is that many grants are budgeted for short-term use. If the group is working on a chronic health issue, they may need to apply for several grants to sustain their efforts. Application and reapplication can create gaps in the project. People working on the grant may leave for more secure, permanently funded positions.

The advantage of grants is that they support collaborations in addressing issues of concern within the community or support researchers in novel research, which could lead to cures, treatments, programs, or enhance knowledge within a particular field. The grant system ensures that the recipients use the award for what it was intended. Grantors are able to set conditions on how funds are used and require regular progress reports to monitor budget and progress. A disadvantage is that grants are easily influenced by politics. In 1990, doctors and researchers at University of Washington Harborview Medical Center released a study comparing suicides in King County, Washington, and Vancouver, British Columbia (Sloan et al., 1990). Data analysis found that while suicide rates did not vary, suicide by firearm was almost six times lower in Vancouver where gun laws were stricter. The researchers concluded that stricter gun laws may reduce suicide among people aged 15 to 24. The research was followed up with another study reviewing household risk factors for homicide (Kellermann et al., 1993). This study found that a gun in the home was more likely to be used to kill a family member or friend than a stranger or home invader. In response to the information, the National Rifle Association (NRA) campaigned to eliminate the Centers for Disease Control and Prevention's National Center for Injury Prevention and pressured Congress to reallocate $2.6 million budgeted for firearm injury research (Jamieson, 2013). The injury center survived. However, the message was clear. Firearm injury prevention research was off limits, and engaging in such research could jeopardize financial support from the federal government. For the next 20 years, research on gun violence was stalled. After the Sandy Hook Elementary School shooting, public attention shifted back to gun violence. In 2013, President Barack Obama released a national plan to "end the freeze on gun violence research" (White House, Office of the Press Secretary, 2013). Restored funding enables researchers to study this critical public health problem, which claims the lives of 30,000 people every year. In order to address some of the most pressing health concerns and to inform effective policies, government agencies must be able to support unbiased scientific research, free from political manipulation.

Grants enable public health agencies to explore pressing health problems, translating federal goals to individuals in homes, communities, and businesses across the nation. Although grants offer a well-established system for allocating and monitoring government funds, the application system is tedious and time consuming. There is also a need to improve the system so that public health scientists may engage in uninterrupted projects without fear of reprisal from powerful political groups.

Sally Kuykendall

See also: Collaborations; Evaluation; *Healthy People 2020*; Intervention; Prevention; Substance Abuse and Mental Health Services Administration; *Controversies in Public Health:* Controversy 1

Further Reading

Jamieson, C. (2013). Gun violence research: History of federal funding freeze. *Psychological science agenda.* Retrieved from http://www.apa.org/science/about/psa/2013/02/gun-violence.aspx.

Kellermann, A. L., Rivara, F. P., Rushforth, N. B., Banton, J. G., Reay, D. T., Francisco, J. T., & Somes, G. (1993). Gun ownership as a risk factor for homicide in the home. *New England Journal of Medicine*, *329*(15), 1084–1091. doi:10.1056/NEJM199310073291506

Sloan, J. H., Rivara, F. P., Reay, D. T., Ferris, J. A., & Kellermann, A. L. (1990). Firearm regulations and rates of suicide: A comparison of two metropolitan areas. *New England Journal of Medicine*, *322*(6), 369–373. doi:10.1056/NEJM199002083220605

U.S. Department of Health and Human Services. (2017). Retrieved from http://www.grants.gov/.

White House, Office of the Press Secretary. (2013). *Now is the time: The president's plan to protect our children and our communities by reducing gun violence.* Retrieved from http://www.washingtonpost.com/wp-srv/politics/documents/gun-proposals/GunViolenceExecutiveSummary.pdf.

GRECO-ROMAN ERA, PUBLIC HEALTH IN THE

The Greco-Roman Era started with the rise of Greek philosophy and ended with the fall of the Roman Empire. This lengthy period of history is particularly relevant to public health because this is when beliefs regarding the causes of disease shifted from the supernatural to the natural and man sought ways to prevent illness. Greek philosopher-physicians encouraged healers to move away from magical potions and instead examine the patient's diet, activity, lifestyle, and environment. As the perceived power of the gods decreased, man's control over health increased. The use of observation, investigation, and logic shifted the locus of control (place of control) from external forces (the gods) to internal (the individual and physician) and created the new field of medicine. Greek philosopher-physicians endowed their wisdom by defining and describing the basic bioethical principles that guide today's medical practice. The early Roman civilization developed their own system of public health, which used engineering and architecture to promote sanitation and hygiene and prevent disease. The numerous philosophical and practical advances passed down from early Greek and Roman civilizations form the foundations of current public health practices.

Historical documents indicate that the ancient Greeks and Romans suffered from numerous infectious diseases, injuries, and chronic illnesses, specifically epilepsy, depression, sciatica, and kidney disease. The average life span in ancient Greece was 35 years and 32 years in ancient Rome (Deevey, 1950). Later investigation suggests longer lives, averaging 72 years and up to 107 years (Montagu, 1994). However, these calculations are based on famous men in history who were not enslaved and probably enjoyed wealth and good fortune. Ancient physicians followed the *humoral theory* of medicine, which supposes that the body consists of four humors: black bile, yellow bile, blood, and phlegm. Each humor reflects a particular natural element, earth (black bile), fire (yellow bile), air (blood), and water (phlegm). Imbalances in the humors resulted in disease or disability. Medical treatment aimed to restore balance through counterbalance or in some cases with the same humor. The Greek approach was both analytical and holistic. The role of the physician was to support the body in natural healing. By the first century CE, the Romans conquered most of Europe. Greek philosophies were saved but given lesser prominence. Naturalistic treatments were considered too passive by Roman standards.

The Greeks did not have a formal system of health care. Itinerant healers traveled from town to town treating the sick. The major disadvantage to this system was that a physician may not be in town when an epidemic struck. Over time, towns organized to pay a regular salary to a physician, encouraging him to stay in the area and treat townspeople regardless of ability to pay. This was the first system of public health care in Western civilization. To earn the privilege of a steady wage, the physician must be both skilled and trustworthy. Skill did not mean that everyone was healed and no one died. It was better for a physician to accurately predict disease outcome, even if the outcome was negative, than to give false hope or promises. Inaccurate prognosis made the physician appear incompetent, greedy, or deceitful. Thus, Greek doctors focused on diagnosing illnesses and accurate prognoses.

Hippocrates of Cos (Kos) is recognized as the Father of Western Medicine for his role in transforming medicine into a science and developing a code of medical ethics. Hippocrates advocated for a formal process of medical care that consisted of (1) patient examination, (2) diagnosis, (3) prognosis, and (4) treatment. As physicians supplanted the gods of healing, Hippocrates also recognized the potential for abuse of power. Trust between physician and the community was critical to quality care. Lying, cheating, or abuse of power not only affected the individual physician, it marred the profession. Hippocrates advised physicians to act with humanity, honesty, and integrity, to respect human life and the power of medicine. The Hippocratic Oath, which was not actually written by Hippocrates, summarizes ethical guidelines for medical practice. Graduating medical students use an updated version of the Hippocratic Oath, vowing to protect the sanctity of human life and to avoid causing pain, injury, or death.

Under the Roman Empire, interest in health was limited to practices that forwarded the agenda of building military might, government, and economy. Maintaining the empire required large armies of strong, healthy men. However, as these large armies moved from area to area, they spread diseases that were once contained within smaller areas. Roman doctors and architects suspected that diseases were caused by contaminated water, foul air, sewage, and lack of hygiene. To prevent diseases, army camps were set up away from swamps and foul odors, or swamps were drained to make room for encampments. Freshwater aqueducts, drains, sewers, public baths, and toilets were built to bring in clean, fresh water and dispose of contaminants. Ill or injured soldiers were treated in military hospitals by army doctors.

Although Greek medical practices fell out of favor with the rise of the Roman Empire, ethical principles were translated into Latin and withstood the test of time. *Primum non nocere* (Firstly do no harm) is reflected in the public health code of ethics, and *Ne quid nimis* (Nothing in excess) is a basic concept of public health prevention. The Hippocratic principles of medicine and medical ethics are the foundation of today's public health, and medical practices and Roman sanitation created ways to ensure the public health of large masses of people living in urban environments.

Sally Kuykendall

See also: Ancient World, Public Health in the; Code of Ethics; Core Competencies in Public Health; Hippocrates

Further Reading

Deevey, E. S. (1950). The probability of death. *Scientific American, 182*, 58–60.

Koloski-Ostrow, A. O. (2015). *The archaeology of sanitation in Roman Italy: Toilets, sewers, and water systems.* Chapel Hill: The University of North Carolina Press.

Magner, L. (1992). *A history of medicine.* New York: Marcel Dekker.

Montagu, J. D. (1994). Length of life in the ancient world: A controlled study. *Journal of the Royal Society of Medicine*, *87*(1), 25.

Rosen, G. (1993). *A History of Public Health* (Expanded ed.). Baltimore: The Johns Hopkins University Press.

Tountas, Y. (2009). The historical origins of the basic concepts of health promotion and education: The role of ancient Greek philosophy and medicine. *Health Promotion International*, *24*(2), 185. doi:10.1093/heapro/dap006

H

HAMILTON, ALICE (1869–1970)

Alice Hamilton was a pioneering physician who used techniques from social medicine, pathology, and epidemiology to create a new field in public health, occupational health and safety. Alice was born in New York City, the second of four girls and a much younger brother. Soon after the girls were born, the family moved to Fort Wayne, Indiana, to live on their grandfather's estate. The estate served as a family compound. Eleven cousins also lived in homes on the estate. The cousins created their own games, social norms, and rules for resolving conflicts. Alice's parents, Montgomery Hamilton and Gertrude Corinne (Pond) Hamilton, did not hold the local public school in high regard and opted to homeschool. The homeschooling focused on what the parents thought was important: literature, languages, and religion. Despite the fact that the family was fairly wealthy and socially isolated, Mr. and Mrs. Hamilton instilled a strong sense of social consciousness, caring for poor and minority groups. The experience of growing up on a compound and a deep commitment to social justice remained with Alice throughout her life.

At the age of 17, Alice attended Miss Porter's School in Farmington, Connecticut. At Miss Porter's, Alice elected to study languages and philosophy. In Fort Wayne, the family fortune was slowly declining, and Alice needed to move toward training, which would bring in a steady income. She decided to become a physician, not because she was good in sciences, but because she would be able to travel. Over the next two years, she studied physics, chemistry, biology, and anatomy to gain entry into medical school. After earning her medical degree from the University of Michigan, Dr. Hamilton interned at Northwestern Hospital for Women and Children in Minneapolis and New England Hospital for Women and Children near Boston. Alice preferred science to clinical medicine, and in 1895 Alice and her sister Edith sailed to Germany to study. Alice planned to study bacteriology and pathology, and Edith planned to study classical literature. (Edith Hamilton later became a famous author.) The women were initially refused admission because German universities did not accept female students. Alice was eventually accepted to study in Munich and at the University of Leipzig under the condition that she kept a low profile and did not disturb the male students. On return to the United States, Alice realized that she would not be able to get a job in pathology and bacteriology. She enrolled at Johns Hopkins University, working in the pathology lab with Dr. Simon Flexner. (Dr. Flexner later became a famous physician-pathologist.)

In 1897, Hamilton was offered a teaching position at Northwestern University in Chicago. Moving to Chicago afforded her the opportunity to join Hull House,

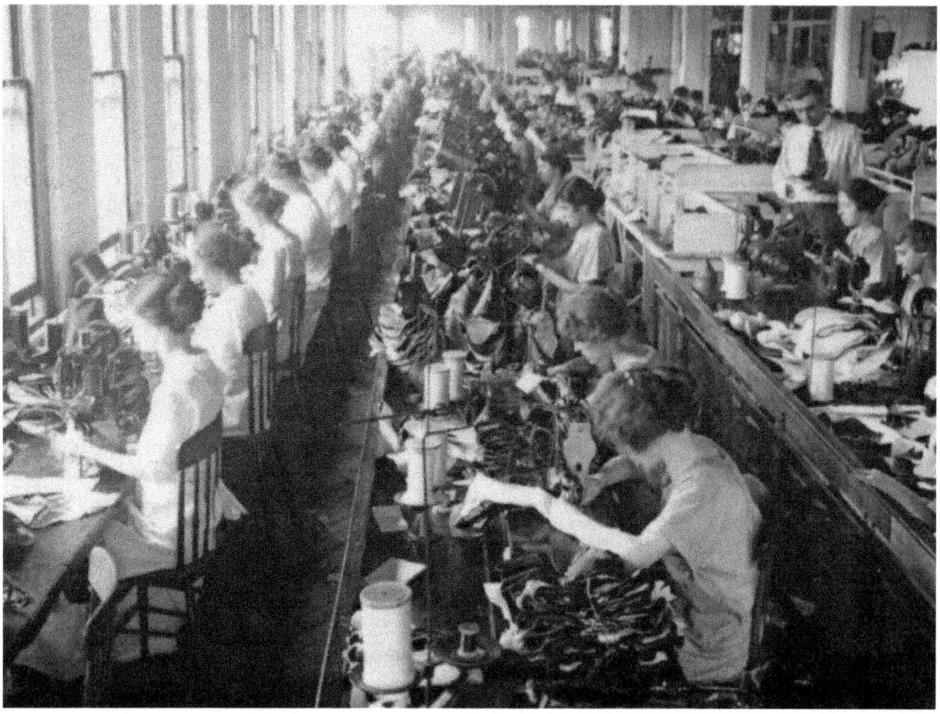

Immigrant factory workers sewing shoes in Syracuse, New York, 1895. Dr. Alice Hamilton noticed unusual illnesses among immigrant residents of Hull House. Her epidemiological investigations created the field of occupational health and safety. (New York Public Library)

an early settlement house founded by Jane Addams and Ellen Gates Starr. The idea of settlement houses originated in London through the social reform movement. In America, settlement houses were houses where people emigrating from Europe could stay while they settled into life and community within the new country. Academic scholars, volunteers, and new immigrants lived, ate, and socialized together. Through day-to-day interactions and planned programs, the academics learned to appreciate the culture, wisdom, and struggles of immigrants and the immigrants learned language, skills, and customs, which helped them to gain employment and blend into American culture. In her autobiography, Hamilton explained, "When I see the varied diet modern mothers give their babies, anything apparently from bacon to bananas, I realize that those Italian women knew what a baby needed far better than my Ann Arbor professor did." The settlement compound served as the center of community life for many, creating social networks, advocating for social justice, and preventing racism. Hull House flourished to include a nursery, kindergarten, public baths, and a playground. While treating and interacting with the immigrants of Hull House, Dr. Hamilton started to notice common ailments: carbon monoxide poisoning, lead poisoning, pneumonia, and rheumatism. People who had come to the United States seeking a better life were suddenly stricken by odd illnesses. Even more troubling was the fact that in the old world, the workers had a network of friends, neighbors, and family members to help them. In the new world, they were alone, and if the main breadwinner became incapacitated and unable to work, the family became destitute.

In 1910, Dr. Hamilton joined a working group led by Professor Charles Henderson, sociologist at the University of Chicago. Henderson received state support to study occupation-related diseases among the working class. The Occupational Disease Commission of Illinois was granted one year and quickly realized that they needed to focus. They decided on occupational poisons, specifically lead. Lead is a highly toxic poison. Symptoms of lead poisoning include headache, abdominal pain, muscle pain, fatigue, radial nerve palsy, delirium, seizures, and coma. To investigate the problem, the researchers interviewed workers, documented symptoms, and hypothesized that toxins in the workplace may cause health problems. Although Hamilton did not have the power to demand entry into workplaces, many business owners willingly let her in. The commission was surprised to learn that lead was used in many different industries, trimming coffins, decorating pottery, as seals on freight cars, cigar wraps, and enamel bathtubs. Hamilton also discovered that employers preferred to hire men with families because family men would continue to work despite poor health. Given that lead workers can bring the toxin home on clothing or skin, not only were workers exposed but also their family members including children. Because of the investigation, Illinois and six other states passed laws requiring employers to develop safety measures to protect workers and to provide regular physical exams to monitor employee health.

By 1911, Dr. Hamilton was a leading authority on industrial toxins and appointed as special investigator for the U.S. Bureau of Labor. While continuing to reside at Hull House, Hamilton traveled the country studying occupational health. She was known for *shoe leather epidemiology*, visiting workshops, construction sites, and factories, observing working conditions, and interviewing workers and employers (Rainhorn, 2012). Through careful, detailed epidemiological investigation, Hamilton created a toolbox of industrial surveys of employee health and safety. Hamilton's family supported her both emotionally and financially during this period of research.

In 1919, Harvard Medical School offered Dr. Hamilton a position teaching industrial medicine. The offer came with conditions. She was not allowed to buy football tickets, proceed with other faculty in the commencement ceremony, or use the Faculty Club. The announcement of the first female professor at Harvard attracted great media attention. The *New York Tribune* headlined, "A Woman on Harvard Faculty—The Last Citadel Has Fallen—The Sex Has Come Into Its Own." Consistent with her spirit of honesty, humor, and seriousness, Hamilton noted, "Yes, I am the first woman on Harvard faculty, but not the first one who should have been appointed!" (Corn, 1999). Until retirement in 1935, Hamilton taught one semester per year. She lived at Hull House and continued her research during the remainder of the academic year. Hamilton never achieved tenure, never progressed beyond the rank of assistant professor, and was only granted a series of three-year contracts.

Hull House was more than a home and research laboratory to Dr. Hamilton. Through Hull House, Hamilton was active in social reform and the women's peace movement. She protested against McCarthyism and the Vietnam War. In 1915, Hamilton attended the International Congress of Women at The Hague with Jane Addams and other influential women. The attendees endorsed a commission of a worldwide organization of nations where conflicts are mediated by neutral nations. Although Hamilton was a pacifist, she advocated for U.S. participation in World War II. After witnessing the racism and cruelty of Nazi Germany, she believed that isolationism would be selfish. By entering World War II, the United States could end the war and Nazi atrocities.

After a period of ill health, Dr. Alice Hamilton died on September 22, 1970, in Hadlyme, Connecticut. Throughout her lifetime, Hamilton was honored with many awards, including the National Achievement Award of the Chi Omega Sorority presented by Eleanor Roosevelt (1935), Men in Science (1944), and Time Woman of the Year (1956). On December 29, 1970, three months after her death, Congress passed the Occupational Safety and Health Act. In 1987, the National Institute of Occupational Safety and Health named its research facility the "Alice Hamilton Laboratory for Occupational Safety and Health." The contributions of this remarkable woman ensure safety for many workers throughout the country.

Sally Kuykendall

See also: Epidemiology; Immigrant Health; Social Determinants of Health

Further Reading

American Chemical Society National Historic Chemical Landmarks. (2002). *Alice Hamilton and the development of occupational medicine.* Retrieved from http://www.acs.org/content/acs/en/education/whatischemistry/landmarks/alicehamilton.html.

Corn, J. K. (1999). Alice Hamilton. *American national biography* (Vol. 9, pp. 910–912). New York: Oxford University Press.

Fee, E., & Brown, T. M. (2001). Alice Hamilton: Settlement physician, occupational health pioneer. *American Journal of Public Health, 91*(11), 1767.

Hamilton, A. (1943). *Exploring the dangerous trades: The autobiography of Alice Hamilton, M.D.* Boston: Little Brown & Co.

Rainhorn, J. (2012). The "shoeleather epidemiology" or the reinvention of medical survey: Alice Hamilton and industrial medicine in early 20th century America. *Gesnerus, 69*(2), 330–354.

Sicherman, B. (2003). *Alice Hamilton: A life in letters.* Cambridge, MA: Harvard University Press.

Windsor, L. L. (2002). *Women in medicine: An encyclopedia.* Santa Barbara, CA: ABC-CLIO.

HANDWASHING

Germs get onto people's hands when they sneeze, cough, handle raw meat, eat contaminated food, defecate, or touch contaminated objects or infected people. Normally, the body has defenses to keep pathogens from attacking the body. However, microorganisms can get past the body defenses when people touch their mouth, nose, or eyes. Germs may also be spread to others through doorknobs, railings, desks, tables, or toys. Handwashing is the easiest and most effective way to prevent germs from entering the body and from being transmitted to other people. Handwashing is an important health practice for everyone and particularly for workers who interact with other people.

The science of handwashing dates back to 1843 when Boston physician Oliver Wendell Holmes Sr. published "The Contagiousness of Puerperal Fever." Puerperal fever is a complication of childbirth caused by bacterial infection. Pathogenic bacteria spread from the uterus, along the fallopian tubes and into the peritoneum, resulting in peritonitis, septicemia, or death. Infants are exposed to the deadly microorganisms during or after childbirth. Holmes believed that puerperal fever was transmitted from patient to patient by doctors and suggested that doctors take precautions. Opponents argued that doctors were gentlemen and gentlemen did not have dirty hands. In 1847, Hungarian obstetrician Ignaz Philipp Semmelweis (1818–1865) served as house officer of two obstetrical wards at the University of Vienna Allgemeine Krankenhaus. Per hospital policy, patients in the First Division ward were cared for by male physicians while patients in the Second Division ward were cared for by nurse midwives. Semmelweis observed:

> Newly admitted patients . . . enter the building in terror, because it is well known to them how large a contingent the institution gives over to death each year . . . That they really dread the First Division can readily be demonstrated, because one must endure heart-rendering scenes, when women, wringing their hands, beg on bended knee . . . for their release, in order to seek admission to the Second Division, after having hit upon the First Division because of unfamiliarity with the place, which the presence of many men made clear to them. Puerperae with uncountable pulse-rates, enormously distended abdomens, dry tongues, i.e. gravely ill with puerperal fever, assured me a few hours before death, that they were entirely well, in order to escape treatment by the physicians, because they realized that such treatment was the forerunner of Death. (Semmelweis & Murphy, 1981, p. 809)

Division One had such an awful reputation in the community that women who were in circulatory shock would beg to be discharged from Division One so that they could be readmitted to Division Two. Semmelweis compared mortality rates of the two divisions for the years 1841–1846. The mortality rate of Division One was 9.9 percent while the mortality rate of Division Two was 3.4 percent (Semmelweis & Murphy, 1981). Semmelweis supposed that many puerperal infections in Division One were related to poor hand hygiene. He observed as medical students and doctors performed autopsies on women who died from puerperal fever and then went straight into the delivery room. Semmelweis recommended that doctors wash their hands in chlorine solution before and after patient care. Although his suggestions were met with resistance, some doctors adopted the practice, and over the next seven months infections in Division One decreased to 3 percent. Dr. Semmelweis is considered the father of hand hygiene.

The Centers for Disease Control and Prevention (CDC, 2016) recommend handwashing before, during, and after preparing food or drinks; before eating; before and after caring for someone who is sick; after using the bathroom, changing diapers, or helping a child to use the bathroom; after sneezing, coughing, or blowing the nose; after touching animals, animal waste, or animal cages, and after feeding animals; after touching garbage; or whenever hands are dirty or greasy. Multiple studies support handwashing as an easy way to reduce the spread of infection and improve individual and community health. Adults who use proper handwashing technique report 31 percent less diarrhea and 21 percent fewer colds (CDC, 2016). The results are even more impressive for people with weakened immune systems among whom good handwashing reduces diarrheal illnesses by 58 percent (CDC, 2016). Handwashing helps children in unexpected ways. Children who are taught to wash their hands achieve developmental milestones in motor movement, interpersonal skills, and communication six months earlier than other children (CDC, 2016). In order to effectively eliminate germs, people must use effective technique. Proper handwashing technique is: (1) Wet both hands with clean running water; (2) use plain liquid soap or bar soap to lather hands, rubbing the soap between both hands; (3) rub the palms, back of hands, and fingers for at least 20 seconds; (4) rinse dirt, grease, and soap off of hands under clean, running water; and (5) dry hands with a clean towel or air dry. If soap and water are not available, alcohol-base sanitizers with at least 60 percent alcohol may be used. Alcohol-based sanitizers are effective against some but not all germs and will not clean dirty or greasy hands.

Handwashing is the simplest and most effective way to prevent illnesses, the spread of germs to others, and to support healthy childhood development. The main advantage of hand hygiene is that anyone can perform this action.

Sally Kuykendall

See also: Antibiotic Resistance; Epidemic; Influenza; Food Safety; Infectious Diseases; Mallon, Mary; Patient Safety

Further Reading

Centers for Disease Control and Prevention (CDC). (2016). *Handwashing: Clean hands save lives.* Retrieved from https://www.cdc.gov/handwashing/index.html.

Global Public-Private Partnership for Handwashing with Soap. (2015). Retrieved http://globalhandwashing.org/.

Semmelweis, I. P., & Murphy, F. P. (1981). Childbed fever. *Reviews of Infectious Diseases*, *3*(4), 808–811. Retrieved from http://www.jstor.org.ezproxy.sju.edu/stable/4452613.

World Health Organization (WHO). (2006). *WHO guidelines on hand hygiene in health care* (Advanced draft). Geneva: World Alliance for Patient Safety. Retrieved from http://www.who.int/patientsafety/information_centre/Last_April_versionHH_Guidelines%5B3%5D.pdf.

HEALTH

In 1946, the World Health Organization (WHO) defined health as "a state of complete physical, mental, and social well-being, and not merely the absence of disease." The WHO definition of health converted the idea of health from physical fitness to a multidimensional concept of biopsychosocial well-being. The inclusion of mental and social health reflected the events and circumstances of the time period. After two world wars, the Great Depression, and the playground movement, the idea of human beings as more than biological creatures was emerging. Sociology and psychology were becoming academic disciplines in their own right. Despite being more than 70 years old, the WHO definition of health is timeless, still used by public health students and professionals today.

Physical, mental, and social health may be understood as simultaneously independent and interdependent. Physical health is how well the body systems function to support movement, oxygenation, fluid and electrolyte balance, hormone regulation, nutrient ingestion, digestion and metabolism, temperature regulation, response to stimuli, protection from the external environment, and excretion of toxins and waste. The body that is physically fit and well nourished is able to respond to potential illness or injury more effectively. Social health is the ability to feel comfortable around others and to enjoy the companionship of friends, family, and colleagues. Humans are social beings. Throughout civilization, individuals depended on one another for survival. People who lived in groups were able to share food, protection, shelter, and work. Individuals who lived alone were susceptible to starvation, harsh elements, or attack from predators, both animal and human. In prosocial societies, most people have an intrinsic need to feel valued, accepted, and belonged. Mental health may be further delineated as emotional, intellectual, and spiritual health. Emotional health is the feelings that one has about self, other people, circumstances, and the surrounding environment. Positive connections with the social and physical world influence the mind and bodily functions. Chronic stress is associated with numerous health problems, including cardiovascular disease, hypertension, substance abuse, obesity, and susceptibility to infection. Intellectual health refers to how people acquire, filter, and use information. People with high intellect gather information from credible sources, are able to critique the quality of the information, and make smart decisions on how to use the information. The person with intellectual health seeking diet changes would use information from reputable sources and avoid sources selling commercial products. Health literacy gives people the ability to make wise choices about their health. Spirituality is the feeling that life is in harmony with one's thoughts, practices, and physical surroundings. Spirituality may be expressed as the belief in higher being(s) or an appreciation of nature, art, literature, gardening, woodworking, or other activity, which allows one to feel interconnected with the world. Spiritual health is achieved when thoughts and actions are in harmony. This means that all of the yoga in the world will not counterbalance lying and cheating others. For spiritual health to occur, thoughts and actions must be consistent. The phrase "state of complete . . . well-being" refers to the overall condition created by the interrelationships of physical, emotional, and social health. Regular walks in beautiful settings can enhance physical, emotional, and social health, lowering blood pressure, increasing high-density lipoproteins (HDL), and building flexibility and balance. Meanwhile, excessive exercising, a form of eating disorder, is associated with anxiety, depression, and amenorrhea. Some experts criticize the WHO definition, claiming that it does not take into account obsessive and harmful health behaviors such as excessive exercising, orthorexia, or obsessive hygiene seen with obsessive compulsive disorder. As scientists explore the complex relationships between physical, mental, and social health, we discover more and more about emotions, the brain, life experiences, and social determinants of health.

According to the WHO, health is *not* the achievement of the perfect physical, emotional, intellectual, social, and spiritual body. Such perfection would be out of reach for many people. Health is a state of wellness based on individual circumstances. People with disease, disabilities, or adverse childhood experiences can achieve health by optimizing those aspects of health that are within their control. History provides numerous examples of people who have overcome physical and mental challenges to achieve incredible accomplishments. Although deaf, Ludwig van Beethoven continued to compose music. Albert Einstein is said to have had a learning disability. Franklin Delano Roosevelt was wheelchair dependent when he served as 32nd president of the United States. Mathematician John Forbes Nash Jr. struggled with paranoid schizophrenia when he was awarded the Nobel Memorial Prize in Economic Sciences (1994). Social scientists purport that disability is not a medical condition. Disability is a socially constructed condition. This means that ability or inability is defined by society. For example, before the Americans with Disabilities Act Accessibility Guidelines (ADAAG), buildings and communities were constructed for people who could walk. Sidewalks, shops, even bathrooms were built for the upright body. People in wheelchairs were limited. Shops, schools, factories, public transportation, sidewalks, and most buildings were not designed to accommodate for wheelchairs. ADAAG did not change the people in the wheelchairs. The act removed barriers established by society, requiring new construction or major renovations to existing facilities to ensure equal access. Similar obstacles exist in social stigmas against people with mental illness. People with paranoid schizophrenia are not accepted by society because society frowns on people who hear voices, suffer from delusions or paranoia, unexplained bouts of anger or anxiety, or detachment from the social group. Health is not simply a reflection of the physical and mental status of the individual. Health is dependent on the built environment, social norms, and cultural values.

Riegelman and Kirkwood (2015) used the mnemonic BIG GEMS to list the numerous factors that influence health and therefore disease. Health determinants are **B**ehavior, **I**nfection, **G**enetics, **G**eography, **E**nvironment, **M**edical care, and **S**ocioeconomic-cultural status. *Behavior* refers to personal actions. Daily exercise and a diet low in concentrated carbohydrates and saturated fats promote well-being. Smoking cigarettes, drinking alcohol, or risky sexual activities threaten health. *Infections*, such as polio, cholera, or malaria are potential health risks, attacking the body and resulting in death or disability. On the other hand, the hygiene hypothesis or alternatively, the microbial deprivation hypothesis, proposes that reduced exposure to germs in early childhood may increase incidence of asthma and allergic diseases. *Genetics* is the genes we inherit from biological parents. Problems occur through hereditary transmission or mutation. Genetic disorders include single gene disorders (such as sickle cell anemia), chromosomal disorders (such as Down syndrome), and complex disorders (such as colon cancer). On the other hand, some genetic conditions provide resistance against disease. Sickle cell carriers infected by parasites with malaria do not succumb to the disease. An enzyme expressed by the sickle hemoglobin produces small amounts of carbon monoxide that protect against malaria. Other genetic disorders that convey resistance are cystic fibrosis and cholera, Tay-Sachs disease and tuberculosis, and myasthenia gravis and rabies. *Geography* influences disease through climate, location, and geological conditions. Hot, wet climates are perfect habitats for wildlife that carry pathogenic organisms. Vast mountain ranges or deserts tend to inhibit disease transmission. *Environment* includes the natural and the man-made world. The World Health Organization (2016) reports that air, water and soil pollution, climate change, ultraviolet radiation, and toxic substances at work and home contribute to more than 100 different health problems. *Medical care* impacts health by providing immunizations against deadly diseases, regular monitoring for early disease identification and treatment, and health education. Conversely, medical care is also responsible for the increase in antibiotic resistant organisms. *Socioeconomic-cultural* determinants of health are level of education, income, and occupation. Poverty is associated with lower life expectancy, higher rates of chronic and acute diseases, and poor mental health. The chronic stress of poverty can lead to decreased white blood cell count, gastrointestinal bleeding, enlargement of the adrenal cortex, and physical deterioration. The BIG GEMS determinants of health suggest opportunities for improving public health as well as challenges to building and sustaining health.

As public health improves, the ability to measure health becomes more important. Historically, health was measured by counting the number of people with a specific disease or the number of infants and people who died each year. Morbidity and mortality rates measure death and disease of a population, not health. The purpose of public health is to promote health, and measuring health is a challenge. Measuring the number of people who remain healthy by not contracting diabetes is impossible unless everyone in the population is regularly screened for diabetes. As health improves, researchers work to develop and refine instruments to measure health. Surveys are used to measure various aspects of health. Instruments exist to gauge social functioning, psychological well-being, functional activity, mental status, pain scale, and quality of life. Ideally, it would be nice if one instrument could be used to measure the health of all individuals under all circumstances in all societies. Such an instrument would enable clear comparisons across groups. Unfortunately, it is unlikely that one instrument, one set of questions will apply to all people and nations. Therefore, measuring health remains an elusive goal for public health researchers.

Health exists as a continuum of interrelated physical, emotional, and social factors. In the seminal work, *The Future of Public's Health in the 21st Century,* the Institute of Medicine (2003, pp. 179–180) noted, "When people are healthy, they are better able to work, learn, build a good life, and contribute to society." The goal of public health, to support the health of all persons, is fundamental to ensuring quality of life, a productive workforce, successful future generations, and global capacity.

Sally Kuykendall

See also: Behavioral Health; Environmental Health; Immigrant Health; Population Health; Prevention; Social Determinants of Health; Spiritual Health

Further Reading

Institute of Medicine. (2003). *The future of the public's health in the 21st Century.* Washington, DC: National Academies Press.

Riegelman, R., & Kirkwood, B. (2015). *Public health 101: Healthy people—healthy populations* (2nd ed.). Burlington, MA: Jones & Bartlett.

World Health Organization (WHO). (1946). *Preamble to the Constitution of the World Health Organization as adopted by the International Health Conference.* New York: Official Records of the World Health Organization. Retrieved from http://apps.who.int/gb/bd/PDF/bd47/EN/constitution-en.pdf?ua=1.

World Health Organization (WHO). (2016). *Environmental health.* Retrieved from http://www.who.int/topics/environmental_health/en/.

HEALTH AND MEDICINE DIVISION OF THE NATIONAL ACADEMIES OF SCIENCES, ENGINEERING, AND MEDICINE

Formerly known as the Institute of Medicine (IOM), the Health and Medicine Division (HMD) of the National Academies of Sciences, Engineering, and Medicine (the National Academies) provides independent, nonpartisan advice to Congress and the White House to ensure that each new or revised policy has a valid scientific basis. The National Academies consist of three private, nonprofit organizations that collaborate with noted experts in various fields. The National Academies and the experts work free of charge so that they can maintain professional and scientific integrity and are not influenced by money or power. The National Academies are consistently recognized for providing valuable information, which benefits the nation and public health.

The National Academies are made up of the National Academy of Sciences (NAS), the National Academy of Engineering (NAE), and the National Academy of Medicine (NAM). The original agency, the NAS, was founded by congressional charter and approved by President Abraham Lincoln on March 3, 1863. The Civil War–era group consisted of 49 experts who were willing to share their knowledge and expertise in ways that advanced the nation. Today, the NAS has more than 3,000 experts, 200 of whom are Nobel Prize winners. The HMD focuses on finding the most effective and efficient ways to alleviate pressing medical and health issues. The division supports medical science by funding research studies and fellowships, rewarding outstanding contributions to the field, and developing collaborations to solve complex problems. In the past, IOM experts addressed malaria, vaccine safety, medical errors, the nursing shortage, public health preparedness, and end-of-life care. Current working groups address global health, food and nutrition, health care services, public health, veterans' health, and children's health. To create expert consensus, HMD develops a formal statement of task that defines the problem scope. A committee of individual experts is convened. Committee members are selected based on their ability to provide expertise, wisdom, and balanced perspectives. All committee members are screened for potential conflicts of interest at the beginning of the project and throughout the project. HMD schedules forums, workshops, roundtables, and committees to collect information on the defined health issue. The committee reviews and critiques information from the meetings, published literature, and their own research to develop a report that summarizes the science and provides objective recommendations. The expert consensus meetings are closed to avoid undue pressure from businesses or other interested groups. Final reports are reviewed by a second group of independent experts who provide feedback to the committee. HMD goes to great lengths to ensure that each report provides valuable, credible, and objective advice that adheres to the highest scientific standards.

HMD promotes effective public health policies by gathering the best and the brightest of the nation's scholars and putting them to work on critical health issues. The resulting recommendations can have widespread utilization. For example, in 2003, the National Academies released the report *The Future of the Public's Health in the 21st Century*. The landmark report described the importance of health determinants, ways to strengthen public health infrastructure and partnerships, improving accountability, and enhancing systems communication. The report is used by the

American Public Health Association (APHA) and Schools of Public Health to educate and prepare the next generation of public health professionals.

Sally Kuykendall

See also: American Public Health Association; Core Competencies in Public Health; Health; Health Disparities; Health Policy; Patient Safety

Further Reading

Institute of Medicine. (2003). *The future of the public's health in the 21st century.* Washington, DC: National Academies Press.

National Academies of Sciences. (2017). *About HMD.* Retrieved from http://www.nationalacademies.org/hmd/About-HMD.aspx.

HEALTH BELIEF MODEL

The health belief model is a diagrammatic representation of the psychological and social factors that influence an individual's willingness and likelihood to take action to prevent disease. The model was developed by public health practitioners to understand the thought processes people go through when deciding whether to use health services. It is now one of the preeminent public health models used to motivate people to adopt disease management activities or healthy behaviors. The model applies to numerous health behaviors from tuberculosis screening to smoking, safe sexual practices, or dental flossing. Benefits of the health belief model are that it provides a deeper understanding of motivation and suggests techniques that can be used to motivate people toward health. Criticisms are that while the model explains motivation, it cannot predict motivation. Further refinement of the model is needed to test and ensure effective application.

The health belief model originated in the 1950s after the U.S. Public Health Service offered mass disease campaigns with limited success. One such campaign was screening services for the deadly infectious disease, tuberculosis (TB). At the time, TB was known as the *white plague.* Mortality rates varied from 6.2 per 100,000 people in Wyoming to 59.6 per 100,000 in Arizona (Division of Chronic Disease and Tuberculosis, 1953). *Mycobacterium tuberculosis* is easily transmitted. Once the bacterium enters the body, it may become latent (noninfectious) *TB infection* or active *TB disease* attacking the lungs and other parts of the body. More than one-third of the world's population currently has latent TB (WHO, 2016). In an effort to combat the disease, public health professionals offered free neighborhood screenings. Mobile X-ray units were dispatched to at-risk communities. The plan was to screen for TB using X-rays and refer cases for antibiotic treatment, thus reducing transmission. Very few people came for screening. Social psychologists decided to explore why people did not come (Hochbaum, 1958; Rosenstock, 1960, 1966, 1974). The researchers focused on people's readiness for screening, beliefs about susceptibility, and perceptions of whether X-ray was an effective method of detection. The studies found that the decision to go for screening was dependent on how susceptible the person believed he or she was to TB and perceptions about the severity of the disease. Since initial conception, behavioral theorists have refined the model to include concepts from cognitive theory, and translational researchers extended application to preventive actions, sick-role behaviors, and disease management.

The key concepts of the health belief model are perceived susceptibility, perceived severity, cues to action, perceived benefits, and perceived barriers. *Perceived susceptibility* is one's belief of vulnerability to the health issue. A simple and common problem, such as oral hygiene, may be used to demonstrate the constructs and value of the health belief model. Dental caries affects 91 percent of U.S. adults, aged 20 to 64 (CDC, National Center for Health Statistics, 2016). The American Dental Association (ADA) recommends using an interdental cleaner (flossing) at least once a day (ADA, 2016). Yet, only 4 out of 10 people floss on a daily basis, and 2 out of 10 people never floss (ADA, 2014). The health belief model outlines demographic and other factors that might influence one's perception of susceptibility. Age, gender, race, socioeconomic status, and education or knowledge may influence how one thinks about his or her vulnerability to cavities. If one recognizes susceptibility, the next question is *perceived severity*. Is the problem serious enough to warrant action? If the person feels that cavities are unimportant and can be easily remedied, then he or she will be less likely to brush and floss. If someone has experienced *cues to action*, the pain of a cavity, difficulty chewing food, the irritating sound of the dental drill, or the inconvenience of Novocaine, perceived threat (severity) increases. Other cues to action are health education in schools or by dental staff, public service announcements, or posting a note on the bathroom mirror to remind self to floss. The final considerations are perceived benefits minus perceived barriers. Decisional balance, weighing advantages (pros) and disadvantages (cons), is a concept used and repeated throughout health. The benefits of flossing are a beautiful smile, the ability to enjoy crunchy foods, and not having to go to the dentist more often than every six months. The disadvantages or barriers to flossing are the additional time that it takes each day (2 to 3 minutes), purchasing and maintaining a supply of floss, and having to clean the particles of food that are projected throughout the area during flossing. The final consideration is, do the benefits outweigh the barriers? If so, the person is likely to take action (floss) to prevent periodontal disease.

In summary, the health belief model proposes that individuals will take action to prevent disease (or injury) if they perceive that they are susceptible to the disease, the disease is severe enough to warrant a course of action, and the benefits of taking action outweigh the barriers to behavioral change. The health belief model is an amazingly basic and easily understood model that can be applied to bicycle helmets, diabetes management, and numerous other health issues.

Sally Kuykendall

See also: Epidemiology; Health Communication; Intervention; Population Health; Social Determinants of Health

Further Reading

ADA. (2014). *Survey finds shortcomings in oral health habits.* Retrieved from http://www.ada.org/en/publications/ada-news/2014-archive/october/survey-finds-shortcomings-in-oral-health-habits.

ADA. (2016). *Federal government, ADA emphasize importance of flossing and interdental cleaners.* Retrieved from http://www.ada.org/en/press-room/news-releases/2016-archive/august/statement-from-the-american-dental-association-about-interdental-cleaners.

Centers for Disease Control and Prevention, National Center for Health Statistics. (2016). *Oral and dental health.* Retrieved from http://www.cdc.gov/nchs/fastats/dental.htm.

Division of Chronic Disease and Tuberculosis. (1953). Tuberculosis mortality by state, 1950. *Public Health Reports, 68*(6). Retrieved from http://www.ncbi.nlm.nih.gov/pmc/articles/PMC2024038/pdf/pubhealthreporig00186-0086.pdf.

Glanz, K., Lewis, F. M., & Rimer, B. K. (1997). *Health behavior and health education: Theory, research, and practice* (2nd ed.). San Francisco: Jossey-Bass.

Hochbaum, G. M. (1958). *Public participation in medical screening programs: A sociopsychological study.* PHS Publication no. 572. Washington, DC: U.S. Government Printing Office.

Janis, I. L., & Mann, L. (1977). *Decision making: A psychological analysis of conflict, choice, and commitment.* New York: Free Press.

Rosenstock, I. M. (1960). What research in motivation suggests for public health. *American Journal of Public Health and the Nation's Health, 50*, 295–302.

Rosenstock, I. M. (1966). Why people use health services. *The Milbank Memorial Fund Quarterly, 44*(3), 94–127.

Rosenstock, I. M. (1974). Historical origins of the Health Belief Model. *Health Education Monographs, 2*, 328–335.

World Health Organization (WHO). (2016). *Tuberculosis.* Fact Sheet No. 104. Retrieved from http://www.who.int/mediacentre/factsheets/fs104/en/.

HEALTH CARE DISPARITIES

Health care disparities refer to inequities experienced by different populations in obtaining medical treatment. Health care disparity is not to be confused with health disparity. Health care disparities refer to "differences between groups in health insurance coverage, access to and use of care, and quality of care" (Artiga, 2016). Health disparity refers to "a higher burden of illness, injury, disability, or mortality experienced by one population group relative to another group" (Artiga, 2016). Health disparity refers to clinical health problems. Certain diseases may be more prevalent in one population group than others due to culture or genetics. Sickle cell disease affects people of African, Hispanic, southern European, Middle Eastern, and Asian backgrounds. Tay-Sachs disease, an autosomal recessive trait, is more common among the Cajun, French Canadian, and the Ashkenazi Jewish populations. On the other hand, health care disparity is a problem of the health care system, thereby making it a social justice concern. Health disparity and health care disparity are closely related because addressing health care disparities naturally closes some of the gap created by health disparities. When a population suffers higher rates of disease, accessing health services is critical for early diagnosis and treatment. Early services can reduce adverse consequences and promote better quality and length of life.

Health care disparity is a persistent sociopolitical problem. People who are Hispanic, black, Native American, Alaskan Native, and Asian/Pacific Islander or low income do not have the same opportunities for services as affluent whites. Race and income are not separate or isolated issues. In 2013, wealth inequality between blacks and whites reached the highest point since 1989. White households are 17 times wealthier than black households (Kochhar & Fry, 2014). Wealth provides privilege, the benefit of insurance, access to services, care by highly qualified medical professionals, diagnostic testing, treatment, and rehabilitation programs. Disparities also exist by age, gender, geographic location, disability, citizenship status, and sexual identity. People aged 65 and older receive worse care than people aged 18 to 44, and residents of rural areas have poorer access to care than urban dwellers (Agency for Healthcare Research and Quality, 2012). Challenges in obtaining medical care are compounded for undocumented immigrants who struggle with language barriers, in low-paying jobs without health insurance, and live in fear that accessing care could lead to jail or deportation.

Beardsley (1992) presents the historical background of racial health care disparities in the United States as three time periods: the era of denial (1900–1930), the era of inclusion (1930–1960), and the era of attempted restitution (1960–?). During the era of denial, many white Americans, including politicians, doctors, sociologists, and respected scholars, believed that black Americans were inherently lazy, ignorant, and self-destructive, and therefore any efforts to improve health were futile. Some white supremacist groups preferred the high mortality rates suffered by black communities. White supremacists feared that treating and preventing diseases among black communities would increase the numbers of black people, displacing white power and privilege. Politicians were pressured *not* to provide services to black communities. As a result, the majority of black people were cared for out of hospital by less qualified community health workers. Those who were able to afford hospitalization were required to use segregated black hospitals. Black hospitals provided primitive care with outdated equipment and poorly trained staff. In some areas, hospitals for black people did not even exist. In South Carolina, the sanatorium to treat black patients with tuberculosis opened five years after the white sanatorium and offered fewer beds, even though rates of tuberculosis were four to five times higher among blacks than whites. The black community had to raise partial funding in order to build the sanatorium. In 1911, malaria was a major health issue throughout South Carolina and affected blacks at rates of two to four times that of whites. When South Carolina state health officer James A. Haynie requested federal support for malaria eradication, he argued on the grounds that eliminating malaria would allow whites to reinhabit South Carolina's fertile coastal lowland regions, areas that were currently inhabited by blacks. Toward the end of the 1930s, small gains were made in improving health care systems for black patients. The Duke Endowment invested millions of dollars to improve Carolina hospitals for both blacks and whites. Dr. Matilda Evans opened the Evans Clinic in Columbia, South Carolina, treating hundreds of patients daily. The Atlanta Project started by Lugenia Hope created a settlement house, medical clinic, nursing clinics, and mobile health clinics.

The Great Depression of the 1930s unraveled many of the advancements achieved during the preceding decade. Yet, mutual suffering also spurred solutions. With high unemployment among both blacks and whites, government officials instituted programs such as the New Deal, Federal Emergency Relief Administration to hospitals, school lunch programs, investments in the public health workforce, and the Social Security Act. The policies did not discriminate between black and white because everyone was struggling. Even the horror of two world wars brought medical advancements. Venereal diseases, which had long been a problem among black communities, became a national priority. Politicians were concerned with the high number of American soldiers contracting syphilis and gonorrhea overseas. The federal government invested in research and treatment. Penicillin was discovered. Effective community-based treatment programs were funded. Perhaps one of the biggest steps toward social justice occurred through Emergency Maternal and Infant Care Program (EMIC), a federal effort to support military families. The federal government realized that in order to support soldiers, they needed to support the men's families on the home front. EMIC subsidized hospital care for wives of military men in the lowest pay grades. Since the lowest pay grades were disproportionately black men, EMIC improved care for black families. EMIC led to the Hospital Survey and Construction Law (1946), a program offering states matched funding for the construction of new hospitals and clinics. A condition of the funding was that the state must plan construction based on needs. In so doing, state health officials were forced to look at the health of populations throughout the state. Despite federal efforts, racism continued at regional levels. Chicago's hospitals designated 315 beds to care for the city's population of 350,000 black residents (Beardsley, 1992). Twelve private hospitals systematically excluded black patients, even those who could afford to pay. Hospital beds designated for white people sat empty while black patients, including expectant mothers, vied for care.

The civil rights movement of the 1960s banned segregation and outright discrimination. Beardsley (1992) suggests that programs such as Medicare, food stamps, and WIC provide attempted restitution. Data from multiple sources contradict this idea. The Centers for Disease Control and Prevention, Office of Minority Health (2016), reports that African Americans have double the infant mortality rate, a 40 percent higher rate of death due to heart disease, and an 80 percent higher rate of diabetes, compared to non-Hispanic whites. Death rates due to HIV/AIDS are seven times higher, and homicide is six times higher among African Americans in comparison to non-Hispanic whites. Other races are not immune from such disparities. Latinos have higher rates of tuberculosis, diabetes, obesity, hypertension, and low birth weight infants. Low birth weight is associated with poor lung development and infant death. Asian and Pacific Islanders suffer from higher rates of cervical cancer, tuberculosis, and hepatitis. Even more alarming is the fact that these disparities cannot simply be ascribed to lifestyle. African American women perform mammography screening at the same rate as white women, yet die of breast cancer at much higher rates. Our health care system continues to fail minority ethnic groups.

Today, public health is actively seeking solutions to health care disparities. The 1998 surgeon general's report, *Tobacco Use among U.S. Racial/Ethnic Minority Groups*, addressed the need for tobacco control measures for the racial/ethnic minority groups and contributed to the enactment of the Minority Health and Health Disparities Research and Education Act of 2000. The act led to the establishment of National Center on Minority Health and Health Disparities (NCMHD), which is now the National Institute on Minority Health and Health Disparities (NIMHD). Investment in health care disparities research has provided further insight in achieving inclusion. Medical researchers have begun to produce significant works on health and health care disparities. The Patient Protection and Affordable Care Act (PPACA) enacted in 2010 will reduce disparities by increasing coverage options for low and moderate income populations. The Department of Health and Human Services Office of Minority Health (HHS) produced the 2011 Action Plan to Reduce Racial and Ethnic Health Disparities under the vision of "a nation free of disparities in health and healthcare." The major focus of the HHS Action Plan is on increasing culturally appropriate health care services for the minority populations by hiring more ethnic-minority health care providers and providing training and language translation services.

The measures discussed so far are a standard, top-down approach, relying primarily on federal and state policies. Inner-city public health clinics are challenged with treating populations who speak different dialects and engage in many different health practices. Community collaborations suggest one possible solution. Each community has unique concerns with unique demographics, and reducing health care disparities sometimes requires dramatically different solutions for different communities. The collaborative approach is an attempt to find solutions through the network of community members, particularly with the help of the community leaders. Community health promotion programs are one way to improve care among impoverished neighborhoods. Under the Emergency Medical Treatment & Labor Act (1986), local hospitals are legally required to medically stabilize patients admitted to their emergency rooms. In many regions, hospital emergency rooms have become clinics for those without health insurance and undocumented immigrants. In Philadelphia, three hospitals of the Mercy Health System hospitals were in a financial quandary regarding how to provide medical services to low income patients. In 2012, Mercy partnered with academics at Saint Joseph's University Institute of Clinical Bioethics (ICB). The group reached out to the community religious leaders and began Health Promoters. Mercy medical residents run free monthly clinics focusing on preventive medicine and nutritional and lifestyle counseling. Goals are to improve the general health of the community and reduce the number of preventable emergency room visits (Ochasi & Clark, 2014). The next steps are evaluation of the project as an evidence-based program. The multifaceted grassroots approach suggests promise in reducing health care disparities.

Through political and social policies and practices, the United States systematically neglected and deprived minorities and low income populations of needed medical care. Today, the U.S. population is becoming increasingly heterogeneous. Each population shares the work of maintaining the nation. Yet, racial minorities and the poor carry a higher burden of injury, disability, and death. Social justice demands shared responsibility and benefits. By 2044, people of color will account for more than half of the population, with the largest growth occurring among people of Hispanic race (Colby & Ortman, 2015). This shift raises questions of how society will look in terms of income, race, and health care expenses. Building equitable health care systems now will ensure success for future generations.

Marvin J. H. Lee and Sally Kuykendall

See also: Affordable Care Act; Care, Access to; Emergency Medical Treatment and Labor Act; Epidemiology; Ethics in Public Health and Population Health; Health Disparities; Population Health; Social Determinants of Health

Further Reading

Agency for Healthcare Research and Quality. (2012). *Disparities in healthcare quality among racial and ethnic groups: Selected findings from the National Healthcare Quality and Disparities Reports.* Washington, DC: U.S. Department of Health and Human Services. Retrieved from http://archive.ahrq.gov/research/findings/nhqrdr/nhqrdr11/minority.html.

Artiga, S. (2016). *Disparities in health and health care: Five key questions and answers.* Washington, DC: Kaiser Family Foundation. Retrieved from http://kff.org/disparities-policy/issue-brief/disparities-in-health-and-health-care-five-key-questions-and-answers/.

Beardsley, E. (1992). Race as a factor of health. In R. Apple (Ed.), *Women, health, and medicine in America: A historical handbook.* New Brunswick, NJ: Rutgers University Press.

Betancourt, J., Green, A., Carrillo, J., & Park, E. (2005). Cultural competence and health care disparities: Key perspectives and trends—Among stakeholders in managed care, government, and academe, cultural competence is emerging as an important strategy to address health care disparities. *Health Affairs*, *24*(2), 499–505.

Bylander, J. (2016). Tackling disparities with lessons from abroad. *Health Affairs (Project Hope)*, *35*(8), 1348–1350. doi:10.1377/hlthaff.2016.0794

Colby, S. L., & Ortman, J. M. (2015). *Projections of the size and composition of the U.S. population: 2014 to 2060.* U.S. Census Bureau. Retrieved from http://www.census.gov/population/projections/data/national/2014/publications.html.

Evans, R. G., Barer, M. L., & Marmor, T. R. (1994). *Why are some people healthy and others not? The determinants of health of populations*. New York: Aldine de Gruyter.

Kochhar, R., & Fry, R. (2014). *Wealth inequality has widened along racial, ethnic lines since end of great recession*. Washington, DC: Pew Research Center. Retrieved from http://www.pewresearch.org/fact-tank/2014/12/12/racial-wealth-gaps-great-recession/.

Ochasi, A., & Clark, P.A. (2014). Mercy health promoter model: Meeting needs of specific immigrant communities. *Health Progress*, 33–37. Retrieved from https://www.chausa.org/publications/health-progress/article/march-april-2014/mercy-health-promoter-model-meeting-needs-of-specific-immigrant-communities.

Office of Minority Health. (2016). *Minority population profiles*. Retrieved from http://minorityhealth.hhs.gov/omh/browse.aspx?lvl=2&lvlid=26.

Purnell, T. S., Calhoun, E. A., Golden, S. H., Halladay, J. R., Krok-Schoen, J. L., Appelhans, B. M., & Cooper, L. A. (2016). Achieving health equity: Closing the gaps in health care disparities, interventions, and research. *Health Affairs (Project Hope)*, *35*(8), 1410–1415. doi:10.1377/hlthaff.2016.0158

HEALTH COMMUNICATION

Health communication is defined as "the study and use of communication strategies to inform and influence individual and community decisions that enhance health" (National Cancer Institute [NCI], 1989). Health communication translates complex scientific information into clear, understandable language in order to enhance health. The discipline draws on knowledge from engineering, psychology, sociology, business, and medicine. And while one would think that policy makers, patients, and members of the general public would be interested in information intended to improve quality and length of life, unfortunately, this is not always the case. Public health communication must overcome skepticism and compete with wealthy businesses trying to sell products or services.

Health communication practice developed from engineering and telecommunications. Dr. Harry Nyquist (1889–1976) was a Swedish American electronics engineer who worked at AT&T and Bell Telephone Laboratories, investigating ways to optimize communications systems. Although the telephone had been invented in 1876, Morse code was still used for critical communication, such as between military bases, ships, and warplanes in World Wars I and II. In researching ways to optimize communications, Nyquist noticed that the most efficient Morse code readers were not translating the procedural signal as alphanumeric characters, but were listening to the rhythm of the signal and translating the code as a language. He noted that how the recipient receives and decodes the message is an important component of telecommunication. Instead of using the term "message," Nyquist used the term "intelligence" to name the information that was transmitted from sender to recipient. Nyquist's work was continued by Dr. Claude E. Shannon, also an engineer at Bell Telephone Laboratories. Shannon developed a diagram outlining five major elements of communication. *Intelligence* starts at the *information source* and is passed to the *transmitter.* The transmitter interprets, writes, or codes the message and selects a *channel*. The channel carries the message to the *receiver* where the message is decoded and reconstructed. The reconstructed message is passed to the *destination*. Since Shannon was an engineer, working in telecommunications, he added a sixth intervening element of *noise*. Noise is something that interferes with transmission between transmitter and receiver. The Shannon-Weaver model or information theory was reprinted and published by scientist and mathematician Dr. Warren Weaver (1894–1978). The model was picked up by social scientists who envisioned application to interpersonal communication. And the model is highly applicable to social sciences in that the psychosocial attributes of the sender and receiver can impact how a message is transmitted or perceived. Social science application also brought criticism because the model is one-directional. The message is transmitted without feedback, acceptance, acknowledgment, or clarification by the receiver. In normal, healthy human relationships, feedback is essential to the communication process.

In 1972, a group of scholars recognized the opportunity to apply communication science to public health. Members of the International Communication Association (ICA) formed the Therapeutic Communication interest group. The group attracted educators, researchers, and practitioners with varied interests in

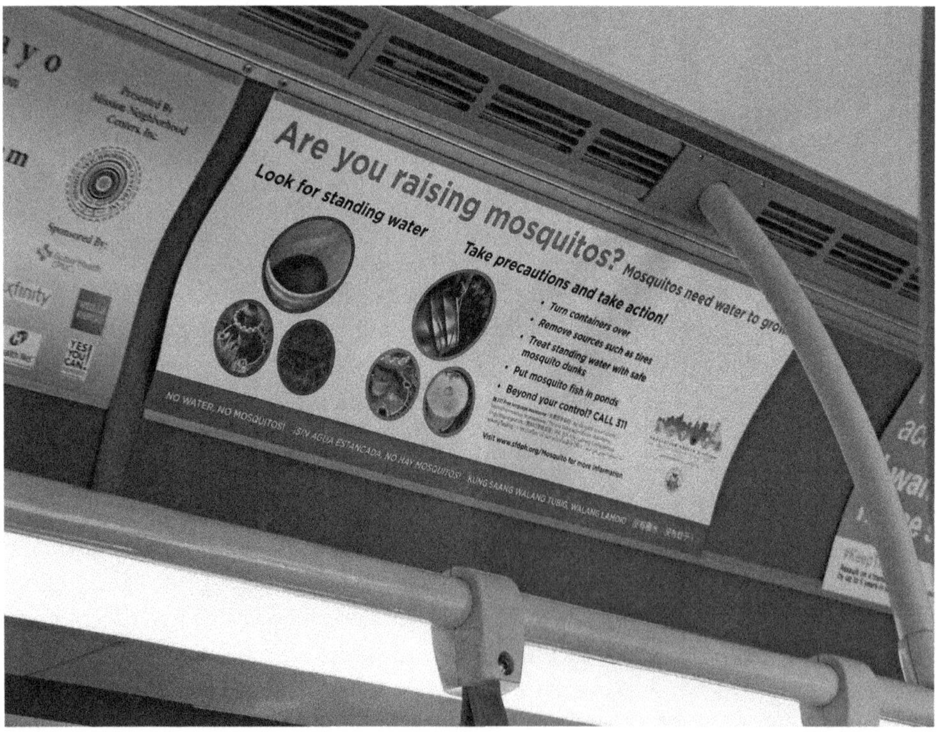
Are you raising mosquitos?
Look for standing water
Take precautions and take action!
NO WATER, NO MOSQUITOS!

Health communication translates complex scientific information into clear, simple, and memorable messages. This public service announcement gives bus riders straightforward tips for mosquito control and where to go for further information. (Sara Ann Kuykendall)

interpersonal communication, mass communication campaigns, and health services. The National Cancer Institute (NCI) quickly embraced health communication as a way to refute common myths about cancer, increase public knowledge, influence attitudes, prompt behavioral changes, advocate for policy, and strengthen health care systems (NCI, 1989). The first professional journal of the field, *Health Communication,* was started in 1989. Seven years later, the Centers for Disease Control (CDC) developed an office of communications. The following year, the American Public Health Association (APHA) formed the Health Communication division. Today, the field of health communication has evolved greatly, employing the media, entertainment industry, interactive technology, and direct patient-provider communication to inform and influence health behavior and decisions.

The task of health communication is onerous and requires a mixed skillset. Health communicators must be able to read, understand, and interpret difficult, tedious, and technical scientific information, identify the key points of interest to different audiences, and translate that information into an easily understandable message, web page, poster, brochure, or tweet. The basic steps in developing health communications are:

- Gather accurate information from reliable sources and identify five or fewer key points.
- Identify the goals or objectives of the communication.
- Identify the target audience.
- Identify the channel or medium to transmit the message.
- Create and pilot test the message.
- Develop a plan for promotion.
- Implement the strategy.
- Evaluate process, impact, and outcome.

Note that the steps include components of the Shannon-Weaver model with the addition of defined goals or objectives, pilot testing, and feedback (evaluation). Health educators must be able to identify what information is most relevant to a particular audience and to tailor the message to the audience. This is where other models or theories are useful. For example, the health communicator could use the health belief model, social cognitive theory, transtheoretical model or diffusion or innovations theory to develop the message. *Healthy People 2010* lists and describes the attributes of effective health communication as accuracy, availability, balance, consistency, cultural competence, evidence base, reach, reliability, repetition, timeliness, and understandability (U.S. Department of Health and Human Services, 2000).

Evaluating the success of health communication programs can be very difficult because mass communication campaigns have little direct follow-up with the recipients. In 2012, researchers at Kings College in London partnered with Cancer Research UK to evaluate England's national smoking cessation campaign, Stoptober. Based on a nationally representative sample of 31,566 smokers, the researchers estimated that Stoptober was related to 350,000 quit attempts and saved 10,400 discounted life years at a cost of £415 per life year (Brown, Kotz, Michie, Stapleton, Walmsley, & West, 2014). Researchers from the CDC evaluated the cost benefit of the National Colorectal Cancer (CRC) Action Campaign, *Screen for Life*. They estimated that if the campaign influenced only 0.5 percent of viewers who did not regularly screen for CRC to get screened, the campaign would lead to an additional 251,000 people getting screened for CRC at a cost of $2.44 per person. If the campaign influenced 10 percent of the population, an additional 5.01 million people would be screened at a cost of $0.12 per person (Ekwueme, Howard, Gelb, Rim, & Cooper, 2014). Finding ways to measure the impact of health communication campaigns can help to create the most effective messages and advance the field of health communications.

Obstacles to health communication include personal attitudes toward the message, competition for public attention, and competition with businesses marketing unhealthy products. Gollust and Cappella (2014) propose that the receiver may reject messages that elicit anger or counterargument or are perceived as weak. Health communicators must walk a line between providing information that empowers people and appearing too weak or too dictatorial. One of the largest obstacles to health communication is competition with business. In 2013, businesses spent $165 billion on advertising (GroupM, n.d.). The tobacco industry spent $244 million and food and beverage companies spent $136 million (Kantar Media & OAAA, n.d.a; Kantar Media & OAAA, n.d.b). In comparison, the CDC budget for chronic disease prevention and health promotion—which includes surveillance, interventions, and research—was $1.1 billion (CDC, 2014). It is difficult to compete with businesses with much deeper pockets. Furthermore, health communicators must work within ethical boundaries, providing honest and accurate information, while businesses are not constrained to the same ethical principles. One highly effective public health campaign was the *Truth* campaign by the American Legacy Foundation. The Truth campaign presented the target audience with facts about tobacco products and the tobacco industry in powerful and memorable advertisements. The campaign successfully deconstructed tobacco marketing to influence youth attitudes and behaviors toward smoking.

Health communication takes difficult to understand information and turns it into easily understandable concepts. The goal is to empower people with the latest science and information so that they can make educated decisions regarding their health. The discipline employs techniques from the fields of science, medicine, psychology, and human development to meet the needs of different audiences.

Sally Kuykendall

See also: Health Belief Model; Health Education; Health Literacy; *Healthy People 2020*; Social Cognitive Theory; Society of Public Health Education; Transtheoretical Model; *Controversies in Public Health:* Controversy 4

Further Reading

Brown, J., Kotz, D., Michie, S., Stapleton, J., Walmsley, M., & West, R. (2014). How effective and cost-effective was the national mass media smoking cessation campaign "Stoptober"? *Drug and Alcohol Dependence*, *135*, 52–58. doi:10.1016/j.drugalcdep.2013.11.003

Centers for Disease Control and Prevention (CDC). (2017). *Gateway to health communication and social marketing practice*. Retrieved from https://www.cdc.gov/healthcommunication/healthbasics/whatishc.html.

Ekwueme, D. U., Howard, D. H., Gelb, C. A., Rim, S. H., & Cooper, C. P. (2014). Analysis of the benefits and costs of a national campaign to promote colorectal cancer screening: CDC's Screen for Life—National Colorectal Cancer Action Campaign. *Health Promotion Practice*, *15*(5), 750–758. doi:10.1177/1524839913519446

Gollust, S. E., & Cappella, J. N. (2014). Understanding public resistance to messages about health disparities. *Journal of Health Communication*, *19*(4), 493–510. doi:10.1080/10810730.2013.821561

GroupM. (n.d.). *Advertising spending in the United States from 2011 to 2017 (in billion U.S. dollars)*. In Statista—The Statistics Portal. Retrieved from https://www-statista-com.ezproxy.sju.edu/statistics/236958/advertising-spending-in-the-us/.

Kantar Media & OAAA. (n.d.a). *Advertising spending of the cigarettes and tobacco industry in the United States in 2013, by medium (in thousand U.S. dollars)*. In Statista—The Statistics Portal. Retrieved from https://www-statista-com.ezproxy.sju.edu/statistics/245332/advertising-spending-of-the-ttobacco-industry-in-the-us-by-medium/.

Kantar Media & OAAA. (n.d.b). *Advertising spending of the food and beverage industry in the United States in 2013, by medium (in thousand U.S. dollars)*. In Statista—The Statistics Portal. Retrieved from https://www-statista-com.ezproxy.sju.edu/statistics/319053/food-beverage-ad-spend-medium/.

National Cancer Institute. (1989). *Making health communications work*. Pub. No. NIH 89-1493. Washington, DC: U.S. Department of Health and Human Services. Retrieved from https://www.cancer.gov/publications/health-communication/pink-book.pdf.

Shannon, C. E., & Weaver, W. (1949). *The mathematical theory of communication*. Urbana: University of Illinois Press.

U.S. Department of Health and Human Services. (2000). *Healthy People 2010* (2nd ed.). Health communication. Washington, DC: U.S. Government Printing Office. Retrieved from http://www.healthypeople.gov/2010/document/pdf/Volume1/11HealthCom.pdf.

U.S. Department of Health and Human Services. (2014). *HHS FY2015 Budget in brief*. Retrieved from https://www.hhs.gov/about/budget/fy2015/budget-in-brief/cdc/index.html.

HEALTH DISPARITIES

The Institute of Medicine defines health care disparities as differences in treatment or access between population groups that cannot be justified by different preferences for services or differences in health (McGuire, Alegria, Cook, Wells, & Zaslavsky, 2006). Health disparities are defined as differences in health outcomes across population groups (Schnittker & McLeod, 2005). Within the United States, much of the focus on health and health care disparities has turned to differences in access and quality across racial and ethnic groups, along with differences in socioeconomic status (SES), especially education and income and factors such as geographic location, gender, and sexuality.

The growth in interest in research about social differences in health and health care disparities was summarized well by the Adler and Rehkopf (2008) review of U.S. disparities in health by examining literature for the term "health disparities. Although this was a key word in only one article in 1980, and fewer than 30 in the 1990s, it went up to more than 400 articles from 2000 to 2004. If the term "health inequalities" was used instead, the pattern of increase was similar. That term is used more often in British studies.

Within the United States, some of these earlier studies led to the now well-known efforts in the United States to examine and try to eliminate health disparities due to race/ethnicity and socioeconomic status in the *Healthy People* series. From the federal government level, one of the pushes for more research on health care inequalities came from the passage of Public Law 106–129, the Healthcare Research and Quality Act of 1999. That law called for two annual reports, one focused on quality and one focused on disparities. Within the work on disparities was a call to track prevailing disparities in health care delivery as they relate to racial and socioeconomic factors among priority populations such as low income groups, racial and

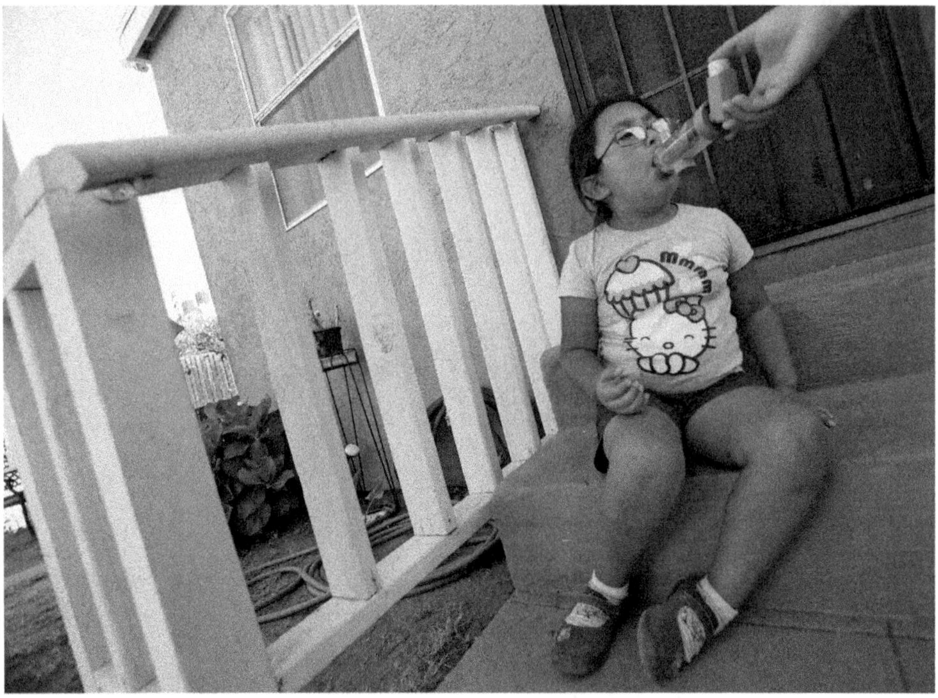

Cuicani Villegas stops playing to use her asthma inhaler. Children in inner city neighborhoods are regularly exposed to industrial pollutants leading to higher burdens among poor black and Hispanic children. (Bob Chamberlin/Los Angeles Times via Getty Images)

ethnic minorities, women, children, the elderly, individuals with special health care needs, the disabled, people in need of long-term care, people requiring end-of-life care, and places of residence (rural communities). A first *National Healthcare Disparities Report* (2004) built on previous efforts in the federal government, especially *Healthy People 2010* (U.S. Department of Health and Human Services, 2000) and the IOM Report, *Unequal Treatment: Confronting Racial and Economic Disparities in Healthcare* (Smedley, Stith, & Nelson, 2003). Elimination of disparities in health was a goal of *Healthy People 2010. Unequal Treatment* extensively documented health care disparities in the United States and focused on those related to race and ethnicity, but not on SES, a weakness of the report. The Institute of Medicine (IOM) report on *Unequal Treatment* also looked at factors related to providers of care and argued that providers' perceptions and, from that, their attitudes toward patients can be influenced by patient race or ethnicity (Smedley, Stith, & Nelson 2003).

The *National Healthcare Disparities Report* (2004) did focus on the ability of Americans to access health care and variation in quality of care. Disparities related to socioeconomic status were included, along with racial/ethnic disparities. Some key findings from the report included that inequality in quality of care continues to exist and that disparities often are particularly true for some more serious health care problems, such as minorities being diagnosed with cancer at later stages, less often receiving optimal care when hospitalized for cardiac problems, and higher rates of avoidable hospital admissions among blacks and poorer patients.

In 2005, the third *National Healthcare Disparities Report* (2005) was released. The 2005 report focused on findings from a set of core report measures and indicated that disparities still existed, but some disparities were diminishing. Disparities remained in areas of access, quality, and across many levels and types of care including preventive care, treatment of acute conditions, and management of chronic disease. This applies to a variety of specific clinical conditions including cancer, diabetes, end stage renal disease, heart disease, HIV disease, mental health and substance abuse, and respiratory diseases.

Major issues of disparity occur for poor people and Hispanics, with lesser but important issues for blacks, American Indians, and Asians. Poor people have worse access to care than high income people for all eight core report measures. Hispanics have worse access for 88 percent of the core report measures, while blacks and American Indians have worse access on half of the measures. Asian Americans have worse access on 43 percent of the measures. The 2005 report also tracks changes in the core measures over time. For racial minorities, more disparities in quality of care were becoming smaller rather than larger, while for Hispanics, 59 percent were becoming larger and 41 percent smaller (*National Healthcare Disparities Report*, 2005).

Federal government focus on these efforts has continued, with the *Healthy People 2020* publication, much of which is now easily obtainable through U.S. government websites through the U.S. Department of Health and Human Services. For the 2020 effort, the report points out that in *Healthy People 2000*, the goal was to reduce health disparities among Americans, and in *Healthy People 2010* the goal was to eliminate, not just reduce, health disparities. By *Healthy People 2020,* that goal was expanded even further: to achieve health equity, eliminate disparities, and improve the health of all groups. *Healthy People 2020* defines health equity as attaining the highest level of health for all people. It points out that both efforts to eliminate disparities and achieve health equity have focused primarily on diseases or illnesses and on health care services.

In the United States, in addition to federal government efforts, some important private foundations such as the Commonwealth Foundation now have programs that focus on health differences and health disparities (Commonwealth Fund, 2013). The goals of the Commonwealth Fund's Program on Health Care Disparities are to improve the overall quality of health care delivered to low income and minority Americans, and to eliminate racial and ethnic health disparities.

Geographical and Place Factors and Disparities

In some ways, it is difficult to discuss the issue of geographical and place factors, since they become so intertwined with SES and race/ethnicity. More recently, there has been a concern to include the environment as part of the social ecological approach (Parcel & Baranowski, 1981, 2002). Social ecological theory emphasizes a holistic approach to environmental factors. There has also been growth in recent years in articles that look at geographic factors as one component of disparity. For example, one article has focused on place and geography for chronic kidney disease (McClellan, Plantinga, & McClellan, 2012). This article was a review article that included geographic attributes such as diversity in the physical environment as well as socioeconomic and medical care characteristics of the environment. Outside of the United States, examining differences between rural and urban areas in terms of health variations has been particularly important in Canada, and a recent article points out that not only are there rural urban differences, but that heterogeneity in health is also found within rural areas (Lavergne & Kephart, 2012).

An important set of studies examining geographic disparities in health care use have been those linked with the Dartmouth Atlas Project (Fisher & Wennberg, 2003; Wennberg, 1984; Wennberg & Gittelsohn, 1973). This project, beginning with early work in the 1970s and continuing into the present, has demonstrated the importance of what were initially called small area variations (focusing on geographic differences) in the types and amounts of health care used within the United States. As the work of this group has expanded, they have looked at cost and quality variations as well, and documented major variations in how medical resources are distributed and used in the United States. Today, the research group maintains a website that provides much greater detail, much of which uses Medicare data to provide information and analysis about national, regional, and local markets, as well as hospitals and affiliated physicians (Dartmouth Atlas of Health Care, 2013).

Cooper argues that meaningful health care reform will need to accept the reality that poverty and its cultural extensions are the major causes of geographic variation in health care utilization and also a major source of escalating health care spending (Cooper, 2011).

Health Problems and Disparities

This section will review a few interesting studies on heart disease related mortality trends, specialty care use with chronic diseases, and also one study that examines functional limitations across states. Looking at the latter issue first, Asada, Yoshida, and Whipp (2013) point out that among the challenges of reporting on health disparities, one often overlooked is how best to report health disparities associated with multiple attributes. They report a general lack of consistency in the rankings of overall and attribute-specific disparities in functional limitation across states. Wyoming has the smallest overall disparity and West Virginia the largest. In their analysis, they found three different disparity profiles across states: (1) the largest contribution from race/ethnicity (34 states), (2) roughly equal contributions of race/ethnicity and socioeconomic factor(s) (10 states), and (3) the largest contribution from socioeconomic factor(s) (7 states).

Two heart disease related studies both use major U.S. databases to examine coronary artery disease mortality trends and stroke mortality trends. The article on coronary heart disease (CHD) mortality trends uses the U.S. mortality files for 1977–2007, as obtained from the Centers for Disease Control and Prevention in the United States (Gillum, Mehari, Curry, & Obisesan, 2012). They found higher death rates for African American men and women as compared to European American men and women. Although rates declined in all groups over the time period studied, in women rates declined more in later years of life. For men, rates declined less for African Americans. Rates were higher in the Ohio and Mississippi River areas. In the study looking at stroke mortality over the same time period, rates declined in all groups, but declined less for African American males (Gillum, Kwagyan, & Obisesan, 2011).

Jennie Jacobs Kronenfeld

See also: Bousfield, Midian Othello; Community Health; Cultural Competence; Disability; Ethics in Public Health and Population Health; Leading Health Indicators; Population Health; Rural Health; Social Determinants of Health

Further Reading

Adler, N. E., & Rehkopf. (2008). U.S. disparities in health: Descriptions, causes and mechanisms. *Annual Review of Public Health*, *29*, 235–252.

Asada, Y., Yoshida, Y., & Whipp, A. M. 2013. Summarizing social disparities in health. *Milbank Quarterly, 91*(1), 5–36.

Commonwealth Fund. (2013). Retrieved from http://www.commonwealthfund.org/Program-Areas/Archived-Programs/Health-Care-Disparities.aspx.

Cooper, R. A. (2011). Geographic variation in health care and the affluence poverty nexus. *Advances in Surgery*, *45*, 63–82.

Dartmouth Atlas of Health Care. (2013). Retrieved from http://www.dartmouthatlas.org/.

Fisher, E. S., & Wennberg, J. E. (2003). Health care quality, geographic variations, and the challenge of supply-sensitive care. *Perspectives in Biology & Medicine*, *46*(1), 69.

Gillum, R. F., Kwagyan, J., & Obisesan, T. O. (2011). Ethnic and geographic variation in stroke mortality trends. *Stroke*, *42*(11), 3294–3296.

Gillum, R. F., Mehari, A., Curry, B., & Obisesan, T. O. (2012, June 6). Racial and geographic variation in coronary heart disease mortality trends. *BMC Public Health, 12*, 410. doi:10.1186/1471-2458-12-410

Lavergne, M., & Kephart, G. (2012). Examining variations in health within rural Canada. *Rural & Remote Health*, *12*(1), 1.

McClellan, A. C., Plantinga, L., & McClellan, W. M. (2012). Epidemiology, geography and chronic kidney disease. *Current Opinion in Nephrology and Hypertension, 21*(3), 323–328.

McGuire, T., Alegria, M., Cook, B. L., Wells, K. B., & Zaslavsky, A. M. (2006). Implementing the Institute of Medicine definition of disparities: An application to mental health care." *Health Services Research,* 41:1979–2005.

National healthcare disparities report: Summary. (2004, February). Agency for Healthcare Research and Quality, Rockville, MD. Retrieved from http://www.ahrq.gov/qual /nhdr03 /nhdrsum03.htm.

National healthcare disparities report. (2005, December). Agency for Healthcare Research and Quality, Rockville, MD. AHRQ Publication No. 06-0017. Retrieved fromwww.ahrq.gov /qual/nhdr05/nhdr05.pdf.

Parcel, G., & Baranowski, T. (1981). Social learning theory and health education. *Health Education, 12,* 14–18.

Parcel, G., & Baranowski, T. (2002). How individuals, environments, and health behavior interact: Social cognitive theory. In K. Glanz, B. Rimer, & F. Lewis (Eds.), *Health behavior and health education: Theory, research and practice* (pp. 165–184). San Francisco: Jossey-Bass.

Schnittker, J., & McLeod, J. D. (2005). The social psychology of health disparities. *Annual Review of Sociology, 31*, 75–103.

Smedley, B. D., Stith, A. Y., & Nelson, A. R. (Eds.). (2003). Unequal treatment: Confronting racial and ethnic disparities in health care. Institute of Medicine. Washington, DC: National Academies Press.

Truman, B. I., Smith, C. K., Roy, K., Chen, Z., Moonesinghe, R., Zhu, J., Crawford, C. G., & Zaza, S. (2011, January 14). Rationale for regular reporting on health disparities and inequalities—United States. *Morbidity and Mortality Weekly Report Supplements, 60*(1), 3–10.

U.S. Department of Health and Human Services. *Healthy People 2010* (2nd ed.). (2000, November). With understanding and improving health and objectives for improving health. Washington, DC: U.S. Government Printing Office.

U.S. Department of Health and Human Services. *Healthy People 2020.* (2013, March). Retrieved from http://www.healthypeople.gov/2020/about/disparitiesAbout.aspx.

Wennberg, J., & Gittelsohn, A. (1973). Small area variations in health care delivery: A population-based health information system can guide planning and regulatory decision-making. *Science, 182*, 1102–1108.
Wennberg, J. E. (1984). Dealing with medical practice variations: A proposal for action. *Health Affairs, 3*(2), 6–32.

HEALTH EDUCATION

Health education is the acquisition of health-enhancing knowledge, attitudes, or skills as a result of planned learning experiences. Health education can occur through a variety of channels, such as books, pamphlets, courses, videos, demonstrations, guided discovery, or social media. The key concepts of health education, as opposed to marketing or other activities that mimic health education, are that the learning is intentional (planned), information is delivered by health educators following a professional code of ethics, and activities utilize health promotion theories and evidence-based practices. Health education follows an established procedure of (1) needs assessment, (2) setting project goals, (3) planning, (4) implementation, and (5) evaluation. Health educators continually assess, revise, and refine activities with the goal of improving programs and services for the people and the communities they serve.

The term "health education" is used to describe any activity or combination of activities designed to encourage, support, or reinforce healthy behaviors. Health education is a form of health promotion in that health education empowers individuals to self-determine their health. However, health promotion is a broader term, which includes health policy, health regulations, social and environmental interventions, and organizations that support health. Health education is also a form of health communication in that health educators use communication strategies to inform people. However, health communication goes beyond health education to address health literacy. Some health communications, such as mass media campaigns, involve one-way communication whereas health education activities tend to take place in formal, interactive settings, delivered as face-to-face, online, lectures, workshops, or seminars. Some advertisers use the guise of health education to market products, programs, or services. A major difference between marketing and health education is that health educators are bound by a code of professional ethics. Professional health educators have a responsibility to act with honesty and integrity in all interactions with communities and individuals. Health educators will not try to sell a product or program that is not beneficial to the client.

The Society of Public Health Educators (SOPHE) is the main professional organization supporting health education practice by school, community, and public health professionals. SOPHE sets standards for professional practice, which include the following:

- Accurate representation of information, products, programs, or services
- Speaking out against ideas, products, or issues that may be harmful to health

- Protecting the dignity and privacy of clients
- Protecting individual right to make his or her own decisions about health
- Maintaining professional competency by staying up to date in the field
- Promoting open criticism and opportunities to improve the profession
- Encouraging diversity in representation, thought, and action
- Reporting unethical behaviors by peers

Ethical standards ensure that health educators work for the benefit of patients, clients, and communities as opposed to personal benefit and interests.

The steps of the health education process are (1) assess health needs of the community or individual, (2) develop learning goals and objectives, (3) plan curriculum and learning activities, (4) implement program and learning activities, and (5) evaluate program effectiveness. The first step, the needs assessment, collects information on the health and education needs of the community, available resources, and opportunities for collaboration. The needs assessment helps the planning committee to establish learning goals and objectives for the project. Goals are broad statements that name the population of interest and what is expected to happen because of the learning activity. Objectives are precise statements that define the steps or tasks necessary to meet the intended goal. Goals and objectives help to focus the project's efforts and keep the planned activities manageable. The next step is to plan learning activities. Effective programs require detailed planning for the allocation of resources, marketing, development of program materials, and needs of the target population. Implementing effective health education programs requires an understanding of how people learn and what motivates people to improve health behaviors. Learning is most effective when the lessons are enjoyable, learning is active and involves multiple senses (visual, auditory, touch, taste, and smell), the learner is prepared and ready to learn, the environment is free of distractions, lessons are appropriately paced, and information progresses from simple to complex with reinforcement of the more difficult concepts through repetition or hands-on activities (McKenzie, Neiger, & Thackeray, 2012). Adult learners are motivated to learn when they understand *why the information is important*, *feel valued* for their ideas, wisdom, and expertise, and the information *relates to life experiences*. The intervention phase can use a variety of learning activities. Common educational activities are presentations, videos, web programs, social media, printed materials, role play, case studies, debates, experiments, and discussion. Evidence-based programs promise the most effective ways to improve behavior or knowledge. Evidence-based programs are health promotion or disease prevention activities that have been tested and proven to work in research. Several federal and nonprofit organizations list and report recommended evidence-based programs. The final stage of the health education cycle is program evaluation. Health educators build evaluation procedures into the program during the planning stage. Simple measures of program evaluation are attendance, participant satisfaction, or key stakeholder satisfaction. Other ways to measure program effectiveness assess changes

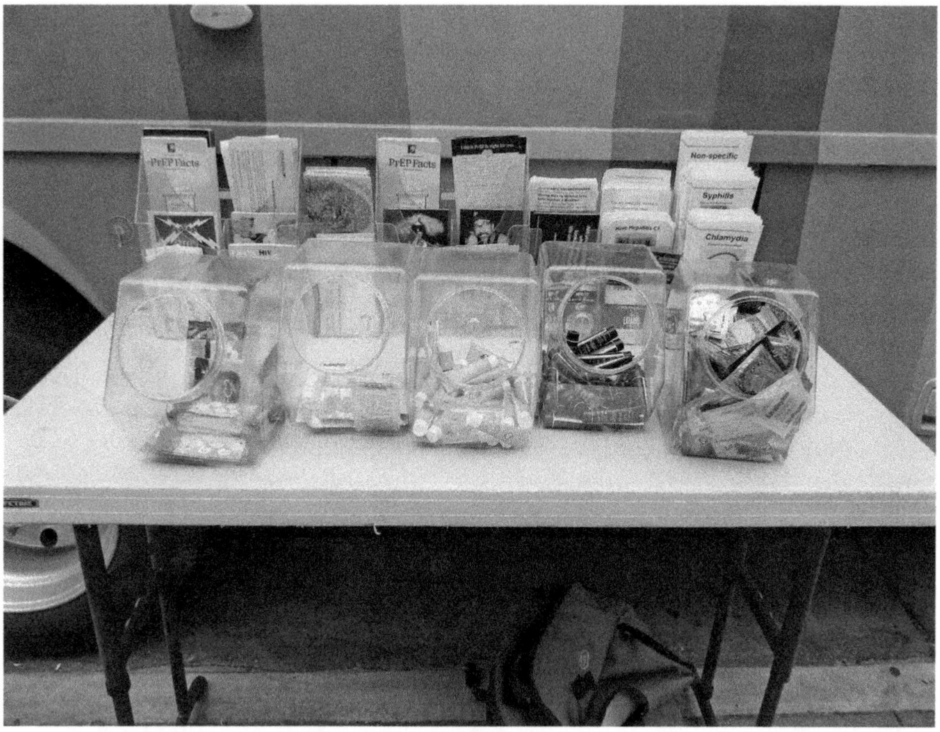

On a Friday evening in the Castro District of San Francisco, community health educators set up health information materials on the street, and offer screening and counseling for sexually transmitted diseases. (Sara Ann Kuykendall)

in knowledge, attitudes, or behavior because of program participation. The results of the evaluation are used to improve the program for future use.

One of the most commonly recognized venues of health education is schools. More than 50 million children attend public schools with classes on nutrition, physical activity, oral health, decision-making skills, healthy personal boundaries, disease, and injury prevention. To promote personal, family, and community health, the American Public Health Association (APHA), the American School Health Association (ASHA), and the Society of Health and Physical Educators (SHAPE) developed standards for school health education. The National Health Education Standards (NHES) identify benchmarks of what children should know by grades 2, 5, 8, and 12. Teachers, administrators, and policy makers can use the standards to select topics, plan curriculum, instruct, and assess learning. Improving the health of children provides academic and social benefits. Studies show improved concentration, memory, and mood, improved academic achievement, increased attendance and graduation rates, and decreased school dropout and behavioral problems among children who are physically active and enjoy a nutritious diet. To support the NHES, the Substance Abuse and Mental Health Services Administration (SAMHSA) offers a searchable database of evidence-based programs, and the

Centers for Disease Control and Prevention (CDC) offers professional development tools for school health educators and the Health Education Curriculum Analysis Tool (HECAT). The School Health Policies and Practices Study suggests additional ways to enhance school health education, such as *not* withholding recess as a punishment for bad behavior, *not* using physical activity (running laps or pushups) as punishment for poor athletic performance, encouraging walking or biking to school, integrating physical activity into the classroom schedule, and providing club or intramural sports programs. Expanding school policies and procedures to support health education lessons supports learning and positive behavioral change.

A major limitation of health education is that giving people the information that they need to act in healthy ways does not necessarily lead to healthy behaviors. People who smoke know that smoking is bad for them. They know that smoking causes cancer, chronic obstructive pulmonary disease, coronary heart disease, stroke, birth defects, rheumatoid arthritis, Type 2 diabetes mellitus, and many other diseases. Yet, people still smoke! Improving knowledge does not mean that people will change behavior. This is where health models and theories are useful. The transtheoretical model, health belief model, social cognitive theory, and diffusion of innovations theory consider the wider array of social, physical, and emotional factors that play a role in personal health behaviors. Health programs that use health theories and models are more successful than programs that rely on conveying information alone.

Health education is a professional field that seeks to improve health behaviors by building accurate knowledge and understanding of health, wellness, and disease prevention. Health educators follow a code of professional ethics, which require them to act in ways that advance the health of others. Health educators plan, develop, and evaluate programs in order to promote individual and community health. Public health can be further enhanced through policy and practices that are consistent with health education.

Sally Kuykendall

See also: Core Competencies in Public Health; Ethics in Public Health and Population Health; Evaluation; Evidence-Based Programs and Practices; Goals and Objectives; Grants; *Healthy People 2020*; Intervention; Logic Model; Society of Public Health Education

Further Reading

American School Health Association. (n.d.). Retrieved from http://www.ashaweb.org/.

Centers for Disease Control and Prevention (CDC). (2016). *CDC training tools for healthy schools: Professional development.* Retrieved from https://www.cdc.gov/healthyschools/trainingtools.htm.

Joint Committee on Health Education and Promotion Terminology. (2012). Report of the 2011 joint committee on health education and promotion terminology. *American Journal of Health Education*, 43, 1.

McKenzie, J. F., Neiger, B. L., & Thackeray, R. (2012). *Planning, implementing, & evaluating health promotion programs: A primer* (6th ed.). New York: Pearson.

SHAPE America. (n.d.). Retrieved from http://www.shapeamerica.org/.

Society of Public Health Educators. (2017). Retrieved from http://www.sophe.org/.

Substance Abuse and Mental Health Services Administration. (2016). *NREPP: SAMHSA's national registry of evidence-based programs and practices*. Retrieved from http://www.samhsa.gov/nrepp.

HEALTH INFORMATION MANAGEMENT (HIM)

In order to ensure the best possible care, patients must be able to report symptoms and attain treatment confident that health care providers will not misuse personal and private information or report a stigmatizing disease to the patient's employer. Under the Health Insurance Portability and Accountability Act (HIPAA) Privacy Rule, patients have the right to such privacy and to determine who has access to their personal health information. This means that public health organizations must have systems in place to secure personal health information. Health information management (HIM) is a field of public health that deals with the documentation, collection, maintenance, organization, and legal adherence in the use, transmission, and management of patient records. The American Health Information Management Association defines HIM as "the practice of acquiring, analyzing, and protecting digital and traditional medical information vital to providing quality patient care" (AHIMA, 2016). HIM oversees medical records including diagnosis, treatment, procedure classification, coding, billing, and reimbursement. The computerization of health records has made the management of health records easier and more accurate, contributing to quality patient care. As methods of recording patient information evolve, the field of HIM also evolves.

Godyson Orji

See also: Administration, Health; Degrees in Public Health; Health Insurance Portability and Accountability Act; Public Health Law

Further Reading

American Health Information Management Association (AHIMA). (2016). *What is health information?* Retrieved from http://www.ahima.org/careers/healthinfo.

Zeng, X., Reynolds, R., & Sharp, M. (2009, Summer). Redefining the roles of health information management professionals in health information technology. *Perspective in Health Information Management, 6*, 1–11. Retrieved from https://www.ncbi.nlm.nih.gov/pmc/articles/PMC2781729/pdf/phim0006-0001f.pdf.

HEALTH INSURANCE PORTABILITY AND ACCOUNTABILITY ACT (HIPAA)

More commonly referred to as HIPAA, the Health Insurance Portability and Accountability Act of 1996, also known as the Kennedy-Kassebaum Act, consists of two parts. The first part, Title I, sets guidelines on how much agencies offering health plans can limit coverage when employees change jobs. To stop people from waiting to purchase health insurance only when they get sick, health insurance companies can refuse to pay for preexisting conditions—health problems the person already knew about. Title I limits how much a plan can restrict paying for preexisting health conditions. If the worker can show consistent credible coverage, as defined by Title I, the insurance company is obligated to cover preexisting conditions with some exceptions. Title II is primarily aimed at preventing health care fraud and abuse by securing the privacy of confidential health information. Title II has far-reaching implications for everyday health care practice. The HIPAA Privacy Rule is a national law ensuring individuals' rights to determine who has access to their personal and private health information, mandating organizations and individuals to have systems in place to secure personal health information, and setting civil and criminal penalties for violations of privacy. HIPAA does not restrict the patient's rights to access information. Patients and their recognized caregiver or legal representative have full access to the protected health information. Patients may review their own medical chart or ask for copies of medical records. A health care provider or administrator will typically sit in on the chart review to answer any questions.

Throughout history, sensitive health information, diagnoses, treatments, or billing have been used to hurt people, socially and financially. The unscrupulous employer who learns that an employee has been diagnosed with HIV could take action to terminate the employee. Colleagues and acquaintances could use sensitive information to coerce a person to do things that they would not normally do. The Privacy Rule controls what information may be shared and whom it may be shared with. Under the law, all "individually identifiable health information" is protected. The patient's name, address, birth date, social security number, and demographic information; past, current, and future physical and mental health issues; treatments; and billing for health services are considered confidential and cannot be shared with outside persons or agencies unless the patient gives express permission or the disclosure is part of the organized system of care or payment. HIPAA is important in public health because patients must be able to seek treatment for health issues without fear that their personal information will be revealed to others. On July 4, 2015, New York Giants' football player Jason Pierre-Paul injured the index finger of his right hand when a firework that he was attempting to light exploded. Hospital workers leaked pictures of the football player's medical chart along with news that the finger was amputated. The personal health information was tweeted to more than 4 million people by ESPN reporter Adam Schefter, and the New York Giants rescinded Pierre-Paul's $60 million contract offer. Pierre-Paul recovered from his injury and uses his experience to educate others on fireworks safety. The leak was traced to two hospital employees, an operating room nurse, and a unit secretary, who were fired. Under HIPAA regulations, the hospital could be fined $50,000 for each violation. ESPN and Schefter are excluded from HIPAA rules because they are not health care organizations or health professionals. The

Privacy Rule only applies to health providers, health plans, health care clearinghouses, and business associates.

There are intentional exceptions to the Privacy Rule. As part of normal operations, health care facilities maintain a list of current inpatients or residents. When a friend, family member, or religious leader calls in person or on the phone, it is assumed that patients want the operator to share their room number and general condition with callers. When the patient is not in a condition to grant permission or make health care decisions, due to stroke, injury, or other illness, the physicians, nurses, or therapists may discuss progress and treatment plans with the primary caregivers. The patient does not need to give permission because the Privacy Rule assumes that the patient would give permission if he or she were able to do so. Protected health information must be disclosed to federal, legal, and local health authorities. The Department of Health and Human Services may access personal health information when performing a compliance review. Health professionals are required to release records to legal authorities where the patient has been the victim of abuse, neglect, domestic violence, or other crime; when a subpoena or court order has been issued for the information; or where there has been a death or a crime. They are also obligated to share necessary information with organ or tissue donation organizations, the Food and Drug Administration, if the patient suffered an adverse reaction to a medication or medical devise, or for the benefit of public health. Public health agencies need to be notified regarding outbreaks of infectious diseases or other events that threaten the public health. In such cases, patient information may be shared fully, partially, or as de-identified information. De-identified information, where the patient cannot be identified, may be shared as long as the knowledge cannot be traced back to the patient. De-identified data allow public health administrators, researchers, or epidemiologists to study trends in health and disease in order to prioritize community efforts. HIPAA rules include companies or individuals who provide or pay for health, dental, vision, prescription, or long-term care services. Companies providing services for health through workman's compensation, motor vehicle, or property insurance are not covered.

This extensive law was implemented not only to protect patients but providers as well. HIPAA provides guidelines of how patient health information should be used, what information may be shared and whom information may be shared with. Other best practices and health laws have developed through HIPAA.

Sally Kuykendall and Leapolda Figueroa

See also: Administration, Health; Health Information Management; Patient Safety; Public Health Law

Further Reading

Health Information Privacy (HHS). (2015). *HIPAA for professionals.* Retrieved from http://www.hhs.gov/hipaa/for-professionals/index.html.

HEALTH LITERACY

Health literacy is the degree to which an individual has the capacity to obtain, communicate, process, and understand basic health information and services to make appropriate health decisions (Centers for Disease Control and Prevention, 2016). Having health literacy does not simply mean being able to read health information. It means being able to use a broad range of skills, including self-advocacy, to make informed health care decisions for oneself, one's family, and one's community (Zarcadoolas et al., 2006). Some reports have noted that at least half of the adults in the United States have difficulty understanding and acting upon health-related information, such as health plan communications, medication instructions, and public health warnings (Nielson-Bohlman et al., 2004; Zarcadoolas et al., 2006). Further, according to the 2003 National Assessment of Adult Literacy, 12 percent of American adults have adequate health literacy; that is, 9 out of 10 adults lack the broad range of skills needed to proficiently manage their health (Department of Health and Human Services).

Health literacy is a growing and dynamic field. For instance, the ability to understand and use health information and services shifts with scientific discovery, urbanization, changes in the education system, and technological and medical advances. The term "health literacy" was first used in 1974 by Scott Simonds, in his argument that it would be good social policy for schools to prioritize health education in all grade levels (Ratzan, 2001). The early use of the term demonstrates the link between health literacy and health education: poor health education is related to poor health literacy (Ratzan, 2001). However, health literacy issues have grown more complex as the health system has become more difficult to navigate. Today, the term is understood in relation to not only health education, but also treatment options, diagnoses, preventive behaviors, and chronic disease management.

Major advances have been made in the field of health literacy, particularly over the past 15 years. In 2003, Louisiana became the first state to enact legislation to improve health literacy, setting the stage for other states to follow (Parker & Ratzan, 2010). In 2007, the National Health Literacy Act, a bill seeking to ensure that Americans have basic health literacy skills, was introduced before the Senate. Moreover, President Barack Obama's Patient Protection and Affordable Care Act, signed into law in 2010, includes the definition of health literacy and formally integrated health literacy into the law (Parker & Ratzan, 2010). A growing body of research in the scientific community continues to inform programs and policies that impact health literacy.

There is ample evidence to suggest that low health literacy impacts a person's health. People with low health literacy may be less likely to use preventive services and have difficulty reading instructions for taking medications, following public health warnings, or reading emergency information (Nielson-Bohlman et al., 2004; Zarcadoolas et al., 2006). People with low health literacy also may have difficulty accessing health care. They may not be able to understand health plan information or medical treatment options. As a result, many chronic diseases, such as heart disease and diabetes, go untreated or undiagnosed (Zarcadoolas et al., 2006).

Low health literacy also affects our health system. When people cannot understand or follow medical regimens, properly take medications, or understand and act upon risk avoidance and health prevention guidelines, they may overuse or misuse the health care system (Zarcadoolas et al., 2006). Some reports have demonstrated that lower health literacy is associated with higher rates of hospitalization and use of emergency services (Nielson-Bohlman et al., 2004). Overall, studies have shown an association between health literacy and health care costs; one analysis estimates that low health literacy in the United States results in $69 billion in additional health spending (Nielson-Bohlman et al., 2004).

Limited health literacy influences all adults, although rates vary by race/ethnicity, education level, age, and insured status. According to the National Assessment of Adult Literacy, 28 percent of white adults had basic or below basic health literacy, compared to 34 percent of those in the "other" category (including Asians, Native Americans, and multiracial adults), 57 percent of black adults, and 65 percent of Hispanic adults (Department of Health and Human Services [DHHS], n.d.). Health literacy tends to increase with higher educational attainment. In the survey, more than 75 percent of adults with less than a high school degree were at the basic or below basic level, compared to 12 percent of college graduates (DHHS, n.d.). Adults 65 or older were more likely to have basic or below basic health literacy skills than those under 65, and those over 75 had the lowest levels (DHHS, n.d.). Finally, adults who were uninsured and those enrolled in Medicare or Medicaid were more likely to have low health literacy; over half of people who were uninsured, on Medicare, or on Medicaid had basic or below basic health literacy, compared to one-fourth of people with employment-based health insurance (DHHS, n.d.).

Health literacy is an important public health issue that requires attention from health care administrators, policy makers, educators, practitioners, researchers, and public health professionals, all of whom can affect people's ability to find, use, and understand health services and information. Although much work has been done in health literacy over recent years, disparities in and levels of health literacy suggest that there is more work to do. Recommendations to advance the field and improve people's health literacy include (1) making accessible and easy to understand health information more widely available; (2) educating health professionals about how to be better communicators; (3) encouraging funding of research that will lead to a better understanding of how to measure, monitor, and improve health literacy levels; and (4) developing health literacy learning standards across the life course that incorporate health literacy into school-based education (DHHS, n.d.; Parker & Ratzan, 2010). These measures and others may help to address the gap that currently exists between health information available and the skills people have to understand and use this information.

Elizabeth Y. Barnett

See also: Health; Health Communication; Health Education

Further Reading

Centers for Disease Control and Prevention. (2016). *Health literacy.* Retrieved from https://www.cdc.gov/healthliteracy/index.html.

Department of Health and Human Services, Office of Disease Prevention and Health Promotion. (n.d.). *Quick guide to health literacy.* Retrieved from https://health.gov/communication/literacy/quickguide/Quickguide.pdf.

Nielson-Bohlman, L., Panzer, A., & Kindig, D. (Eds.). (2004). *Health literacy: A prescription to end confusion.* Washington, DC: National Academies Press.

Parker, R., & Ratzan, S. (2010). Health literacy: A second decade of distinction for Americans. *Journal of Health Communication, 15*(S2), 20–33.

Ratzan S. (2001). Health literacy: Communication for the public good. *Health Promotion International, 16*(2), 207–214.

Zarcadoolas, C., Pleasant, A. F., & Greer, D. S. (2006). *Advancing health literacy: A framework for understanding and action.* San Francisco: Jossey-Bass.

HEALTH POLICY

Policy refers to the overall goals, principles, actions, or practices by the government or on behalf of the government. Policies guide decision making for laws and allocating resources. Policy makers are responsible for designing plans to accomplish intentional goals. In public health, overall goals are to promote good health through physical and social environments, childhood development, and lifestyle choices, in order that all people may enjoy long lives free of disease, disability, and injury (Office of Disease Prevention and Health Promotion, 2016). In the United States, policy occurs at the federal, state, tribal, territorial, and local levels of government. Any significant reform to health policy can have important economic and political implications by altering the health care system that comprises both individuals and private stakeholders. Health professionals, health insurance companies, pharmaceutical companies, hospitals, and patients are all impacted by changes in health policy. Comprehensive policy analysis requires not only assessing the technical content of a health policy document but also understanding the historical context and politics that influence the policy design process.

Health policies are created through a systematic process of conceptualization, development, adoption, and evaluation (Centers for Disease Control, 2014). The policy process starts with problem identification. Data are collected and analyzed to determine the nature of the problem. Policy developers examine how people and society are impacted and determine the severity of the problem. Childhood obesity may be examined as one such critical issue that could be reduced through health policy. The health consequences of obesity are heart disease, diabetes, stroke, and some types of cancers. For many, obesity starts in childhood. Children who are obese are more likely to become obese as adults. Experts estimate that obesity adds $19,000 per person over a lifetime of direct medical costs (Finkelstein, Wan Chen Kang, &

Malhotra, 2014). In 1998, 10.5 percent of youth, aged 2 to 19, were obese (National Center for Health Statistics, 2016). Within less than 20 years, obesity increased to affecting twice as many youth (20.5 percent) with the highest rates among African American females (24.4 percent) and males (20.9 percent), Mexican females (24.2 percent) and males (22.8 percent), and Hispanic or Latino females (22.8 percent) and males (22.7 percent). Youth who live below the poverty line had rates of up to 25.7 percent.

The second step of policy development is to identify possible options, considering the economic and health impact of each potential policy. This is achieved by reviewing scholarly literature. Kristensen and colleagues (2014) compared the cost benefit analysis of three commonly proposed obesity prevention policies: after-school programs encouraging physical activity, ban on fast food marketing targeting children, and a one cent per ounce excise tax on sugar-sweetened beverages. The scholars predicted that after-school activity programs would reduce childhood obesity by 1.8 percentage points among children who would most likely participate in such programs. For example, if 20 percent of the population of children aged 6 to 12 is obese, after-school activity programs would reduce obesity to 18.2 percent. A ban on fast food advertisements would reduce obesity by 0.9 percentage points. An excise tax on sugar-sweetened beverages would reduce obesity by 2.4 percentage points among adolescents, 13 to 18 years of age. All three policies would have a greater impact on children of minority race, which means the policies would have an added benefit of reducing racial disparities in health. Consistent with the Kristensen et al. analysis, Ludwig, Peterson, and Gortmaker (2001) found that risk of obesity increases 60 percent for each additional soda or pop that a child drinks daily, and Wang, Coxson, Shen, Goldman, and Bibbins-Domingo (2012) estimated that a penny-per-ounce tax on sugar-sweetened beverages would prevent 26,000 premature deaths, 95,000 cardiac events, 8,000 strokes, and 2.4 million years of individuals living with diabetes. Thus, the cost-benefit analyses suggest that an excise tax on sugar-sweetened beverages of $0.01 per ounce would have a significant impact on overall health.

The third step of policy development is developing a vision of what the policy will look like in reality. During this stage, strategic planners examine how the policy will be applied and the key people who can implement the policy. The proposed tax on sugar-sweetened beverages would need to be communicated to grocery and convenience store owners as well as the general public through letters, news releases, and media notices. People debate health policies that they perceive as impacting personal rights. A tax on sugar-sweetened beverages is criticized as government overreach and impacting those who least can afford higher grocery bills. Beverage manufacturers claim that obesity is a multifactorial issue, people should be able to enjoy their product, and that policy should focus on physical activity. Others may question the science behind the policy, especially when businesses finance their own studies countering unhealthy foods as a cause of increasing obesity. The fourth step to policy development is enactment, writing the regulation and passing it through the law approval process. This phase might include setting up the administrative systems to collect the sugar-sweetened beverage tax. The fifth step is policy implementation. During implementation, the administrators must ensure sufficient capacity to implement and sustain the policy. This stage is the nuts and bolts of implementation, how the taxes are collected, where the funds go, and monitoring effectiveness of the policy and the system. Stakeholder engagement and education are critical to each phase of policy development. Public health policy experts do not only partner with those who support the policy, but they must also engage with those who are against the policy. Understanding and respecting objections facilitates communication between groups and ensures plans can move beyond potential barriers. Formal evaluation of the policy is also important. If the sugar-sweetened beverage tax does not reduce obesity, public health professionals may need to consider changing the policy or using other policies.

Although policies can be highly effective in addressing public health issues, policy development can be complex, and the intended outcomes may be difficult to achieve. Systems often resist change due to path dependence, the concept that people make decisions based on past habits, behaviors, and perceptions. Obesity prevention has been a goal of national health policy since 1980. The first *Healthy People* report (1979) targeted individual behavior by focusing on healthy eating and increased physical activity. Yet, over the late 1980s and 1990s, obesity rates continued to escalate (Mokdad et al., 1999). Reasons for the failure of the original guidelines are multifaceted. Historically, public health policy focused too narrowly on individual behaviors and paid less attention to wider societal factors such as access to safe recreational areas, obesogenic environments, and the difference in cost between nutritious foods and unhealthy, affordable fast foods. Eating healthily may pose an economic hardship for low income populations. Politics has been a further deterrent; the U.S. Congress has been unwilling to allocate significant resources to support obesity prevention policy, and the fast food and soda industries oppose health policy reforms when these measures threaten company profits. In 2013, beverage manufacturers spent $866 million advertising unhealthy drinks to youth (Rudd Center for Food Policy & Obesity, 2014). Spanish-speaking youth are targeted disproportionately by advertising. Policies, alone, are not sufficient to impact multifactorial health problems. Solutions require socially responsible, balanced approaches that respect the health and welfare of all communities.

Recent policy guidelines by federal health agencies (U.S. Department of Health and Human Services, and Office of Disease Prevention and Health Promotion, 2010) have begun to embrace ambitious proposals to address obesity. At the federal level, provisions to address obesity are included in the ACA. Former First Lady Michelle Obama's Let's Move campaign raises the public profile of childhood obesity. States, in turn, are developing guidelines for providing obesity-related services to adults and children on Medicaid. Finally, municipalities are reforming urban policies to encourage physical fitness and improve access to healthful foods. This interagency collaboration traversing federal, state, and local levels reflects how policy makers are learning from past mistakes by actively engaging with stakeholders to address the problem.

Catherine van de Ruit and Sally Kuykendall

See also: Administration, Health; Affordable Care Act; Body Mass Index; Health Resources and Services Administration; Motor Vehicle Safety; Public Health Law; Social Security Act; Winslow, Charles-Edward Amory

Further Reading

American Public Health Association. (n.d.). *Taxes on sugar-sweetened beverages.* Retrieved from https://www.apha.org/policies-and-advocacy/public-health-policy-statements/policy-database/2014/07/23/13/59/taxes-on-sugar-sweetened-beverages.

Berwick, D. M., Nolan, T. W., & Whittington, J. (2008). The triple aim: Care, health, and cost. *Health Affairs, 27*(3), 759–769.

Centers for Disease Control and Prevention (CDC). (2014). *Using evaluation to inform CDC's policy process.* Atlanta: Centers for Disease Control and Prevention, U.S. Department of Health and Human Services. Retrieved from http://www.cdc.gov/policy/analysis/process/docs/usingevaluationtoinformcdcspolicyprocess.pdf.

Davis, K., Stremikis, K., Squires, D., & Schoen, C. (2014). *Mirror, mirror on the wall mirror: How the performance of the U.S. health care system compares internationally.* New York: The Commonwealth Fund. Retrieved from http://www.commonwealthfund.org/~/media/files/publications/fund-report/2014/jun/1755_davis_mirror_mirror_2014.pdf.

Finkelstein, E. A., Wan Chen Kang, G., & Malhotra, R. (2014). Lifetime direct medical costs of childhood obesity. *Pediatrics, 133*(5), 854–862. doi:10.1542/peds.2014-0063

Healthy People: The Surgeon General's report on health promotion and disease prevention. (1979). Department of Health, Education, and Welfare, Public Health Service, Office of the Assistant Secretary for Health and Surgeon General. Washington, DC: For sale by the Superintendent of Documents, U.S. Government Printing Office.

Kristensen, A. H., Flottemesch, T. J., Maciosek, M. V., Jenson, J., Barclay, G., Ashe, M., & Brownson, R. C. (2014). Reducing childhood obesity through U.S. federal policy: A microsimulation analysis. *American Journal of Preventive Medicine, 47*(5), 604–612. doi:10.1016/j.amepre.2014.07.011

Let's move: America's move to raise a healthier generation of kids. (2017). Retrieved from http://www.letsmove.gov/.

Ludwig, D. S., Peterson, K. E., & Gortmaker, S. L. (2001). Relation between consumption of sugar-sweetened drinks and childhood obesity: A prospective, observational analysis. *Lancet, 357*(9255), 505–508.

Mokdad, A. H., Serdula, M. K., Dietz, W. H., Bowman, B. A., Marks, J. S., & Koplan, J. P. (1999). The spread of the obesity epidemic in the United States, 1991–1998. *Journal of the American Medical Association, 282*(16), 1519–1522.

National Center for Health Statistics. (2016). *Health, United States, 2015: With special feature on racial and ethnic health disparities.* Hyattsville, MD. Retrieved from https://www.cdc.gov/nchs/data/hus/hus15.pdf#053.

Office of Disease Prevention and Health Promotion. (2016). *Healthy People 2020.* Retrieved from https://www.healthypeople.gov/.

Rudd Center for Food Policy & Obesity. (2014). *Sugary drink F.A.C.T.S.: Food advertising to children and teens score.* Retrieved from http://www.sugarydrinkfacts.org.

Starr, P. (1982). *The social transformation of American medicine.* New York: Basic Books.

United States Census Bureau. (2011). *Income poverty and health insurance coverage in the United States: 2010.* Washington, DC: U.S. Government Printing Office.

United States Census Bureau. (2014). *2013 and 2014 current population survey reports.* Washington, DC: U.S. Government Printing Office.

United States Department of Health and Human Services, and Office of Disease Prevention and Health Promotion. (2010). *Healthy People 2020.* Retrieved fromhttps://www.healthypeople.gov/.

Wang, Y. C., Coxson, P., Shen, Y. M., Goldman, L., & Bibbins-Domingo, K. (2012). A penny-per-ounce tax on sugar-sweetened beverages would cut health and cost burdens of diabetes. *Health Affairs, 31*(1), 199–207.

Weissert, C. S., & Weissert, W. G. (2008). *Governing health: The politics of health policy.* Baltimore: Johns Hopkins University Press.

HEALTH RESOURCES AND SERVICES ADMINISTRATION (HRSA)

The U.S. Health Resources and Services Administration (HRSA) is the federal agency responsible for ensuring that people who are geographically isolated, economically disadvantaged, or medically vulnerable are able to access quality health care. In other words, HRSA ensures that people who live in isolated areas, such as rural Alaska or the Pacific Islands, and people who are disabled or who have HIV/AIDS are able to get the care that they need in a timely manner. To achieve this mission, HRSA responsibilities range from supporting health workforce development, identifying at-risk groups, to improving access to quality care services. HRSA also protects the public and those who are working on behalf of the public, by monitoring organ, bone marrow, and cord blood donation, compensating people who have been harmed by vaccinations, and preventing malpractice, fraud, or abuse by health care providers. The overall vision of the agency is to reduce health inequities and to build healthy communities.

HRSA roles and responsibilities are managed by five bureaus and 11 offices. The Bureau of Health Workforce (BHW) supports training and development of health professionals through scholarships, loans, and loan repayment programs and connects graduates to communities with health professional shortages. The BHW manages the National Health Service Corps, NURSE Corps, Native Hawaiian Health Scholarship Program, and other health professional scholarship and loan programs. More than 11 million people live in underserved communities and benefit from BHW-supported health professionals (HRSA, 2017). The Bureau of Primary Health Care (BPHC) funds 1,400 health clinics and centers delivering primary and preventive health care services to over 24 million people (HRSA, 2017). The Healthcare Systems Bureau (HSB) manages specific health programs, including organ donation and transplantation programs, the C. W. Bill Young Cell Transplant

Program, Poison Control Program, 340B Drug Pricing Program, the National Vaccine Injury Compensation Program, the Countermeasures Injury Compensation Program, and the National Hansen's Disease (Leprosy) Program. Each year, HRSA's transplantation programs facilitate more than 33,000 organ transplants and 6,000 bone marrow and cord blood transplants (HRSA, 2017). The HIV/AIDS Bureau (HAB) manages the Ryan White HIV/AIDS Program that provides primary medical care and support services to more than 500,000 economically disadvantaged people each year (HRSA, 2017). The Maternal and Child Health Bureau (MCHB) funds programs, research, and clinical practices that support medical and mental health care to women, infants, and children, promote optimal child development, and reduce health disparities. More than 50 million women and children benefit from MCHB programs. The Federal Office of Rural Health Policy (FORHP) provides grant funding to support quality health services within rural communities. An estimated 57 million people living in isolated communities benefit from access to health centers and hospitals (HRSA, 2017). The Office of Communications manages internal and external communications, responding to media queries, updating the HRSA website, and creating health communications for the agency. The Office of Civil Rights, Diversity, and Inclusion ensures fair and just distribution of HRSA grants and funds. The Office of Federal Assistance Management monitors grant programs to ensure honest, effective, and efficient use of funds. The Office of Global Health (OGH) safeguards health by supporting border health programs, advancing United Nations Sustainable Development Goals, and strengthening global health systems to address acute and chronic diseases and conditions. The Office of Health Equity works to reduce health disparities experienced by minority racial groups, people with disabilities, and rural and urban communities. The Office of Legislation provides information to congressional committees preparing HRSA-related legislative proposals. The Office of Operations manages the finances, human, and material resources of HRSA bureaus and offices. The Office of Planning, Analysis, and Evaluation (OPAE) prioritizes issues and initiatives, analyzes public policies related to health care financing and regulation, supports evaluation and research of HRSA programs, and manages quality improvement. The Office of Regional Operations (ORO) provides regional outreach and technical assistance to support local, state, and federal partnerships. The Office of Women's Health (OWH) supports health-related policies, programs, and outreach and education for women and girls who are geographically isolated and economically or medically vulnerable. OWH focuses on three priority areas: preventive services, violence prevention, and trauma-informed care.

HRSA services support health professional training, public health clinics, specialized programs, such as the Poison Control Center, and rural hospitals and ensure that millions of people who are disadvantaged by finances, geography, or medical condition are able to obtain needed medical care.

Sally Kuykendall

See also: Centers for Disease Control and Prevention; Children's Health; Community Health Centers; Cutter Incident, The; Food and Drug Administration; Maternal Health; U.S. Department of Agriculture; U.S. Department of Health and Human Services

Further Reading

Health Resources and Services Administration (HRSA). (2017). *HRSA Agency overview.* Retrieved from https://www.hrsa.gov/about/budget/hrsabudgetoverview-2017.pdf.

HEALTHY PEOPLE 2020

When the U.S. Public Health Services released *Healthy People: The Surgeon General's Report on Health Promotion and Disease Prevention* in 1979, the report was the first of its kind to identify goals for the health of the nation. Previous government reports focused on the number of people who died and the leading causes of death. *Healthy People* looked forward, toward preventing illness and injuries. *Healthy People* (1979) was followed by *Promoting Health/Preventing Disease* (1980). This second report identified 226 health objectives to be achieved within 10 years. Identifying, naming, and disseminating goals and objectives proved to be a valuable tool. *Healthy People* defined direction for the resources and efforts of government organizations, nonprofit agencies, businesses, workers, health professionals, and communities. The goals and objectives brought diverse groups together to collaborate toward a common goal. The tradition of developing and reporting 10-year goals continued with *Healthy People 2000, Healthy People 2010*, and *Healthy People 2020* published by the Office of Disease Prevention and Health Promotion (ODPHP). Although the objectives change with advancements in science and medicine, evolving health behaviors and emerging diseases, the overall vision of increasing quality of life and length of life remain unchanged. The nation is making progress toward *Healthy People* goals. Over the past decade, the number of children who received vaccinations according to schedule increased 54 percent, adults who were physically active increased 13 percent, homicides decreased 13 percent, and children exposed to secondhand smoke decreased 20 percent (Office of Disease Prevention and Health Promotion, 2017). *Healthy People* continues to influence public policy, education, and community efforts in increasing years of potential life and improving quality of life in the United States.

Over the past century, life expectancy in the United States increased dramatically. In 1900, the average life expectancy was 47 years (National Center for Health Statistics, 2016). Many people died from the communicable diseases, pneumonia, influenza, tuberculosis, and diarrhea. Discoveries in public health, microbiology, virology, and medicine improved sanitation, created immunizations, and eliminated many infectious diseases. By 2014, the average life expectancy was 79 years (NCHS, 2016). However, the advantages were not equally dispersed. Men have lower life expectancy (76 years) than females (81 years), and people with dark skin color have lower life expectancy (76 years) than people with light skin color (79 years). Average life expectancy for black men is 73 years, 8 years less than white women who have a life expectancy of 81 years (NCHS, 2016). *Healthy People* sets the goal of increasing life expectancy for all people with a special focus on disadvantaged populations. In addition to reducing health disparities related to ethnicity and gender, *Healthy People* seeks to reduce health disparities based on sexual identity, disability status, and geographic location.

Each health objective listed in *Healthy People* is grouped by health indicator or health topic. For example, under the health topic of heart disease and stroke (HDS), the second objective (HDS-2) is to "reduce coronary heart disease deaths." Objectives are expressed clearly and concisely. The targeted change is quantified by incidence, prevalence, or mortality rate. For example, coronary heart disease (CHD) accounted for 129.2 deaths per 100,000 people in the baseline years of 2007–2009. The ODPHP selects a reasonable target that is achievable within the 10-year period. In the case of CHD, the nation seeks to reduce deaths by 20 percent (2 percent per year). Therefore, the aim is to reduce CHD mortality to 103.4 deaths per 100,000 people. *Healthy People* outlines ways to achieve the various objectives. CHD may be reduced by increasing the number of adults who can recognize and respond to the early warning signs of heart attack, increasing the number of adults who can perform cardiopulmonary resuscitation (CPR) in the community, increasing the number of people who receive electrical shock within the first six minutes of a heart attack, and increasing the number of heart attack victims who receive artery-opening treatment. By outlining secondary objectives, *Healthy People* suggests practical areas for collaboration by community groups, nonprofit organizations, local emergency response associations, and individuals.

Funding for the goals of *Healthy People* presents a challenge. Although U.S. citizens enjoy some of the best medical care in the world, other countries enjoy better quality and length of life at a lower cost. Health care accounts for 17.1 percent of the U.S. gross domestic product (GDP). The average U.S. citizen spends $9,403 per year on health care. People in Sweden spend $6,808 per person and have a life expectancy of 82 years. People in Canada spend $5,292 per person and have a life expectancy of 82 years. Denmark has the same life expectancy as the United States but spends $6,463 per person and consistently ranks as the happiest country on earth. So, while the United States spends more on health care than many other countries, the nation does not have the best value for the money. The United States ranks 42nd in life expectancy, between the Virgin Islands at 41 and the Turks and Caicos Islands at 43 (CIA, 2016). Achieving *Healthy People* goals will require a reevaluation of how health care dollars are spent.

The scientific, medical, and public health advancements of the 20th century substantially increased life expectancy and changed the focus of public health from reducing deaths to preventing illnesses and injury. *Healthy People* establishes a roadmap for the nation and calls on individuals, community groups, businesses, and state and local governments to collaborate in disease prevention and health promotion. The *Healthy People* reports are now recognized as one of the most important public health documents in the nation, providing direction and focus.

Sally Kuykendall

See also: Goals and Objectives; Health Care Disparities; Health Disparities; School Health; Violence

Further Reading

Central Intelligence Agency. (2016). Country comparison: Life expectancy at birth. *The world fact book*. Retrieved from https://www.cia.gov/library/publications/the-world-factbook/rankorder/2102rank.html.

National Center for Health Statistics (NCHS). (2016). *Health, United States, 2015: With special feature on racial and ethnic health disparities*. Hyattsville, MD. Retrieved from https://www.cdc.gov/nchs/data/hus/hus15.pdf#053.

Office of Disease Prevention and Health Promotion. (2017). *Healthy People 2020*. Retrieved from https://www.healthypeople.gov/.

World Bank Group. (2017). *Health expenditures per capita (current US$)*. Retrieved from http://data.worldbank.org/indicator/SH.XPD.PCAP?end=2014&start=1995&view=chart&year_high_desc=true.

HEALTHY PLACES

The homes, buildings, and neighborhoods where people live, learn, work, and play control health and wellness. Physical, mental, and spiritual health are enhanced by walking, bicycling, and communing in nature. When isolated, sporadic developments replace farms, woods, parks, and other recreational areas, physical activity decreases and reliance on motor vehicles increases. A lack of safe places to exercise and play increases risk of obesity, hypertension, diabetes, asthma, pedestrian injuries, and some cancers. Increased motor vehicle traffic causes air, land, and water pollution and creates global warming. The inability to walk in one's neighborhood and regularly interact with neighbors undermines social integrity, leaving individuals feeling isolated and powerless. Urban sprawl can be minimized and reversed by thoughtful planning. The Centers for Disease Control and Prevention's (CDC) Built Environment and Health Initiative (Healthy Places) is a resource for local township officials and community members to assist in designing and planning communities that support and enhance health. Creating safe spaces for physical activity yields a valuable return on investment. Dr. Gotschi (2011) of the University of Zurich, Switzerland, analyzed the cost benefit of one project creating bicycle paths in Portland, Oregon. Results showed that by 2040, an investment of $138 to $605 million would save $388 to $594 million in health care costs, $143 to $218 million in fuel, and $7 to $12 billion in the value of statistical lives. Every dollar spent on bicycle paths saved $1.2 to $3.8 in health care and fuel. Prevention experts calculate that designing urban and suburban infrastructures for physical activity could reduce the national cost of treating the obesity-related diseases by $147 billion per year (in 2008 dollars) (Finkelstein, Trogdon, Cohen, & Dietz, 2009).

Healthy Places partners with many other nonprofit, government, and business agencies to assist with local community planning. The main public health strategies are to minimize pedestrian and motor vehicle injuries, reduce global warming, reduce air and water pollution, and promote physical activity, mental health, and access to nutritious foods. The American Planning Association (2002) defined the tenets of smart growth as planning, developing, or revitalizing communities in a way that fosters a sense of uniqueness, preserves natural and cultural resources, ensures just distribution of costs and benefits, promotes public health, honors sustainability, and enhances housing, employment, and transportation in a fiscally responsible manner. The National Park Service offers the *Parks, Trails, and Health Workbook* (CDC and National Park Service, 2015). This workbook presents steps and resources to planning trails and recreational areas:

- Community health profile
- Site assessment
- Site planning
- Park and trail system planning
- Monitoring and evaluation

The community health profile gathers data on population density, socioeconomic status, disease prevalence, and potential partners. Potential sources of data are the census bureau, county or local public health departments, hospitals, and other local health agencies. The U.S. Department of Transportation provides data comparing health and transportation within and between specific regions and states. Site assessment maps existing geographic conditions, existing resources, potential hazards, and sites of cultural or historic significance. Site planning is the more detailed planning, of planning amenities, entry and exit points, signage, water features, shade protection, areas for social interaction, and security. Park and trail system planning refers to a larger network of linked trails. As new developments are proposed, local planners can identify ways to link existing or future parks. Monitoring and evaluation help determine whether a project met the intended objectives. Tools to evaluate successes include case studies, photo voice, regular site inspections, and a variety of audit instruments. In addition to promoting physical activity and healthy areas to live and recreate, Healthy Places encourages town and city planners to consider an equal and fair share of burdens and benefits. This means that poor or minority neighborhoods do not carry the burden of heavy traffic, sparse recreational facilities, and limited educational and job opportunities while wealthy neighborhoods enjoy taxpayer-funded, protected open spaces.

A health impact assessment (HIA) is a tool used to assist local officials in evaluating the potential health effects of a proposed policy or project. In Antwerp, Belgium, researchers used an HIA to assess the Ringland Project, a proposal to replace the current open air ring road with a filtered tunnel ring road. The HIA predicted that the filtered tunnel would reduce air particulate matter, $PM_{2.5}$ (a measure of air pollution), and save 21 lives each year out of 352,000 inhabitants. The predicted impact on lung cancer mortality and myocardial infarctions was less than expected with a reduction of 0.1 per 100,000 inhabitants (Van Brusselen et al., 2016). Using an HIA empowers local township and city planners to make smart, long-range decisions regarding community design and improvement. The Pew Charitable Trusts and Robert Wood Johnson Foundation developed and offer an HIA that identifies potential health considerations, assesses risks and benefits, provides recommendations, and facilitates reporting and project evaluation.

Urban sprawl results from unplanned or poorly planned growth. In an effort to encourage communities to support public health, Healthy Places provides a variety of tools, resources, and suggestions. The general suggestions for community design or redesign are to maximize the use of the existing infrastructure, encourage the cleanup and renovation of brownfields, urban centers, and older towns, plan for mixed-use communities that integrate residential and business and serve people of varied socioeconomic status, integrate walking paths and bicycle routes, and preserve open spaces (National Center for Environmental Health, n.d.). The long-term cost benefit of developing walkable and bicycle rideable communities are enormous in terms of reducing disease and disability and enhancing physical, emotional, and social health.

Sally Kuykendall

See also: Environmental Health; Obesity; Physical Activity; Social Determinants of Health; Social Ecological Model

Further Reading

American Planning Association. (2002). *APA policy guide on smart growth.* Retrieved from https://www.planning.org/policy/guides/adopted/smartgrowth.htm.

Centers for Disease Control and Prevention. (2013). *Addressing obesity disparities.* Retrieved from https://www.cdc.gov/nccdphp/dnpao/state-local-programs/health-equity/framing-the-issue.html.

Centers for Disease Control and Prevention and National Park Service. (2015). *Parks, trails, and health workbook.* Washington, DC: National Park Service. Retrieved from https://www.nps.gov/public_health/hp/hphp/press/Parks_Trails_and_Health_Workbook_508_Accessible_PDF.pdf.

Finkelstein, E., Trogdon, J., Cohen, J., & Dietz, W. (2009). Annual medical spending attributable to obesity: Payer- and service-specific estimates. *Health Affairs, 28*(5), W822–W831.

Gotschi, T. (2011). Costs and benefits of bicycling investments in Portland, Oregon. *Journal of Physical Activity & Health, 8,* S49–S58.

National Center for Environmental Health. (n.d.). *Healthy community design: Fact sheet series.* Centers for Disease Control and Prevention. Retrieved from https://www.cdc.gov/healthyplaces/factsheets/healthy_community_design_factsheet_final.pdf.

The Pew Charitable Trusts. (2017). *Health impact project.* Retrieved from http://www.pewtrusts.org/en/projects/health-impact-project.

Van Brusselen, D., Arrazola de Oñate, W., Maiheu, B., Vranckx, S., Lefebvre, W., Janssen, S., & . . . Avonts, D. (2016). Health impact assessment of a predicted air quality change by moving traffic from an urban ring road into a tunnel: The case of Antwerp, Belgium. *Plos ONE, 11*(5), 1–19. doi:10.1371/journal.pone.0154052

HEART DISEASE

Heart disease is the leading cause of death in the United States and is also the leading global cause of death. Although in the past, many people thought of heart disease as more of a male disease, it is the leading cause of death for both men and women in the United States. It is also the leading cause for most racial/ethnic groups in the United States, including African Americans, Hispanics, and whites. It is the second leading cause of death for Asian Americans or Pacific Islanders and American Indians or Alaska Natives (second to cancer) (CDC, 2017a). Among the most important risk factors for heart disease overall are high blood pressure, high LDL cholesterol, and smoking. Almost half of Americans (49 percent) have at least one of these three risk factors) (CDC, 2017a). In addition to these three factors, some other lifestyle choices and related health problems also increase the probability of the occurrence of heart disease. This includes diabetes, obesity and overweight, poor diet, physical inactivity, and excessive alcohol use.

In some ways, it is a simplification of the complexity of heart disease to discuss it as one term. One of the first issues in any discussion of heath disease is what do we mean by the term and what aspects of the term are being covered in this entry. Heart disease as a term can be used to describe a broad range of conditions that affect the heart. Typically, diseases under the heart disease umbrella include blood vessel diseases, such as coronary artery disease and heart rhythm problems (arrhythmias). Sometimes people also include heart defects a person is born with (congenital heart defects), but this entry will not cover congenital heart defects. In addition to the question of how broadly one can interpret the term "heart disease," another complication is that the term is sometimes used interchangeably with the term "cardiovascular disease." Cardiovascular disease most typically refers to conditions that involve narrowed or blocked blood vessels that can lead to a heart attack, chest pain (angina), or stroke. Other heart conditions, such as those that affect a heart's muscle, valves, or rhythm, at times are also considered forms of heart disease. This entry will focus on coronary artery disease, heart rhythm problems, and stroke.

Coronary Artery Disease (Blood Vessel Problems)

The most common type of heart disease in the United States is coronary artery disease, which affects the blood flow to the heart (Kochanek, Murphy, Xu, & Arias, 2014). Coronary artery disease is a result of plaque buildup in the arteries.

Arteries in young people start out as smooth and elastic, but over time they can acquire plaque on their inner walls, which can make them more rigid and narrowed. Plaque can inflame the walls and raises the risk of blood clots and even heart attacks. Plaque makes the inner walls of vessels sticky, allowing things such as inflammatory cells, lipoproteins, and calcium to also travel in the bloodstream. As more of these inflammatory cells join in, along with cholesterol, plaque increases, both pushing the artery walls outward and growing inward. That makes the vessels narrower. This process is often known as atherosclerosis, or a buildup of the fat plaque in the arteries. As these fat deposits build up, they put too much pressure on the artery, which restricts the blood flow in the body.

Thus, blood flow to the heart can be restricted, and the arteries can become starved of oxygen. Over time, this plaque can even rupture, leading to a heart attack or sudden cardiac death. Cardiac ischemia can occur when plaque and fatty matter narrow the inside of an artery so much that it cannot supply enough oxygen-rich blood to the heart. Heart attacks can occur either with or without chest pain and other symptoms.

Arrhythmias (Heart Rhythm Problems)

Heart rhythm problems (heart arrhythmias) occur when the electrical impulses that coordinate heartbeats do not work properly. This causes the heart to beat inappropriately, either too fast, too slow, or irregularly. Heart arrhythmias can be relatively harmless and merely feel like a fluttering or racing heart or more serious. Most of those considered harmless are not treated. Some heart arrhythmias cause bothersome and at times life-threatening signs and symptoms. These can be managed by heart arrhythmia treatment to control or eliminate fast, slow, or irregular heartbeats. Often, troublesome heart arrhythmias do not occur alone, but are either made worse or in some cases even caused by a weak or damaged heart. Therefore, some of the same preventive efforts to deal with other aspects of heart disease may also be helpful with heart arrhythmias. One solution to heart rhythm problems is a pacemaker, a small device that helps the heart beat more regularly. A pacemaker uses electrical stimulation to help control heartbeat. Generally, pacemakers are put under the skin in the chest and hooked to the heart with very small wires. Some people only need these devices for a short time, such as after a heart attack and for this there are external devices, but other people live with these for many years.

One particular type of health rhythm problems is atrial fibrillation (AFib). This is an irregular heartbeat where the atria beat too fast. Generally, AFib keeps the atria and ventricles from working together normally. Typically, the heart contracts and relaxes to a regular beat. In atrial fibrillation, the upper chambers of the heart (the atria) beat irregularly (quiver) instead of beating effectively to move blood into the ventricles. As a result, blood can clot in the atria, and if part of a clot breaks free, that part could break off and enter the bloodstream and then travel to the brain and lead to strokes. There are medical treatments with blood thinning drugs that are used to treat this problem, or pacemakers can be used, depending on a variety of clinical factors. About 15to 20 percent of people who have strokes have this heart arrhythmia.

Stroke

A stroke occurs when there are blood supply problems to the brain, such as the blood supply being blocked or a blood vessel within the brain rupturing. In either case, the blood supply to part of the brain is interrupted or severely reduced, depriving brain tissue of oxygen and nutrients. A stroke is a medical emergency because within minutes, brain cells begin to die. Thus, immediate treatment is critical. Early action can minimize the danger to the brain and some of the more serious complications of stroke. Since the beginning of the 21st century there have been improved ways to prevent stroke and treat strokes if detected early enough. Given this, the death rate from stroke has been decreasing in the United States. Since 2010, the death rate from stroke in the United States has fallen about 34 percent, and the number of stroke deaths has dropped about 18 percent. Despite these improvements, stroke is still the fifth leading cause of death overall in the United States. For African Americans, stroke is the third leading cause of death. In the world, stroke is now the second leading cause of death (American Heart Association, 2017). Stroke is a leading cause of disability and the leading cause of preventable disability in the United States.

There are three different kinds of strokes: ischemic strokes, hemorrhagic strokes, and transient ischemic attacks (TIAs), also known as ministrokes. Ischemic strokes are caused by a narrowing or blocking of arteries to the brain. They are the most common type of stroke, accounting for about 85 percent of all strokes. Hemorrhagic strokes are caused by blood vessels within or around the brain bursting or leaking. Treatment varies by the type of stroke. Ischemic strokes can be treated with "clot-busting" drugs such as tissue plasminogen activators (TPAs), but these drugs must be given within 4.5 hours of the beginning of the stroke, which is one of the reasons why rapid treatment is so critical. Hemorrhagic strokes are generally treated with surgery to repair or block blood vessel weakness. Healthy lifestyles are one of the most effective ways to prevent strokes. TIAs are different from the other two types of strokes because the flow of blood to the brain is only briefly interrupted. Nevertheless, they are also medical emergencies even if the blockage of the artery is temporary. They are also viewed as important warning signs for future strokes, and about one-third of people who have a TIA will have a major stroke within a year if they do not receive further treatment. It is estimated that about 10 to 15 percent of people who have a TIA will have a major stroke within three months (CDC, 2017b).

Jennie Jacobs Kronenfeld

See also: Air Pollution; Body Mass Index; Diabetes Mellitus; Environmental Protection Agency; Heart Truth® (Red Dress) Campaign, The; Hypertension; Leading

Health Indicators; Men's Health; National Heart, Lung, and Blood Institute; Nutrition; Physical Activity; Prevention; Women's Health

Further Reading

American Heart Association. (2017). *Heart disease, stroke and research statistics at-a-glance.* Retrieved from http://www.heart.org/idc/groups/ahamah-public/@wcm/@sop/@smd/documents/downloadable/ucm_480086.pdf.

Centers for Disease Control and Prevention (CDC). (2017a). *Heart disease fact sheet.* Retrieved from https://www.cdc.gov/dhdsp/data_statistics/fact_sheets/fs_heart_disease.htm.

Centers for Disease Control and Prevention (CDC). (2017b). *Stroke.* Retrieved from https://www.cdc.gov/stroke/.

Kochanek, K. D., Murphy, S. L., Xu, J., & Arias, E. (2014). *Mortality in the United States, 2013.* NCHS data brief, no 178. Hyattsville, MD: National Center for Health Statistics, Centers for Disease Control and Prevention, U.S. Department of Health and Human Services.

HEART TRUTH® (RED DRESS) CAMPAIGN, THE

More women die of heart disease each year than of stroke, chronic obstructive pulmonary disease, Alzheimer's disease, and diabetes, combined. Despite the high mortality rate (one in four), heart disease was not always recognized as a disease of women. Early investigations of cardiovascular disease focused on men who were believed to be at higher risk due to work stressors. Misperceptions and misinformation resulted in medical neglect and misdiagnosis. Meanwhile, many women suffered sudden, premature, and unnecessary deaths. The Heart Truth® is a public health program to prevent and reduce heart disease among women. Program objectives are to:

1. Increase awareness of heart disease as the number one cause of death among women.
2. Increase awareness of risk factors for heart disease.
3. Increase awareness of the severity of heart disease.
4. Increase perceived susceptibility to heart disease.
5. Increase the number of women who act to reduce risk factors and prevent heart disease. (National Heart, Lung, and Blood Institute)

The campaign combines health behavior theory, specifically the health belief model, with branding strategy from social marketing. Using the red dress logo, The Heart Truth®/Red Dress Campaign partners with airports, schools, worksites, health care organizations, faith-based organizations, stores, and shopping malls to hold fashion displays and rallies with health screenings and health education programs. Within the first four years of implementation, program developers reported an outreach of 348 events with over a quarter of a million participants (Long, Taubenheim, McDonough, Austin, Wayman, & Temple, 2011).

Early physicians believed that heart disease primarily affected men. In summarizing an 1872 lecture by the preeminent physician Sir Richard Quain to the British College of Physicians, the *British Medical Journal* reported:

> Enlargement of the heart, one of the most distressing and fatal diseases, is more than twice as frequent in males as in females, the precise proportion being 8 to 3. This remarkable liability to enlargement of men's hearts, as compared to those of women, is, he [Quain] thinks, unquestionably due to the greater amount of work and anxiety which, under the present dispensation, falls upon men. Ladies may take this fact to heart, and reflect whether, in claiming the rights of women, they may not at the same time incur the risks of men, and with them a new and unexpected form of disability. They might do wisely to rest content for their sex, with hearts suffering, it may be, from those tender affections which often pain, but never kill. (Influence of Sex on Heart-Disease, 1872, p. 347)

Thus, the world's most respected medical professionals not only supposed that women were immune to heart disease, but they used the argument to suppress equal rights of women. Over the next century, misconceptions influenced research, diagnoses, and treatment of heart disease. Women who complained of heart palpitations or chest discomfort were misdiagnosed or labeled as hysterical. It was not until several large-scale surveys identified high rates of heart disease among women that experts started to take notice. Despite epidemiological data, public misperceptions continued. The majority of women were unaware of heart disease risk factors and symptoms. This means that when a woman experienced palpitations or moderate chest discomfort, she may very likely ignore the signs and subsequently die of sudden cardiac arrest or she might go to the doctor or hospital only to be told that she had indigestion or bronchitis. Doctors who believed that women were less likely to suffer from heart disease neglected to order EKGs or cardiac enzyme tests. Without treatment, a second, more serious heart attack was highly likely.

Beyond lack of awareness, another major obstacle to screening and prevention was lack of time. The highest risk age group, women 40 to 60 years of age, compose the *sandwich generation,* responsible for caring for aging parents while also caring for children and partners. Multiple demands for time, resources, and emotional support interfere with self-care. In 2001, the National Heart, Lung, and Blood Institute partnered with Ogilvy Public Relations Worldwide to develop a national social marketing campaign to increase public awareness of women and heart disease. With a special focus on minority women (the highest risk group for heart disease), the program planners undertook formative research to identify and develop a public health program. Focus group participants preferred the name The Heart Truth® because it was strong, clear, and simple. The play on words with the phrase "the hard truth" was easy to remember. The women overwhelmingly preferred the red dress logo. As one participant noted, "The red color of the dress catches your eye, and the message is very clear. Heart disease doesn't discriminate" (Wayman et al., 2008, p. 44). Through alliances with businesses and nonprofit organizations, The

Heart Truth®/Red Dress Campaign was sent out into communities and was quickly embraced by top designers at New York Fashion Week and America's First Ladies. In addition to The Heart Truth® website, the program is represented on national wear red day (the first Friday in February), heart healthy cereal boxes, and by the iconic red dress pins available in a simple version from the American Heart Association, with dazzling Austrian crystal beads, or as a Native American buckskin tunic from the Association of Black Cardiologists.

The program motto "Heart Disease Doesn't Care What You Wear—It's the #1 Killer of Women" was and is highly effective. The percentage of women who recognized that heart disease was the leading cause of death among women increased from 30 percent in 1997 to 56 percent in 2012 (Mosca et al., 2013). Despite progress, racial disparities exist where many at-risk minority women do not recognize their own susceptibility to heart disease. Although 65 percent of white women recognize heart disease as the leading cause of death, only 36 percent of women of color recognize the problem. The Heart Truth®/Red Dress Campaign is a model for other public health programs. The key components of formative research, program branding, successful campaign launch, widespread outreach, and maintaining program integrity with partners can be applied to other public health problems.

Sally Kuykendall

See also: Body Mass Index; Diabetes Mellitus; Health Belief Model; Heart Disease; Hypertension; Leading Health Indicators; National Heart, Lung, and Blood Institute; Nutrition; Obesity; Physical Activity; Prevention; Women's Health

Further Reading

Centers for Disease Control. *Heart disease fact sheet.* Retrieved from https://www.cdc.gov/dhdsp/data_statistics/fact_sheets/fs_heart_disease.htm.

Influence of Sex on Heart-Disease. (1872). *The British Medical Journal, 1*(587), 347–347. Retrieved from http://www.jstor.org.ezproxy.sju.edu/stable/25231769.

Long, T., Taubenheim, A. M., McDonough, S., Austin, P., Wayman, J., & Temple, S. (2011). Delivering The Heart Truth® to women through community education. *Social Marketing Quarterly, 17*(4), 24–40. doi:10.1080/15245004.2011.620682

Mosca, L., Albert, M. A., Hammond, G., Harvey-Berino, J., McSweeney, J., Mochari-Greenberger, H., & . . . Bezanson, J. L. (2013). Fifteen-year trends in awareness of heart disease in women results of a 2012 American Heart Association National Survey. *Circulation, 127*(11), 1254–1263. doi:10.1161/CIR.0b013e318287cf2f

National Heart, Lung, and Blood Institute. The Heart Truth®. Retrieved from https://www.nhlbi.nih.gov/health/educational/hearttruth/

Thomas, J. L., & Braus, P. A. (1998). Coronary artery disease in women. *Archives of Internal Medicine, 158*(4), 333.

Wayman, J., Long, T., Ruoff, B. A., Temple, S., & Taubenheim, A. M. (2008). Creating a women and heart disease brand: The heart truth campaign's red dress. *Social Marketing Quarterly, 14*(3), 40–57. doi:10.1080/15245000802279409

HEPATITIS

Hepatitis is the inflammation, swelling, and irritation of the liver. Because hepatitis may be a severe and fatal disease, public health practitioners focus on prevention of the disease.

The liver is an organ that is essential for life, performing almost 500 tasks in the body (Zakim, 2003). The liver is able to achieve these many, many functions because it is highly vascular. Blood cells pick up nutrients and toxins from the stomach and intestines and travel through the liver before flowing to the heart to be pumped out to the entire body. The liver helps break down food components, process and store nutrients, break down toxic chemicals, and helps blood to clot or fight infections (Maton, 1993). Hepatitis can interfere with these functions by impairing the blood flow through the liver. Left untreated, hepatitis can progress to more serious health problems and death.

Hepatitis may be "acute" or "chronic." Acute hepatitis is a new onset or rapid onset of liver inflammation. Most cases of acute hepatitis resolve, or go away without treatment or long-term damage to the liver. In rare cases, acute hepatitis may escalate to severe damage or even death (Ryder & Beckingham, 2001). Chronic hepatitis is liver inflammation that perseveres for more than six months. It can continue for many, many years and usually lasts until the factors causing the inflammation are eliminated. Chronic hepatitis may result in serious liver damage, liver cancer, cirrhosis, and death (Dienstag, 2012). Cirrhosis—scarring of the liver—is a serious complication. As the liver tissue scars, the liver cells can no longer clean or process the blood.

Hepatitis affects millions of people around the world. It is difficult to accurately predict how many people live with hepatitis because many cases go undiagnosed and untreated. About 1 million people die each year from cirrhosis, and liver cancer has become the third most common type of cancer worldwide (WHO, 2008). Some regions of the world have higher rates of hepatitis than others.

There is no one, specific cause of hepatitis. Inflammation is caused by many different factors. Most cases of hepatitis are viral hepatitis, due to viral infections such as mononucleosis. The most common viruses are hepatitis A virus (HAV), which causes hepatitis A; hepatitis B virus (HBV), which causes hepatitis B; and hepatitis C virus (HCV), which causes hepatitis C. Excessive consumption of alcohol can cause alcoholic hepatitis. Autoimmune hepatitis is a form of hepatitis that occurs when the body attacks its own immune system, including the liver cells. Bacterial or parasitic hepatitis are caused by bacteria and parasites, respectively. Toxin-induced hepatitis is caused by chemicals, including some over-the-counter and prescription medicines. Ischemic hepatitis is caused by reduced blood flow to the liver. Other known causes of hepatitis include excess fat in the liver (steatosis); inherited conditions, such as diseases that allow a buildup of iron or copper in the liver; and complications during pregnancy (Jacobsen & Wiersma, 2010). The major causes of hepatitis vary from region to region and often reflect the public health problems of the region.

Worldwide, HAV infects 119 million people and results in 34,000 deaths each year (Jacobsen, 2010). In 2012, there were approximately 3,500 cases of HAV in the United States (CDC, 2015). Typically, a person becomes infected with HAV after swallowing viral particles. Infected people shed the virus in their feces. Other people become infected when food, water, or surfaces are contaminated with particles of the infected feces. This is more common in areas with poor sanitation and hygiene, but it can happen anywhere. Concern about hepatitis A is one reason you see signs in restaurant restrooms reminding employees to wash their hands thoroughly before returning to work. There is a vaccine for hepatitis A, and it is recommended that all babies born in the United States receive this vaccine during infancy or early childhood.

HBV has infected more than 2 billion people worldwide, and 240 million remain chronically infected (WHO, 2015). HBV is responsible for 500,000 deaths annually (WHO, 2008). In the United States, between 1 and 2 million people have chronic HBV (CDC, 2015). It can be transmitted to others through contact with an infected person's bodily fluids or blood. This may happen during sexual intercourse, childbirth, or sharing needles. It may also happen if instruments for health care, tattoos, or piercing are not sterilized (CDC, 2015). It's recommended that all newborn babies in the United States receive the vaccine for HBV.

More than 150 million people have chronic HCV infections, and worldwide roughly 350,000 people die from HCV-related liver damage annually (WHO, 2008). In the United States, 3.2 million people have chronic HCV (CDC, 2015). HCV can be passed to others if they come in contact with the blood or some types of bodily fluid from an infected person. This may occur when people inject drugs, experience childbirth, or have sexual intercourse. It may also take place during health-care procedures, tattooing, and piercing. There is no vaccine for HCV.

Because many people with hepatitis have no symptoms, it is referred to as a "silent" condition. In fact, most people with hepatitis don't know it. They feel fine. People may appear and feel healthy, as the liver is being damaged and while cirrhosis or cancer set in. If symptoms do appear, they may be mild and similar to other illness, or they may be severe and debilitating. The symptoms of hepatitis are generally the same, regardless of the cause. The most common symptoms include tiredness, loss of appetite, low-grade fever, nausea and vomiting, or weight loss. Less common symptoms are pain or bloating in the belly, dark urine and light-colored feces, itching, or yellowing of the skin or eyes, a condition known as jaundice (Jacobsen & Wiersma, 2010).

It is important to identify hepatitis before liver damage occurs and to help prevent transmission of communicable particles to others. Even if a person has no symptoms, hepatitis may be identified through physical exams with blood tests. Health care providers check the upper right side of the abdomen, just under the ribs, for signs of liver enlargement. Blood tests look for signs of liver inflammation, poor function, or viruses. People who drink alcohol regularly, work with hazardous chemicals, or take medicines known to affect the liver should be routinely monitored for hepatitis and cirrhosis. People with exposures to viruses, bacteria, and parasites known to cause hepatitis should be tested for infections. The risks of exposure vary by type of bacteria, virus, or parasite.

The major risk factors for hepatitis include the following:

- Travel to countries where hepatitis is common
- Being born in or to parents from a country where hepatitis is common, particularly Asian and Pacific Island countries
- Having family members with hepatitis
- Consuming food or water that may be contaminated
- Engaging in unprotected sex or having multiple sexual partners
- Being a man having sex with another man
- Using drugs, particularly injecting drugs
- In the United States, being born between 1945 and 1965
- Receiving blood transfusions before 1992
- Exposure to blood or body fluids of other people who are infected, such as sharing needles or syringes or unintentional needle sticks among health care workers. (CDC, 2015)

If hepatitis is suspected, health care providers usually try to identify the cause, determine the amount of liver damage, and consider what treatment is most appropriate. The first step is to screen patients through interview. To determine the cause, the health care provider will ask the patient about recent travel, family history, medications, exposure to chemicals, sexual practices, and drug and alcohol use. Blood tests, laboratory, and imaging tests, like ultrasound and MRI, may be used to determine the degree of liver damage. Treatment varies by cause and severity of the damage. Some patients will need no treatment at all. Some patients may need to change their diet or reduce alcohol or chemical exposure. Some patients may need medications or procedures like dialysis or surgery to support the liver or other organs. Some medications are available to treat infectious hepatitis. Patients with severe liver damage may need a liver transplant. Those with liver cancer may need medications and surgery.

Treatment of viral hepatitis varies according to the type of virus involved. Infections may eventually go away untreated. This usually happens with hepatitis A, hepatitis E, and the virus that causes mononucleosis. Hepatitis B and D infections may go away after a few months, or stay and become chronic infections. Children are more likely than adults to develop chronic hepatitis B and D. Medications that try to keep the infection under control may be prescribed. Most people with hepatitis C (80 percent) become chronically infected. Hepatitis C can be treated with medications, and many people treated with these medicines will be cured. Treatment works for many people, but some patients do die from the effects of hepatitis. Risk of liver failure and cancer can be reduced if people are diagnosed early and get proper care.

Prevention of hepatitis is an important public health care initiative. Hepatitis may be prevented by avoiding or limiting alcoholic beverages; using medicines only as directed; accurately reporting all current medicines, even vitamins and nutritional supplements, to health care providers and pharmacists so that they may consider the potential cumulative effects of on the body; wearing protective clothing and equipment when working with hazardous chemicals; getting vaccinated against hepatitis A and B; using condoms or other barriers during sexual intercourse; washing hands before food preparation and consumption; and avoiding drug use. If someone is already using drugs, harm-reduction actions such as using only sterile needles and syringes may reduce the risk of hepatitis. Make sure to follow the warnings of health officials when drinking water or eating food from areas that are contaminated with hepatitis-causing organisms. To avoid contracting hepatitis in areas where the disease is more common, travelers are advised to check the official safety recommendations for that area. The Centers for Disease Control and Prevention maintains a website for traveler information (http://wwwnc.cdc.gov/travel/page/traveler-information-center).

Amy Jessop

See also: Addictions; Alcohol; Behavioral Health; Centers for Disease Control and Prevention; Dritz, Selma Kaderman; Global Health; Infectious Diseases; Prevention; Syringe Service Programs; Vaccines; Waterborne Diseases; World Health Organization

Further Reading

Boyer, T. D., Manns, M. P., & Sanyal, A. J. (2012). *Zakim and Boyer's hepatology: A textbook of liver disease* (6th ed.). Philadelphia: Saunders Elsevier.

Centers for Disease Control and Prevention (CDC). (2015, January 5). Surveillance for viral hepatitis—United States, 2012. *Weekly Epidemiological Record.* Retrieved from http://www.cdc.gov/hepatitis/Statistics/2012Surveillance/Commentary.htm#hepA.

Centers for Disease Control and Prevention (CDC). (2015, May 31). *Hepatitis B information for health professionals.* Retrieved from http://www.cdc.gov/hepatitis/hbv/StatisticsHBV.htm.

Centers for Disease Control and Prevention (CDC). (2015, May 31). *Hepatitis C FAQ's for health professionals.* Retrieved from http://www.cdc.gov/hepatitis/hcv/hcvfaq.htm#section1.

Dienstag, J. L. (2012). *Harrison's principles of internal medicine* (18th ed.). New York: McGraw-Hill.

Jacobsen, K. H., & Wiersma, S. T. (2010). Hepatitis A virus seroprevalence by age and world region, 1990 and 2005. *Vaccine, 28*, 6653–6657.

Maton, A. (1993). *Human biology and health.* Englewood Cliffs, NJ: Prentice Hall.

Ryder, S. D., & Beckingham, I. J. (2001). Acute viral hepatitis. *British Medical Journal, 322*, 151–153.

World Health Organization (WHO). (2008). *The global burden of disease: 2004 update.* World Health Organization Press. Retrieved from http://www.who.int/healthinfo/global_burden_disease/GBD_report_2004update_full.pdf?ua=1.

World Health Organization (WHO). (2015, July). *Hepatitis B.* Retrieved from http://www.who.int/mediacentre/factsheets/fs204/en/.

Zakim D. (2003). *Hepatology: A textbook of liver disease* (4th ed.). Philadelphia: Saunders.

HINTON, WILLIAM AUGUSTUS (1883–1959)

Dr. William Augustus Hinton was a physician who specialized in microbiology and pathology. Hinton set milestones in public health history as the first African American to publish an American medical textbook and the first African American professor at Harvard University. Hinton's most important contribution to public health was developing a convenient, inexpensive, and accurate test to detect syphilis.

William Hinton was born in Chicago, Illinois, to Marie Clark and Augustus Hinton. Both parents were former slaves. William's father worked as a railroad porter, a job that required long hours of service without additional pay. While William was young, the family moved to Kansas City, Kansas. At the age of 16, he entered the premedical program at University of Kansas and after two years, he transferred to Harvard University. Harvard offered him a scholarship designed specifically to support students of color. Hinton turned the offer down so that he could apply for a more competitive scholarship. He earned the scholarship and graduated with a bachelor of science degree in 1905. Lacking funds to go directly to medical school, Hinton taught at Meharry Medical College (1905–1909). Meharry was the first historically black medical school in the southern states. He also taught at Agricultural and Mechanical College in Langston, Oklahoma, and took summer courses in bacteriology and physiology at the University of Chicago. In Langston, Hinton met and married Ada Hawes. In 1909, Hinton returned to Harvard to attend medical school and graduated within three years.

Laws segregating patients and medical practitioners by the color of their skin prohibited Dr. Hinton from interning in Boston. Instead, he volunteered as a research assistant at the Wasserman Laboratory, a clinical laboratory of Harvard Medical School and Massachusetts General Hospital. The Wassermann Laboratory was founded by August von Wassermann, inventor of the first blood test for syphilis. Syphilis is a disease that has both plagued and perplexed mankind for centuries. Syphilis is a sexually transmitted disease caused by the bacterium *Treponema pallidum*. The disease follows a very unusual clinical progression. Initial symptoms appear 3 to 90 days after direct contact with *Treponema pallidum*. The primary stage, known as Stage 1, is characterized by the eruption of one or more chancres at the site where the bacteria entered the body (mouth, genitals, or anus). Chancres are firm, painless ulcers. Within about three weeks, the chancre will disappear without treatment. During the secondary stage, a rash develops across the body with telltale rough, reddish brown spots on the palms of the hand or the soles of the feet. The infected person may also experience wart-like lesions in moist areas of the body (groin, mouth, or under the arms) along with signs of infection, fever, swollen lymph glands, sore throat, muscle aches, fatigue, and weight loss. The symptoms will again go away at which point the disease progresses into the latent phase. The person may not have symptoms during the latent phase. However, the infection is still alive and the person can infect others. The latent phase can last for many years. This is a problem as the person may not be aware they are infected and can pass the disease on to sexual partners and unborn children. Tertiary syphilis occurs 10–30 years after first exposure. The disease attacks the nervous system, brain, heart, liver, bones, and eyes resulting in paralysis, dementia, permanent blindness, stroke, meningitis, aneurysm, multisystem organ failure, and death. Syphilis transmitted to unborn infants results in miscarriage, stillbirth, or neonatal death. The transient symptoms and differing stages of syphilis make it a challenging disease to diagnose. Victims may be too embarrassed to seek treatment or may think that they no longer have the disease when symptoms disappear. Official records from the Department of Commerce (1922) report the 1915–1920 mortality rates due to syphilis as 8.6–10.4 deaths/100,000 people. However, the report also clarifies, "The data for syphilis . . . are presented largely as a matter of record, for it is generally recognized that certification of syphilis has been and is still so incomplete that death rates from this cause are almost valueless" (Department of Commerce, 1922, p. 89). The actual death rates are estimated at 16.3–19.8 deaths/100,000 population (Department of Commerce, 1922). Wassermann's test enabled a diagnosis of syphilis, albeit, with a high percentage of false positives. False positives are people who test positive who are, in fact, negative. False positives raise questions regarding the credibility of scientists and doctors and may lead to unnecessary treatment. Hinton's duties included performing autopsies on patients suspected of dying of syphilis. Supervisors were impressed by his skill and knowledge, and he was eventually offered a part-time paid position, which progressed to a full-time position. When the lab was transferred to the Massachusetts Department of Public Health in 1915, Hinton was named assistant director and later, director. In 1927, Hinton developed a simple, quick, and highly replicable test for syphilis that was 98 percent accurate and could be used for mass public health screenings.

For the remainder of his work life, Hinton served as director of the Massachusetts Department of Public Health Laboratory studying syphilis, tuberculosis, influenza, and other venereal diseases. The laboratory was responsible for all syphilis testing in the state of Massachusetts, a requirement for a marriage license. Hinton partnered with John Davies to create an even more accurate test for syphilis, the Davies-Hinton test. He also taught at Harvard University Medical School, earning promotion to professor in 1923. Despite ground-breaking discoveries in medicine and public health, Hinton kept a low profile. He joined professional organizations but did not attend conferences. He feared that his research would be dismissed or demeaned because of the color of his skin. Colleagues at Harvard aided his anonymity, knowing that racism could thwart the scientific progress that Hinton had worked so hard to achieve. In 1936, Hinton published the first medical textbook written by an African American physician, *Syphilis and Its Treatment*. When awarded the prestigious Springarn Medal from the National Advancement of Colored People (NAACP) in 1939, Hinton refused to accept.

Dr. William Augustus Hinton saved thousands of lives by developing accurate tests to diagnose syphilis. Throughout his lifetime, he published 21 articles in professional journals and served as consultant to the U.S. Public Health Service. In 1974, the Massachusetts Department of Public Health in Boston dedicated their new clinical laboratory building in his name. To empower other scientists, Hinton bequeathed funds for the Eisenhower Scholarship at Harvard University in memory of his parents.

Sally Kuykendall

See also: Bousfield, Midian Othello; Health Disparities; Tuskegee Syphilis Study

Further Reading

Centers for Disease Control and Prevention. (2017). *Sexually transmitted diseases: Syphilis.* Retrieved from https://www.cdc.gov/std/syphilis/default.htm.

Cobb, W. M. (1957). William Augustus Hinton, M.D., 1883–. *Journal of the National Medical Association*, *49*(6), 427–428.

[Dedication: William Augustus Hinton]. (2007). *The Journal of Blacks in Higher Education*, (58), 1. Retrieved from http://www.jstor.org.ezproxy.sju.edu/stable/25073801.

Department of Commerce. (1922). *Mortality statistics 1920.* Washington, DC: U.S. Government Printing Office. Retrieved from https://www.cdc.gov/nchs/data/vsushistorical/mortstatsh_1920.pdf.

Ferguson, J. H., & Greenfield, E. C. (1929). Value of the Hinton test in the serum diagnosis of syphilis in comparison with the Kahn and Wassermann reactions. *The British Medical Journal*, *1*(3558), 492–494.

Hinton, W. A. (1936). *Syphilis and Its treatment.* New York: Macmillan.

HIPPOCRATES (460–375 BCE)

Hippocrates II, also known as Hippocrates of Cos, was a Greek physician who lived during the Age of Pericles, the Greek classical period. Many ancient civilizations believed that disease and disability were caused by angry gods as punishment for human transgressions. People used magic, mysticism, and sacramental rites to please the gods into healing the sick or injured. Hippocrates argued that if disease was based on one's ability to please the gods, then wealthy people should have less disease than poor people since wealthy people had more to sacrifice to the gods. However, the wealthy also suffered illness. So Hippocrates proposed that disease is caused by biological imbalance related to the person's diet, activity, lifestyle, or living environment. Hippocrates traveled extensively throughout Greece and Asia Minor, teaching student physicians to use the medical procedure of patient examination, diagnosis, prognosis, and treatment. His philosophy and approach shifted medicine from a theurgical or supernatural practice to a scientific discipline. As physicians supplanted the gods of healing, Hippocrates recognized the potential for abuse of power. He advised physicians to act with humanity, honesty, and integrity, and to respect human life and the power of medicine. The Hippocratic Oath is a vow physicians make to follow strict ethical standards. No business makes such an earnest promise to put the people whom they serve before their own needs. The Hippocratic principles of medicine and medical ethics are the foundation of today's public health and medical practices. Hippocrates is recognized as the Father of Western Medicine for his role in transforming medicine into a science and developing a code of ethics for physician-healers.

Hippocrates was born on the Island of Cos (Kos) in the southeastern Aegean Sea. According to legend, Hippocrates's mother, Praxitela (also referred to as Phenaerete), descended from Hercules, son of Zeus. His father, Heraclides, descended from Asclepius, god of medicine. Hippocrates's father, grandfather (Hippocrates I), two sons, and son-in-law were all physicians. Plato referred to Hippocrates as "Hippocrates the Asclepiad of Cos." The Asclepiad was a family of well-known physicians. It is unclear whether Plato was referring to a biological family or a professional society, similar to a religious order.

Little is known of Hippocrates's life. He is believed to have learned medicine by working as an apprentice with his father, formal study at the Asklepieion of Kos, and studying with the physician Herodicus of Selymbria. Consistent with the philosophy of the time, Hippocrates subscribed to *humoral theory*. The physical body consisted of four humors: black bile, yellow bile, blood, and phlegm. Diet, activity, season, the environment, and vapors created imbalances or deficits in the humors that caused disease or disability. Each humor was associated with a particular element: earth (black bile), fire (yellow bile), air (blood), and water (phlegm). Medical treatment aimed to restore balance with counterbalance. For example, swollen lymph nodes indicated excessive phlegm (water). Balance was restored with hot and drying (yellow bile/fire) treatments, such as mustard seed poultice.

Hippocrates's writings demonstrate diagnosis and treatment of many different types of injuries, diseases, and infections, including sepsis, epilepsy, depression, tetanus, sciatica, and kidney disease. His approach was a balance of analytic and holistic. The role of a physician was to support the body to allow natural healing to occur. The Latin phrase attributed to Hippocrates, *natura sanat, medicus curat* translates to "the physician treats, nature heals." Hippocratic treatments, in order of preference, were medication, surgery, and cautery. He cautioned against aggressive treatments that caused harm to the patient.

With the benefit of generations of medical knowledge, Hippocrates advocated for a formal process of medical care that consisted of examination, diagnosis, prognosis, and treatment. Patient examination consisted of interviewing the patient, learning about the patient's diet, behavior, and living environment and performing a physical examination. Physical examination included auscultation and listening to the lungs and other organs. Accurate diagnosis and prognosis were equally important. The Greeks did not have a formal system of health care. Physician-healers traveled from town to town, treating the sick. This was a very hit-or-miss form of care because a physician may not be in town when an epidemic struck. Over time, some towns organized to pay a regular salary to entice a physician to stay in the area. Hence, the ancient Greeks started public health! To earn the privilege of a steady salary, the physician must be both skilled and trustworthy. Skill did not mean that everyone was healed and no one died. It was better for a physician to accurately predict disease outcome, even if the outcome was negative, than to give false hope or promises. Inaccurate prognosis made the physician appear incompetent, greedy, or deceitful. Trust between physician and the community was a critical part of care. Lying, cheating, or abuse of power not only affected the individual physician, but it also created a stain on the profession. The Hippocratic Oath is a vow taken by doctors to protect the sanctity of human life and to avoid causing pain, injury, or death. The oath was not written by Hippocrates but contains the ideas of the time.

Much of what is known about Hippocrates and classical Greek medicine is drawn from the *Hippocratic Corpus* or *Corpus Hippocraticum*. The *Hippocratic Corpus* is a collection of 72 books gathered by the Museum of Alexandria, Egypt, almost a century after Hippocrates's time. The works carry Hippocrates's name. However, experts believe that only the first 28 were actually written by Hippocrates. Differences in writing style and conflicting ideas suggest different authors, possibly some of Hippocrates's students. The topics vary greatly. For example, *Epidemics* presents weather and weather-associated diseases with case examples and treatment; *Diseases* describes health problems, symptoms, prognosis, and treatment, moving from head to feet; and *On the Physician* describes how physicians should conduct themselves. The works believed to be written by Hippocrates include *On Ancient Medicine*; *On Airs, Waters, and Places*; *On Fractures*; *Nutriments*; *On the Nature of the Child*; *Epidemics 1 and 3*; *Prognostics*; *On the Injuries of the Head*; *On the Articulations*; *Aphorisms*; *On the Sacred Disease*, and *On Humors*. Overall, the body of work describes Greek medicine in simple and direct terms without technical jargon. The treatises (written arguments) present strong support for new medical ideas or theories and convey an earnest desire to help people. What is particularly amazing is how much the ancient Greeks knew about the body. Since dissection was taboo, any knowledge of anatomy or physiology came from direct experiences of treating patients with a specific injury or illness. The *Hippocratic Corpus* presents an amazing degree of anatomical detail and physiological accuracy. For example, the brain is described as two halves, filled with fluid, and surrounded by the meninges. Notes report that injury on one side of the brain may affect movement on the other side of the body. The work even describes coup contrecoup injury—injuries caused when the brain impacts one side of the skull and bounces back to hit the other side of the skull. The coup injury is at the site of impact, and the contrecoup injury is on the opposite side of the brain. The *Hippocratic Corpus* demonstrates how dedicated early Greek physicians were to share their knowledge and help people who were suffering.

When the Roman Empire rose in power, Greek philosophies were saved but given lesser prominence. The Romans focused on the military, the government, and the economy. They believed that the naturalistic medicine was akin to a death watch, and Hippocratic methods fell out of favor. The image of Hippocrates carried on through fictional literature, linking him to historical events in Kos and Greece. These stories exaggerated his achievements and required medical historians to work diligently to discern an image of the true Hippocrates. The Latin translations of Hippocratic philosophy apply to public health practice today. *Ne quid nimis* (Nothing in excess) can apply to the public health recommended diet of low fat, low salt, and low concentrated carbohydrates. *Primum non nocere* (Firstly do no harm) is reflected in the public health code of ethics.

Sally Kuykendall

See also: Ancient World, Public Health in the; Code of Ethics; Core Competencies in Public Health; Ethics in Public Health and Population Health; Greco-Roman Era, Public Health in the

Further Reading

Breitenfeld, T., Jurasic, M., & Breitenfeld, D. (2014). Hippocrates: The forefather of neurology. *Neurological Sciences*, *35*(9), 1349–1352. doi:10.1007/s10072-014-1869-3

Scarborough, J. (2002). Hippocrates and the Hippocratic ideal in modern medicine: A review essay. *International Journal of the Classical Tradition*, 9(2), 287–297.

Suvajdžić, L., Đendić, A., Sakač, V., Čanak, G., & Dankuc, D. (2016). Hippocrates: The father of modern medicine. *Vojnosanitetski Pregled,* *73*(12), 1181–1186. doi:10.2298/VSP150212131S

HOME SAFETY

Home safety refers to the ability to identify and address the potential dangers within and surrounding the household that may result in injury, or in extreme cases death, to occupants or visitors. Approximately 18,000 individuals, including 2,200 children, die from unintentional home injuries each year in the United States (Mullins, 2009; Safe Kids Worldwide, 2016). Children and the elderly are at highest risk. Approximately 3.5 million children go to the emergency department each year due to unintentional injuries (Safe Kids Worldwide, 2016). Injuries are one of the leading public health problems and easily preventable. To change public perceptions of the problem, public health professionals refer to events that result in physical or emotional harm as injuries, rather than accidents. The term "accidents" suggests that the event was unavoidable. Intentional and unintentional injuries are avoidable if people are equipped with safety knowledge. A variety of organizations and educational efforts focus on providing individuals with training to increase awareness of dangers in the home. Public health education in fall prevention, poisoning, fire, burns and scalds, gun safety, safe sleep, and carbon monoxide poisoning can mitigate and prevent injuries and prevent many unnecessary deaths or disability.

Fall Prevention

Unintentional falls are the leading cause of nonfatal injuries treated in hospital emergency departments and the third leading cause of injury death for all ages in the United States (Mullins, 2009). Although falls impact people of all ages, they are the most common in young children and older adults; falls are the leading cause of death among older adults and are the leading nonfatal injury in all age groups under the age of 15. Factors such as muscle weakness, impaired vision, sensory and perception issues, side effects of medications, and other medical conditions may put older adults at an increased risk for falls. Falls in the home can be prevented with secure stair railings, good lighting, eliminating clutter, and using age appropriate child gates at the top and bottom of the landings. Be aware that not all child gates are appropriate to use at the top of the stairs. Mats, decals, handrails in the tub and shower, and anti-slip rugs may also help prevent falls. Organizations, such as the University of Southern California (USC) Leonard Davis School of Gerontology (http://stopfalls.org/), collaborate with service providers, individuals, families, researchers, and educators to reduce falls among the elderly.

Poisoning

The second leading cause of home injury death is poisoning (Mullins, 2009). The Centers for Disease Control (CDC) estimates that in the United States, 2 children die and more than 300 others are treated in the emergency department as a result of poisoning-related injuries. Unintentional poisoning is in the top 10 causes of death for children 5 to 24 years of age in the United States (CDC, 2015). Poison Help (https://poisonhelp.hrsa.gov/) is a resource of the Health Resources & Services Administration (HRSA), which provides information on poisonings and connects individuals with poison control experts in their local area.

Laundry Detergent

One form of ingested poisoning can occur when children ingest laundry detergent. Specifically, laundry detergent pods, which are single-use capsules of concentrated detergent introduced in the United States in 2010, are quickly becoming a case for concern. From 2013 to 2014, there was a 17 percent increase in cases reported to poison control centers of children who ingested laundry detergent packets (CDC, 2012a). Children under five years of age are at high risk for digesting pod and non-pod detergent. Laundry pods may be attractive to children because they resemble candy. Digestion of detergent may result in adverse effects such as gastrointestinal and respiratory complications, altered mental status, and in the most serious cases, death. Recommendations are to keep detergents out of sight and reach, teach children the dangers of toxic substances, and keep a close eye on children, especially in areas of the house where household cleaning products are stored.

Medication

Poisoning can also occur from ingestion of medication or medicines. Given frequent use of over-the-counter medications, the potential of unintentional overdose also increases. It is estimated that roughly 70,000 children under the age of 18 visit the emergency department annually because of unintentional medication overdoses (CDC, 2012b). To prevent unintentional overdoses in children, medications should be stored out of reach and sight. Adults must not refer to medicine as being or tasting like candy, as this may encourage children to ingest the medication. Individuals should also be cautious about taking multiple medications at the same time, as they may result in unplanned side effects or lethal combinations. Lastly, even if the medications in your home are securely stored, be aware that guests may enter the house with unsecure belongings. The best way to prevent unintentional medication ingestion is close supervision.

Fire, Burns, and Scalds

Home fires and burns are the third leading cause of accidental home injury deaths and claim approximately 3,000 lives each year (Mullins, 2009). The American Red Cross recommends installing smoke detectors on each floor of the residence and testing them on an annual basis. Members of the household should know how to and practice more than one way to escape from the house. If clothing catches on fire, individuals should stop, drop, and roll to extinguish a fire. House fires can be prevented through safe cooking practices such as monitoring food while it is cooking, wearing clothing that will not catch fire (e.g., tight fitting, rolled sleeves) while preparing food, and ensuring that grills are a safe distance from the house.

According to data from the American Burn Association from 2016, approximately 486,000 burn injuries require medical treatment each year. A scald injury is an injury that occurs when an individual comes into contact with a hot liquid or steam. The populations at the highest risk for liquid burn injuries are children under 5, adults over 65 years of age, and individuals with disabilities. Common house locations of scald injury include the kitchen, dining area, and bathroom. Home safety recommendations to avoid childhood scald injury are to designate "kid-free zones," turn pot and pan handles toward the back of the stove and away from reach of children, and not leave hot liquids unattended where they could be knocked over or within reach of children. Children need to be supervised while they are using the microwave to prepare quick meals in an effort to prevent scald burns, but they should also have limited mobility within the kitchen area where hot objects are commonly found. Hot water heaters should be adjusted so that the maximum temperature of water is 120°F, and water temperature should always be checked before placing a child in the tub. The U.S. Fire Administration (USFA) works with local fire departments, the media, and researchers to prevent home fires (https://www.usfa.fema.gov/index.html).

Gun Safety

Suicide and homicide by firearm are the fourth and fifth leading causes of violence-related deaths in the United States, respectively. One-third of homes with children under the age of 18 report having a firearm in the residence, and approximately 75 percent of children aged 5 to 14 report knowing where these firearms are kept (Grodzinski, 2015). The U.S. General Accounting Office estimates that approximately 31 percent of unintentional deaths caused by firearms may have been prevented if gun owners used both a child-proof safety lock and a loading indicator. Recommendations to reduce suicides and homicides in the household are to not keep a gun in the home or to provide safe storage using a cable lock, trigger lock, lock box, or gun safe, store the ammunition in a separate location, and disassemble the gun when not in use. For many years, laws prohibited federally funded research and education in firearm injury prevention. Despite the ban, several organizations, such as the Harvard Injury Control Research Center at the T. H. Chan School of Public Health (https://www.hsph.harvard.edu/hicrc/) and the Brady Campaign to End Gun Violence (http://www.bradycampaign.org/about-gun-violence) worked to understand and prevent homicides, suicides, and injuries due to firearms.

Safe Sleep

Approximately 3,500 infants die every year from sleep-related deaths in the United States. Sleep-related deaths can occur from sudden unexpected infant death (SUID) and sudden infant death syndrome (SIDS). SUID is an unexpected death, whether explained or unexplained, that occurs during infancy. Specifically, SIDS refers to infant deaths that cannot be explained, even after thorough investigation. Identified risk factors for SUID and SIDS are bed-sharing, prone sleeping, smoke exposure, and the use of blankets and bedding in the sleep area. Although there are devices on the market that claim to make bed-sharing safe and monitor a sleeping baby, these devices have not been thoroughly tested or evaluated. The American Academy of Pediatrics recommends that parents engage in the following behaviors to promote safe sleep: place baby on back on a firm surface with a tight-fitting sheet, avoid soft bedding (e.g., bumpers, blankets, pillows, and toys) in the crib, do not share the same sleep surface, but do share a bedroom (for at least six months), avoid exposure to smoke, alcohol, and drugs, and offer a pacifier. Safe to Sleep is a public health campaign administered by the Eunice Kennedy Shriver National Institute of Child Health and Human Development. Formerly known as the Back to Sleep program, the campaign reminded parents, grandparents, and caregivers to place babies on their backs to sleep. The program reduced SIDS rates by 50 percent (Trachtenberg et al., 2012).

Carbon Monoxide

Carbon monoxide (CO) is an odorless, colorless gas that may specifically impact infants, the elderly, and individuals with breathing issues. CO is produced by burning fuels in cars, trucks, heaters, and even fireplaces. Common symptoms of CO poisoning are headache, dizziness, weakness, upset stomach, vomiting, chest pain, and confusion. High levels of CO poisoning along with increased time of exposure may result in more severe symptomatology. Approximately 400 Americans die annually from CO poisoning, and close to 25,000 have encounters that lead them to visit the emergency department, and in severe cases undergo hospitalization (CDC, 2015). Ways to prevent CO fumes from building up in the home include regularly servicing appliances powered by gas, coal, or oil; purchasing gas equipment that has been tested by a nationally certified agency; and making sure heating devices are approved for use inside the home and used in properly ventilated areas. To avoid CO poisoning from an automobile, be sure to regularly inspect your exhaust system and never run your car inside your garage, especially if it is attached to your house. Battery-operated detectors can be purchased to detect the amount of CO present in the home and alert the homeowner.

For most people, the home is a place of safety and refuge. Unfortunately, there are many hidden dangers in the home. Many public health professionals and organizations work together to educate the public on home hazards and ways to effectively improve home safety for all.

Autumn Nanassy and Rochelle Thompson

See also: Adverse Childhood Experiences; Aging; Children's Health; Infant Mortality; Injuries; Intervention; National Center for Injury Prevention and Control

Further Reading

American Academy of Pediatrics. (2016, October 24). *American Academy of Pediatrics announces new safe sleep recommendations to protect against SIDS, sleep-related infant deaths.* Retrieved from https://www.aap.org/en-us/about-the-aap/aap-press-room/pages/american-academy-of-pediatrics-announces-new-safe-sleep-recommendations-to-protect-against-sids.aspx.

Centers for Disease Control and Prevention (CDC). (2012a, October 19). Health hazards associated with laundry detergent pods—United States. *Morbidity and Mortality Weekly Report.* Retrieved from https://www.cdc.gov/mmwr/preview/mmwrhtml/mm6141a1.htm.

Centers for Disease Control and Prevention (CDC). (2012b). *The PROTECT initiative: Advancing children's medication safety.* Retrieved from https://www.cdc.gov/medicationsafety/protect/protect_Initiative.html.

Centers for Disease Control and Prevention (CDC). (2015). *Carbon monoxide poisoning.* Retrieved from https://www.cdc.gov/co/faqs.htm.

Centers for Disease Control and Prevention (CDC). (2016). *Poisoning prevention.* Retrieved from https://www.cdc.gov/safechild/poisoning/index.html.

Grodzinski, A. (2015). *University of Michigan Injury Center: Parents' guide to home firearm safety.* Retrieved from http://yvpc.sph.umich.edu/parents-guide-home-firearm-safety/.

Mullins, L. (2009, August 9). The top 5 causes of accidental home injury deaths—and how to prevent them. *U.S. News & World Report.* Retrieved from http://money.usnews.com/money/blogs/the-home-front/2009/08/31/the-top-5-causes-of-accidental-home-injury-deathsand-how-to-prevent-them.

Safe Kids Worldwide. (2016). *We work to prevent injuries in the home.* Retrieved from https://www.safekids.org/general-home-safety.

Trachtenberg, F. L., Haas, E. A., Kinney, H. C., Stanley, C., & Krous, H. F. (2012). Risk factor changes for sudden infant death syndrome after initiation of Back-to-Sleep campaign. *Pediatrics, 129,* 630–638. Retrieved from http://pediatrics.aappublications.org/content/early/2012/03/21/peds.2011-1419.abstract.

HUMAN IMMUNODEFICIENCY VIRUS (HIV) AND ACQUIRED IMMUNE DEFICIENCY SYNDROME (AIDS)

Human immunodeficiency virus (HIV) infection and acquired immune deficiency syndrome (AIDS) refer to a disease that attacks the immune system. This entry will first present the etiology and prevalence of the disease. Next, the history of HIV/AIDS will be discussed, focusing on historical trends of cultural perception of HIV in the United States. Finally, this entry will discuss the contributing factors and determinants of HIV, concluding with evidence-based prevention methods. Biological, social, and psychological factors play significant roles in the prevalence and epidemic of HIV and AIDS. In the United States, 1.2 million people are expected to be living with HIV (Welcome to AIDS.gov).

HIV is disease that targets the immune system in humans, ultimately resulting in AIDS if left untreated. HIV/AIDS is primarily spread through sexual behaviors and needle or syringe use (Vermund, 2014). Needle sharing allows for contact of bodily fluids that may be already infected by HIV. Bodily fluids must enter the bloodstream for disease transmission using needles or syringes (Welcome to AIDS.gov). In addition, HIV may be transmitted through sexual contact, blood, drug usage, breastfeeding, and blood transfusions, to name a few. HIV targets cells within the immune system and eventually leads to immunodeficiency and serious health consequences. Over time, many cells die, thus rendering the body incapable of fighting infections or diseases. Although HIV is treatable, it is a lifelong disease, meaning that once someone has HIV, it becomes chronic. Approximately 12 percent of HIV-positive individuals are unaware that they carry the disease (Welcome to AIDS.gov). Furthermore, about one in four new HIV infections is among young people aged 13–24 (Welcome to AIDS.gov). From 2006 to 2009, HIV infections among 21 to 29-year-olds increased by 21 percent; this increase demonstrated how youth populations in the United States are gradually becoming more at risk for developing HIV (Prejean et al., 2011). Although the disease can be treatable, more than 675,000

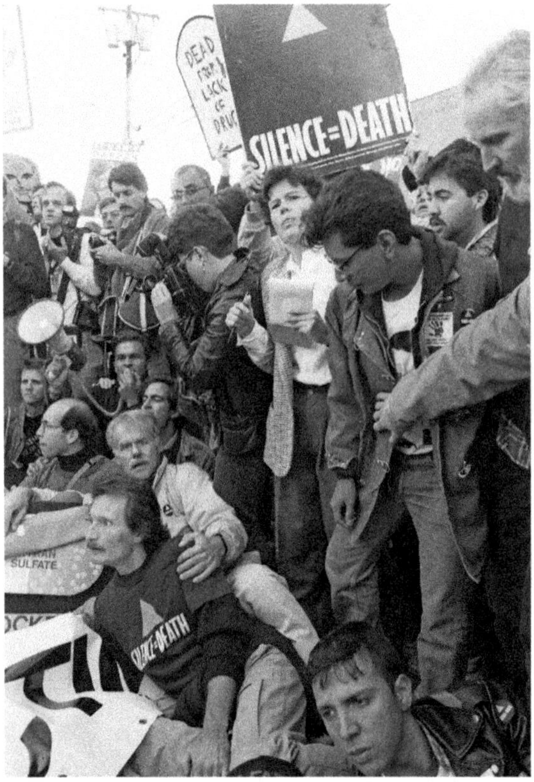

ACT UP (AIDS Coalition to Unleash Power) protesters demonstrate at Food and Drug Administration (FDA) headquarters to call attention to slow, tedious, and elitist clinical drug trials. Later social movements model the thoughtful, creative, and highly effective strategies of early AIDS groups. (Catherine McGann/Getty Images)

people have died of AIDS in the United States since the 1970s (Centers for Disease Control and Prevention, 2016). Due to its prevalence and death rates, HIV is considered a serious epidemic, which must be both treated and prevented.

Documentation of HIV/AIDS has existed in the United States since the 1970s. Scientists believe the virus came about from chimpanzees in West Africa. It is believed that humans obtained the disease when coming into contact with these chimpanzees by means of hunting, as early as the 1800s (CDC, 2017). Over time, the disease spread across Africa and eventually reached countries all over the world. Historically, AIDS has been a controversial topic in public and social media. During Ronald Reagan's presidency in the 1980s, for example, political and governmental involvement in the AIDS epidemic was essentially nonexistent. As tens of thousands of Americans developed both HIV/AIDS during these years, there was little federal attention; and as a result, more than 30,000 Americans died of AIDS during Reagan's presidency. Today, HIV/AIDS is recognized as a global epidemic that must be both researched and prevented. For example, in July 2015, the White House released a Federal Action Plan to update the national strategy to combat HIV/AIDS. This plan included more than 170 action items intended to achieve strategy goals and prevent the spread of HIV/AIDS (Welcome to AIDS.gov). Effective planning strategy includes understanding populations at risk, as well as making compassionate medical care and increasing social awareness accessible to all Americans, regardless of socioeconomic status, gender, race, or sexual orientation.

Certain social determinants explain how HIV incidence may be more prevalent within specific social groups and demographics. Specifically, sexual orientation, race, and socioeconomic status all impact the likelihood of developing HIV. Populations at the greatest risk for developing HIV/AIDS include members of the gay, bisexual, and transgender communities, especially those of color. In 2011, men who have sex with men accounted for 54 percent of all people living with HIV in the United States (CDC, 2015). Therefore, it is recommended that sexually active gay and bisexual men get tested for HIV as often as every three to six months to prevent the spread of HIV (CDC, 2015). As for the transgender community, it was reported that 90 percent of trans women diagnosed between 2007 and 2011 were African American/black or Latina (CDC, 2015). Race also plays a significant role; black and African American people are the greatest at-risk population for developing HIV among all racial groups. This group made up 44 percent of new HIV/AIDS infections in 2010 (Welcome to AIDS.gov). Socioeconomic status plays an additional role; low income communities are also at a greater risk for developing the disease. For example, studies have shown that inadequate access to housing puts individuals at great risk for developing HIV (Aidala et al., 2016). Members of lower socioeconomic status experience less economic and social equality, as exemplified by both racial and housing inequality. As a result, these groups of people are less likely to receive adequate education and awareness of how HIV is both caused and prevented.

Biological factors that put people at risk for HIV include contact and transmission of bodily fluids. Ways that HIV can spread sexually include through semen, rectal fluid, and vaginal fluid. Among the sexual methods of transmission, anal intercourse is the highest risk sexual behavior for developing HIV/AIDS. The second highest risk sexual behavior for transmitting HIV is vaginal intercourse (Welcome to AIDS.gov). HIV is not spread by saliva, air, or casual contact such as shaking hands. These are common misconceptions of HIV transmission.

The interplay of biological and social factors additionally contributes to poor mental health, which many people living with HIV develop. For example, HIV-positive individuals are at great risk for abusing substances and developing mental disorders such as depression (Cramer, 2015). HIV-positive young men who have sex with men, for example, demonstrate disproportionate rates of depression compared to heterosexual HIV-positive young individuals (Salomon et al., 2009). Depressive symptoms may be explained by the effects of experiencing HIV stigma. One example is stereotypes that include assumptions of immorality about people with HIV/AIDS. For example, people with HIV are less likely to get tested for the disease due to social misconceptions and stigma. HIV-positive individuals may develop poor mental and physical health in efforts to escape certain forms of prejudice. Forms of prejudice against people with HIV/AIDS include social isolation or lack of comprehensive health care. In 1988, the United States banned workplace discrimination against people infected with HIV (Welcome to AIDS.gov). Public policy such as this is needed to combat

HIV/AIDS because it prevents the systematic discriminatory perpetuation of the disease.

Despite increasing the likelihood for poor mental and physical health outcomes, HIV and AIDS may both be prevented. Intervention programs that attempt to spread awareness and prevent the spread of HIV range from the individual level to a more systematic governmental level. Condom distribution is an example of individual-level intervention aimed at preventing the disease from spreading. At a more systemic level, evidence-based interventions include the most effective methods of public health strategies based on scientific literature (CDC, 2015). For example, the CDC Division of HIV/AIDS prevention plans to fund programs targeted for young men of color who have sex with men and young transgender persons of color because these two groups are at such high risk for HIV (CDC, 2015). Furthermore, social awareness and intervention programs aimed at high-risk communities are needed to help prevent the spread of HIV. One benefit of the Internet is accessibility to information that may prevent the spread of HIV. Studies show that the use of technology as a prevention method may be useful; prevention interventions on the Internet include enhancing HIV testing, increasing the likelihood to seek treatment, and awareness of how HIV can be spread (Rietmeijer & Shamos, 2007). Testing for HIV is also considered a form of HIV prevention as it additionally decreases the chances of developing AIDS if the disease is diagnosed in time. Regular testing for HIV may also benefit high-risk populations because their primary care provider can supply useful information about how HIV can be both treated and prevented.

Studies suggest that an additional effective method of preventing the spread of HIV is treatment itself (Vermund, 2014). Those receiving treatment for HIV can expect to live a normal life span; however, if untreated, people living with AIDS have a life expectancy of about three years. Treatment for HIV is called antiretroviral therapy (ART), which includes taking daily medicines, also known as an HIV regimen. If taken correctly and daily, ART can slow or prevent the disease from progressing to the next stage. Benefits of ART include reduction of HIV in the blood, reduction of HIV-related illness, and reduction of spreading the disease to others (CDC, 2015). Currently, there are 31 antiretroviral drugs approved by the Food and Drug Administration designed to treat HIV infection (National Institute of Allergy and Infectious Diseases, 2015).

Resilience factors should also be taken into account when examining causes and consequences of HIV/AIDS. For example, HIV-positive people who have viable sources of support are more likely to overcome the negative effects of HIV stigma, and may, in turn, develop positive mental health and well-being. Moreover, both HIV/AIDS-positive individuals and high-risk populations such as gay and bisexual men who develop resilience may be more likely to seek treatment or develop physical, emotional, and functional well-being (Fang et al., 2015). Individuals living with

HIV/AIDS therefore have the ability to live normal, healthy lives despite social stigma and prejudice.

Caitlin Monahan and Nadav Antebi-Gruszka

See also: Affordable Care Act; Care, Access to; Community Health Centers; Dritz, Selma Kaderman; Epidemic; Global Health; Lesbian, Gay, Bisexual, and Transgender Health; National Institutes of Health; Substance Abuse and Mental Health Services Administration; Syringe Service Programs

Further Reading

Aidala, A. A., Wilson, M. G., Shubert, V., Gogolishvili, D., Globerman, J., Rueda, S., & Rourke, S. B. (2016). Housing status, medical care, and health outcomes among people living with HIV/AIDS: A systematic review. *American Journal of Public Health, 106*(1).

Centers for Disease Control and Prevention. (2016). *HIV surveillance report, 2015* (Vol. 27). Retrieved from https://www.cdc.gov/hiv/pdf/library/reports/surveillance/cdc-hiv-surveillance-report-2015-vol-27.pdf.

Centers for Disease Control and Prevention. (2017). *HIV/AIDS.* Retrieved from https://www.cdc.gov/hiv/.

Cramer, R. J., Colbourn, S. L., Gemberling, T. M., Graham, J., & Stroud, C. H. (2015). Substance-related coping, HIV-related factors, and mental health among an HIV-positive sexual minority community sample. *AIDS Care, 27*(9), 1063–1068.

Fang, X., Vincent, W., Calabrese, S. K., Heckman, T. G., Sikkema, K. J., Humphries, D. L., & Hansen, N. B. (2015). Resilience, stress, and life quality in older adults living with HIV/AIDS. *Aging & Mental Health, 19*(11), 1015–1021.

Fumaz, C. R., Ayestaran, A., Perez-Alvarez, N., Muñoz-Moreno, J. A., Moltó, J., Ferrer, M. J., & Clotet, B. (2015). Resilience, ageing, and quality of life in long-term diagnosed HIV-infected patients. *AIDS Care, 27*(11), 1396–1403.

HIV/AIDS. (2015, July). Retrieved January from http://www.mayoclinic.org/diseases-conditions/hiv-aids/basics/definition/con-20013732.

National Institute of Allergy and Infectious Diseases. (2015, December 23). Retrieved January 6, 2016, from https://www.niaid.nih.gov/topics/hivaids/Pages/Default.aspx.

Prejean, J., Song, R., Hernandez, A., Ziebell, R., Green, T., Walker, F., & Lansky, A. (2011). Estimated HIV incidence in the United States, 2006–2009. *PLoS One, 6*, e17502.

Rietmeijer, C. A., & Shamos, S. J. (2007). HIV and sexually transmitted infection prevention online: Current state and future prospects. *Sexual Research and Social Policy, 4*, 65–73.

Salomon, E. A., Mimiaga, M. J., Husnik, M. J., Welles, S. L., Manseau, M. W., Montenegro, B., & Mayer, K. H. (2009). Depressive symptoms, utilization of mental health care, substance use and sexual risk among young men who have sex with men in EXPLORE: Implications for age-specific interventions. *AIDS and Behavior, 13*, 811–821.

U.S. Department of Health and Services. (2015, December 7). Centers for Disease Control and Prevention. Retrieved December 30, 2015, from http://www.cdc.gov/hiv/.

Vermund, S. H. (2014). Global HIV epidemiology: A guide for strategies in prevention and care. *Current HIV/AIDS Reports, 11*(2), 93–98. Retrieved January 13, 2016.

Walensky, R. P., Auerbach, J. D., Office of Aids Research Advisory Council, Carpenter, C. J., Auerbach, J. D., Agosto-Rosario, M., . . . Walensky, R. P. (2014). Focusing National Institutes of Health HIV/AIDS Research for Maximum Population Impact. *Clinical Infectious Diseases, 60*(6), 937–940.

Welcome to AIDS.gov. (n.d.). Retrieved December 9, 2015, from https://www.aids.gov/.

HUMAN TRAFFICKING

Human trafficking is a form of slavery where individuals are forced to perform labor or sexual acts against their will. The Trafficking Victims Protection Act defines *sex trafficking of children* as "the recruitment, harboring, transportation, provision, or obtaining of a person for the purpose of a commercial sex act, in which the commercial sex act is induced by force, fraud, or coercion or in which the person induced to perform such act has not attained 18 years of age" (U.S. Department of State, 2014). *Labor trafficking* is defined as "the recruitment, harboring, transportation, provision, or obtaining of a person for labor or services, through the use of force, fraud, or coercion for the purpose of subjection to involuntary servitude, peonage, debt bondage, or slavery" (U.S. Department of State, 2014). Both types of trafficking happen at the global, national, and local levels. Victims may be brought from other countries into the United States, exported from the United States to other countries, transported to different locations within the United States, or kept in close vicinity to where they were initially trafficked. Human trafficking is a serious human rights violation. Public health clinicians work to identify victims during diagnostic health screenings, provide education and resources for victims, reduce the demand for human trafficking, empower survivors to engage in prevention and intervention activities, and change cultural norms that promote abusive relationships.

Because human trafficking is a heinous crime, it is hard to get clear statistics on the exact number of victims. Across the globe, an estimated 2 million children are exploited by sex traffickers (UNICEF, 2005). Nationally, an estimated 105,000 children are victims of sex trafficking (Estes & Weiner, 2002, as cited in Clayton, Krugman, & Simon, 2013). The average age of "turning out" or entry into sex trafficking is 12 to 14 years old for females and 11 to 13 years old for males (Estes & Weiner, 2001). Children who are victims of sex traffickers may age into adult sex work. However, the health issues of sex trafficked victims, violence, substance abuse, and sexually transmitted diseases significantly reduce life span. The majority of victims (98 percent) are women and girls (ILO, 2005). Youth who identify as lesbian, gay, bisexual, transgender/transsexual, queer (LGBTQ) are five times more likely to be trafficked than heterosexual youth (USDHHS, 2013). Seventy to 90 percent of sex trafficked youth have a history of child sexual abuse (AYCF, 2013). Little is known about sex trafficked males because many victims either do not self-identify as victims or do not seek help due to shame, stigma, lack of screening, limited outreach, and limited resources (AYCF, 2013).

Internationally, 15.4 million adults and 5.5 million children are victims of labor trafficking (ILO, 2012). Labor traffickers disproportionately target foreign nationals (Family and Youth Services Bureau, 2016). The majority of labor trafficked foreign nationals are legal immigrants. However, by the time they escape victimization, 69 percent are undocumented or have expired documentation (Bañuelos et al., 2014). In the United States, two-thirds of all victims are male (Bañuelos et al., 2014). Further research on incidence, prevalence, and risk factors for trafficking can help to prevent and reduce the problem.

Traffickers may be a relative, friend, intimate partner, neighbor, or stranger (Smith et al., 2009). The perpetrator targets vulnerable individuals, people who are homeless, abusing substances, rejected by family, socially isolated, or experiencing intimate partner violence or economic hardship. To gain control, the trafficker targets the person's vulnerabilities, using physical or psychological needs to manipulate the intended victim (Smith et al., 2009). Victims are lured by charisma, flattery, unctuousness, promises, threats, or intimidation (Estes & Weiner, 2001). Once the trafficker controls the relationship, the victim is isolated from potential social supports. The victim's sense of self-worth and autonomy are commandeered by the abuser (Smith et al., 2009). Control is maintained by mental, physical, or sexual abuse.

Although trafficking victims can be hard to identify because they represent different genders, sexual orientations, citizenships, or socioeconomic statuses, health screenings provide one opportunity for identification and intervention. Victims of labor and sex trafficking suffer from many negative health outcomes and may appear at health clinics or emergency rooms for treatment. Physically, victims suffer from traumatic brain injury, broken bones, fractures, strangulation, bruising, and other trauma due to physical abuse by the traffickers or patrons. Victims of sex trafficking are traumatized by sexual abuse. They may present with sexually transmitted diseases, pelvic pain, rectal trauma, or urinary difficulty (Ark of Hope for Children, 2016). Psychologically, victims experience depression, anxiety, and shame. Psychosomatic disorders can arise, such as stomachache, headache, or backache. Sex trafficking victims in particular may move into addiction. Addictions stem from the abuser drugging the victim or from the victim using drugs as a form of self-medication to cope with the abuse. In either case, addiction compounds other health problems. Sex trafficked youth have difficulty achieving key developmental tasks (developing independence and trusting relationships) needed to transition into adulthood (Clayton et al., 2013). If sex trafficking victims reach adulthood, they have a high mortality rate. Women who have been trafficked for sex have mortality rates almost 200 times greater than their demographic counterparts (Shively et al., 2012). The most common causes of death in sex trafficked victims include, in order of frequency: homicide, suicide, drug and alcohol-related problems, HIV infection, and unintentional injuries (Shively et al., 2012).

The League of Nations, which convened after World War I, was the first international organization of nations to address human trafficking. In 1921, *The International*

Convention for the Suppression of Traffic in Women and Children was signed by 33 countries. However, this legislation only covered trafficking for the purposes of sexual exploitation and prostitution. In 1949, after the League of Nations transitioned into the United Nations (UN), the UN created the first legally binding international agreement on human trafficking, titled *The United Nations Convention for the Suppression of the Traffic in Persons and of the Exploitation of the Prostitution of Others*. As of 2015, only 66 nations ratified the agreement. International law and the laws of 134 countries criminalize sex trafficking (Equality Now, 2016). In the United States, the use of children in commercial sex trade is prohibited by law and statute (U.S. Department of State, 2014). In 2007, Polaris created the National Human Trafficking Resource Center (NHTRC) as a clearing house and hotline for victims and survivors of trafficking (NHTRC, 2016). When a call is placed to the hotline at 1-888-373-7888, the caller is directed to resources and assistance in their local area. In addition, NHTRC and Polaris compile statistical data from their callers, providing insight into the scope of the problem. This national resource, along with local resources across the country, is a first step in helping victims and survivors leave the violence.

Current approaches to human trafficking focus on arrest and criminal prosecution of traffickers and victim support. There is the need and potential to expand efforts, using the framework of public health. Knowing risk and protective factors for victimization can identify at-risk youth and adults and suggest prevention strategies. Education of health care workers in early diagnosis, screening, and intervention can intercept and connect victims with available resources. Listening and empowering survivors can help identify best practices in anti-trafficking intervention and prevention. Human trafficking can only exist in cultures with deep-rooted feelings of entitlement, hierarchy, privilege, and inequity. The most effective way to stop this slavery is by addressing the social dynamics that enable perpetrators to feel entitled to take and abuse the lives of other men, women, and children.

Julia Hanes and Maria DiGiorgio McColgan

See also: Children's Health; Immigrant Health; Violence; Women's Health

Further Reading

Ark of Hope for Children. (2016). *Child trafficking statistics: U.S. and international*. Retrieved from http://arkofhopeforchildren.org/child-trafficking/child-trafficking-statistics.

Bañuelos, I., Breaux, J., Bright, K., Dank, M., Farrell, A., Heitsmith, R., McDevitt, J., Owens, C., & Pfeffer, R. (2014). *Understanding the organization, operation, and victimization process of labor trafficking in the United States*. Washington, DC: Urban Institute/Northeastern University.

Clayton, E. W., Krugman, R. D., & Simon, P. (Eds.). (2013). *Confronting commercial sexual exploitation and sex trafficking of minors in the United States*. Washington, DC: National Academies Press.

Equality Now. (2016). *Global sex trafficking fact sheet.* Retrieved from http://www.equalitynow.org/traffickingFAQ.

Estes, R., & Weiner, N. (2001). *The commercial sexual exploitation of children in the U.S., Canada, and Mexico.* Philadelphia: University of Pennsylvania.

Family and Youth Services Bureau. (2016). *Identification of domestic labor trafficking.* Webinar.

International Labour Office (ILO). (2005). *Minimum estimate of forced labour in the world.* Geneva: ILO.

International Labour Office (ILO). (2012). *ILO global estimate of forced labour: Results and methodology.* Geneva: Special Action Programme to Combat Forced Labour (SAP-FL).

National Human Trafficking Resource Center (NHTRC). (2016). *Mission.* Retrieved from https://traffickingresourcecenter.org/mission.

Shively, M., Kilorys, K., Wheeler, K, & Hunt, D. (2012). *A national overview of prostitution and sex trafficking demand reduction efforts.* Washington, DC: National Institute of Justice.

Smith, L., Vardaman, S., & Snow, M. (2009). *The national report on domestic minor sex trafficking: America's prostituted children.* Vancouver, WA: Shared Hope International.

UNICEF. (2005). *Children out of sight, out of mind, out of reach: Abused and neglected, millions of children have become virtually invisible.* New York: Brodock Press.

U.S. Department of Health and Human Services, Administration for Children, Youth, and Families. (2013). *Guidance to states and services on addressing human trafficking of children and youth in the United States.* Retrieved from http://www.acf.hhs.gov/programs/cb/resource/human-trafficking-guidance.

U.S. Department of State. (2014). *What is trafficking in persons? Fact sheet.* Retrieved from at https://www.state.gov/j/tip/rls/fs/2014/233732.htm.

HYPERTENSION (HTN)

Hypertension (HTN) is a medical condition where the pressure exerted by blood against the arterial walls is higher than normal and, if left untreated, will cause major organ damage. High blood pressure harms the arterial walls causing serious damage to the delicate arterioles that feed the kidneys, heart, eyes, and brain. The damaged surfaces attract low density lipoproteins (LDL), known as bad cholesterol. Over time, a thick, hard deposit builds up to create partial or complete blockage. The consequences of HTN are heart attack, stroke, heart failure, vision loss, sexual dysfunction, and kidney disease. Certain conditions, such as diabetes, aggravate the onset and seriousness of HTN. In the United States, one out of three adults has HTN. The disease has few warning signs, which means many people do not realize that they have high blood pressure. Fortunately, the condition is highly preventable. Public health efforts focus on patient education, early detection and treatment, creating healthy communities, building collaborative partnerships, and supporting research, policies, and programs to prevent heart disease.

Blood pressure consists of two numbers: systolic and diastolic. Systolic pressure is the maximum force against the walls of the arteries, the pressure created when the heart contracts and pumps blood into the arteries. Diastolic pressure is the resting pressure, the force against the walls of the arteries when the heart is filling with blood, preparing for the next contraction. Both systolic and diastolic pressures are measured in millimeter of mercury (mmHg), the standard unit of pressure in scientific disciplines. Blood pressure varies with circadian rhythm, activity, emotion, and hydration but typically stays within a range of 15 mmHg throughout the day. In 2014, the National Heart, Lung and Blood Institute (NHLBI) convened a panel of medical experts to review and update the clinical guidelines for diagnosis and treatment of HTN (James et al., 2014). Physicians use clinical guidelines to determine need and type of treatment. According to national guidelines, *normal blood pressure* is defined as a systolic pressure of less than 120 mmHg and a diastolic pressure of less than 80 mmHg. *Prehypertension*, an indication that someone is bordering on hypertension, is a systolic pressure of 120 to 139 mmHg or diastolic pressure of 80 to 89 mmHg. *HTN Stage 1* is a systolic pressure of 140 to 159 mmHg or diastolic pressure of 90 to 99 mmHg. *HTN Stage 2* (severe HTN) is a systolic pressure of 160 mmHg or higher or diastolic pressure of 100 mmHg or higher. Treatment is based on the overall health status of the individual and any comorbidity. *Hypertensive crisis* is a systolic pressure higher than 180 mmHg or a diastolic pressure higher than 110 mmHg. Hypertensive crisis is a medical emergency. The patient needs immediate medical treatment to allay stroke, heart attack, or other irreversible organ damage.

An estimated 75 million people in the United States have high blood pressure. Major risk factors are related to lifestyle, aging, heredity, and stress. An unhealthy diet, physical inactivity, excessive body weight, tobacco use, and alcohol abuse increase risk of HTN. Diets high in saturated fat and sugar act directly and indirectly. Obesity and atherosclerosis force the heart to work harder and increase vascular resistance through atherosclerosis. As people age, the blood vessels lose elasticity. Arteriosclerosis builds and causes a further narrowing of the arteries. Men are at higher risk until age 45 after which risk levels due to gender equalize. After age 64, women are at higher risk. Race is also a critical factor. More than 40 percent of African Americans are hypertensive, and the condition tends to have earlier onset and greater severity among certain minority populations. Racial differences may be related to salt sensitivity. Salt sensitivity is a genetic trait that causes the individual to retain sodium in the body. Scientists believe salt sensitivity evolved as a mechanism for survival (Campese, 1997). Populations that suffered periods of famine, such as Africans, Pima Indians, Asian Indians, Micronesians, and Polynesians developed physiological mechanisms to store sodium and calories. Today, the gene is not necessary due to changes in food availability. However, the physiological mechanism has not changed, and mechanisms that once protected and helped with survival now increase risk for HTN, diabetes, and obesity. People with salt sensitivity respond to salt intake with abnormally high blood pressure increases. Stress increases blood pressure by triggering the fight or flight reaction of the sympathetic nervous system. When people use tobacco or alcohol to self-medicate stressors, these may also increase blood pressure. Tobacco causes vasoconstriction, temporarily increasing blood pressure, and both tobacco and alcohol increase risk of atherosclerosis.

Public health clinics address HTN through early detection, patient education, evidence-based treatments, and prevention. Blood pressure is routinely measured and assessed at every health care visit. Patients who meet the criteria for treatment are prescribed antihypertensive or other medications according to the recommended guidelines. Antihypertensive medication reduces the risk of organ damage. Unfortunately, many people do not take their blood pressure medicine due to cost or undesirable side effects. Helping patients to know what the systolic and diastolic pressures mean and discussing obstacles to treatment can help improve medication compliance and to achieve adequate blood pressure control. The economic cost of medical treatment is high. In 2011–2012, hypertension-related hospitalizations, health care, medication, and lost productivity totaled $48.6 billion per year (Mozaffarian et al., 2016). When the costs of heart disease and stroke are included in the overall cost, direct and indirect costs total $316.6 billion per year.

Preventing HTN could potentially save billions of dollars each year and save countless lives. Risk factors, such as diet, exercise, and lifestyle, are easily modifiable. To control or prevent HTN, experts recommend the following:

- the DASH (dietary approaches to stop hypertension) eating plan: a low-sodium, low-fat diet high in fresh fruits and vegetables,
- maintaining a healthy weight: maintaining a healthy body mass index (18.5 to 24.9 for adults),
- physical activity: two hours and thirty minutes of moderate-intensity aerobic activity each week plus muscle-strengthening activities on two days of each week,
- no tobacco,
- no alcohol or alcohol in moderation, and
- healthy stress management practices.

The recommendations support normotensive blood pressure by reducing the buildup of cholesterol and reducing demand on the heart. These recommendations have the added benefit of reducing risk of other chronic and acute health conditions, such as cancer, chronic obstructive pulmonary disease (COPD), diabetes, heart disease, and stroke.

Cardiovascular diseases (CVD) are the leading cause of death in the United States. There is a lot that individuals can do to reduce their risk of CVD, and numerous government and nonprofit organizations are working to reduce or prevent the problem. The American Heart Association offers brochures, newsletters, fact sheets, and other educational materials for patients and health care providers. The website features recipes that adhere to the DASH eating plan as well as a support network for those recovering from the devastating effects of CVD and caregivers who support them. The NHLBI is an institute of the National Institute of Health (NIH) with the mission of promoting the prevention and treatment of heart, lung, and blood diseases through research and education. In addition to advancing the science of heart, lung, and blood diseases, the NHLBI works with patients, families, advocacy, and community groups to translate the latest research findings into practice. The American Society of Hypertension (ASH) is a professional network of physicians, researchers, pharmacists, and health care professionals working in the diagnosis, treatment, and prevention of HTN and HTN-related diseases. Future efforts seek to increase self-monitoring of blood pressure, reduce the high costs of treatment, and support obesity prevention programs.

Hypertension is a chronic health problem that can cause irreversible organ damage. Over time, the condition can lead to heart attack, stroke, aneurysm, or kidney failure. Treatment is available, but many people with high blood pressure have difficulty controlling the disorder. Fortunately, many cases are preventable through individual, systems, and population-based approaches. Individuals can reduce risk by following the DASH eating plan, getting the recommended amount of exercise, and abstention from smoking and excess alcohol. Health care systems can reduce the prevalence of HTN by offering regular screening and encouraging patients and providers to engage in healthy behaviors. Population-based approaches use policies or target schools, workplaces, and communities for environmental and behavioral changes. Comprehensive approaches to HTN offer promise in reducing the cost of the disease and reducing complications.

Sally Kuykendall

See also: Body Mass Index; Health Disparities; Healthy Places; Heart Disease; National Heart, Lung, and Blood Institute; Nutrition; Obesity; Physical Activity

Further Reading

American Heart Association. (2017). *High blood pressure.* Retrieved from http://www.heart.org/HEARTORG/Conditions/HighBloodPressure/High-Blood-Pressure_UCM_002020_SubHomePage.jsp.

American Society of Hypertension. (2017). Retrieved from http://www.ash-us.org/.

Campese, V. M. (1997). Why is salt-sensitive hypertension so common in blacks? *Nephrology, Dialysis, Transplantation: Official Publication of the European Dialysis and Transplant Association—European Renal Association, 12*(3), 399–403.

Centers for Disease Control and Prevention. (2014). *High blood pressure.* Retrieved from https://www.cdc.gov/bloodpressure/.

James, P. A., Oparil, S., Carter, B. L., Cushman, W. C., Dennison-Himmelfarb, C., Handler, J., & . . . Ortiz, E. (2014). 2014 Evidence-based guideline for the management of high blood pressure in adults: Report from the panel members appointed to the Eighth Joint National Committee (JNC 8). *Journal of the American Medical Association, 311*(5), 507–520. doi:10.1001/jama.2013.284427

Mozaffarian, D., Benjamin, E. J., Go, A. S., Arnett, D. K., Blaha, M. J., Cushman, M., & . . . Turner, M. B. (2016). Heart disease and stroke statistics—2016 update: A report from the American Heart Association. *Circulation, 133*(4), e38–e360. doi:10.1161/CIR.0000000000000350

National Heart, Lung, and Blood Institute. (2017). Retrieved from https://www.nhlbi.nih.gov/.

I

IMMIGRANT HEALTH

According to the Department of Homeland Security (DHS), immigrants, refugees, and migrants to the United States make up a significant portion of the American public. This population is composed of 13.2 million legal permanent residents, 11.4 million unauthorized immigrants, and 1.7 million nonresident visitors (U.S. Department of Homeland Security, 2016). Health concerns among these groups vary due to the large number of countries that refugees and immigrants originate from. In order to improve and maintain the health of immigrants, refugees, migrant workers, and Americans that immigrant people come in contact with on a daily basis, the Centers for Disease Control and Prevention (CDC) provides guidelines for screening, intervention, and services for immigrants and refugees (Centers for Disease Control and Prevention, 2017). Additionally, the CDC tracks, reports, and responds to communicable diseases within these populations. Refugees and immigrants applying for a visa are required to have a medical examination prior to admission. Immigration officers and overseas consular officers have the power to require that temporary visitors have medical examinations if there is suspicion of a health-related condition (Centers for Disease Control and Prevention, 2017). Some diseases, such as cholera, diphtheria, infectious tuberculosis, viral hemorrhagic fever, and influenza warrant quarantine. Cases of polio, plague, severe acute respiratory syndrome, smallpox, yellow fever, and pandemic flu are reported as a public health emergency of international concern.

The United States is a nation of immigrants. The first humans inhabited North America approximately 13,000 years ago when nomadic hunter-gatherers migrated from Siberia to Alaska and later to the Pacific Northwest, Canada, and South America. Population migration allows pathogens that are endemic to one area to be carried to new groups of susceptible hosts. Depending on the severity of the pathogenic strain and the vulnerability of the new population, the disease could have serious repercussions. Spanish explorers brought smallpox to the New World. European immigrants brought the bubonic plague, cholera, diphtheria, scarlet fever, smallpox, typhoid, typhus, tuberculosis, and sexually transmitted diseases. Likewise, travelers can carry pathogens back to the place of origin. Some scholars propose that syphilis was first present in the new world and introduced to Europe by Columbus's crew. In colonial America, early efforts to control the transmission of communicable diseases were haphazard, regulated by state or local governments. In 1647, Boston passed an ordinance requiring all arriving ships to stop at the harbor entrance for inspection. In 1663, New York City passed a law requiring people arriving from areas with smallpox to be reviewed by sanitary officials before entering the city. Seventy-five years later, New York City established a quarantine station at Bedloe's Island. The station isolated immigrants, travelers, and sailors who may be carrying smallpox or yellow fever.

Today, immigration health is regulated under the Division of Global Migration and Quarantine, part of the Centers for Disease Control and Prevention's National Center for Emerging and Zoonotic Infectious Diseases. Immigration personnel review the origin of each traveler to assess health risk and determine the appropriate response. Although these measures help to ensure that the health of legal permanent residents and visitors is serviced, many barriers exist for unauthorized immigrants to attain health services in the United States (Wallace et al., 2013). The majority of people in the United States with health care have access to their plans through their employers. Many unauthorized immigrants work in industries that do not provide health insurance. Unauthorized immigrants are not eligible for public health insurance. They may therefore be required to wait until their conditions have worsened to attain care at emergency rooms, made possible by the Emergency Medical Treatment and Active Labor Act (Caplan & Bateman-House, 2017). Fear of deportation by Immigration and Customs Enforcement may prevent unauthorized immigrants from seeking care. Health care facilities requiring proof of income or residence prior to treatment may also prevent unauthorized immigrants from receiving the care they need. Language is another barrier. Many unauthorized immigrants do not speak English as a primary language, hampering communication between patients and their public health providers (Portes & Fernández-Kelly, 2012). In order to minimize the obstacles to medical treatment and encourage personal responsibility for health, some cities have adopted sanctuary policies. Sanctuary cities are towns and cities that limit reporting of undocumented immigrants in order to encourage illegal immigrants to report crimes and to use health, social, and educational services.

The Centers for Disease Control and Prevention promotes immigrant, refugee, and migrant health by providing guidelines for disease screening and treatment, tracking and reporting communicable diseases, offering leadership, expertise, and care during public health emergencies, and by partnering with immigrant and refugee groups to enhance health among migrant people.

Matthew Black

See also: Affordable Care Act; Association of State and Territorial Health Officials; Baker, Sara Josephine; Epidemic; Global Health; Hamilton, Alice; Human Trafficking; Indian Health Service; Infectious Diseases; Quarantine; Sanger, Margaret Louise Higgins; U.S. Department of Agriculture; World Health Organization; *Controversies in Public Health:* Controversy 5

Further Reading

Biswas, D., Toebes, B., Hjern, A., Ascher, H., & Norredam, M. (2012). Access to health care for undocumented migrants from a human rights perspective: A comparative study of Denmark, Sweden, and the Netherlands. *Health and Human Rights*, *14*(2), 49.

Caplan, A. L., & Bateman-House, A. (2017, July). "Alien" health care. *American Journal of Public Health*, 1029–1030. doi:10.2105/AJPH.2017.303850

Centers for Disease Control and Prevention. (2017). *Immigrant and refugee health*. Retrieved from https://www.cdc.gov/immigrantrefugeehealth/index.html.

Edward, J. (2014). Undocumented immigrants and access to health care: Making a case for policy reform. *Policy, Politics, & Nursing Practice*, *15*(1–2), 5–14. doi:10.1177/1527154414532694

Portes, A., Fernández-Kelly, P., & Light, D. (2012). Life on the edge: Immigrants confront the American health system. *Ethnic & Racial Studies*, *35*(1), 3–22. doi:10.1080/01419870.2011.594173

U.S. Department of Homeland Security. (2016). *Population estimates*. Retrieved from https://www.dhs.gov/immigration-statistics/population-estimates.

Wallace, S. P., Rodriguez, M., Padilla-Frausto, I., Arredondo, A., & Orozco, E. (2013). Improving access to health care for undocumented immigrants in the United States. *Salud Pública De México*, *55*, S508–S514.

INDIAN HEALTH SERVICE (IHS)

In 1787, the U.S. federal government recognized the inherent rights of the first people of North America by granting unique legal status. Article I, Section 8 of the Constitution mandates that Native American tribes are *domestic dependent nations* with parallel sovereignty within the federal government. This means that the federal government has a duty to protect Native American and Alaskan Native people *and* indigenous tribes have the power of self-determination. Federal, state, or local governments have no authority over tribal land or tribal matters. This unusual proclamation was made in an attempt to amalgamate the many formal treaties between the U.S. government and Native American tribes. Because the Native Americans suffered from numerous communicable diseases, treaties for Native American land, supplies, and services often included the provision of medical care. The Indian Health Service (IHS) is an agency within the U.S. Department of Health and Human Services (DHHS) responsible for fulfilling the nation's obligation to provide community health services and primary health care to 2.2 million indigenous Americans from 567 tribes. The mission of IHS is to ensure access to culturally competent, quality health care. Participation in IHS programs does not exclude individuals from participating in other federally supported health care programs.

The first humans inhabited North America approximately 13,000 years ago. Anthropologists believe that nomadic hunter-gatherers migrated from Siberia to Alaska and later trekked to the Pacific Northwest, Canada, and South America. Ancient North America civilizations created their own communities, architecture, art, and culture. DNA analysis of ancient human skeletons matches the DNA of living Native American people. In the late 1700s, Europeans discovered the new world. Without regard for the current inhabitants, Spanish and English explorers claimed the land and resources as their own. Native American tribes were massacred, forced into slavery, and exposed to infectious diseases for which they had no natural immunity. European immigrants transmitted the bubonic plague, cholera, diphtheria, scarlet fever, smallpox, typhoid, typhus, tuberculosis, and sexually transmitted diseases to vulnerable populations. Catholic priests enslaved natives to build missions along the California coast. Death by malnutrition, suicide, and homicide were common among the forced laborers. Given the rate of disease and violence suffered by the indigenous people, peace and land treaties often included some promise of protection from harm or provision of health services. In some regions, military physicians provided care to the people of neighboring tribes. Maintaining the health of indigenous people reduced communicable diseases and protected early settlers. In 1832, Congress allocated $12,000 for smallpox vaccination of Native Americans. Four years later, the federal government started a formal health service program for members of the Ottawa and Chippewa tribes.

As European immigrants moved westward, they violated treaties and encroached on land owned and inhabited by the first people. In 1828, the state of Georgia attempted to seize Cherokee tribal land. The case of the *Cherokee Nation v. Georgia* went to the Supreme Court. The Court ruled that the Cherokee Nation was a sovereign nation and the state of Georgia had no authority over Cherokee land. Chief Justice John Marshall compared the relationship between tribes and the federal government as that of a legal guardian relationship. The federal government is legally obligated to act as a guardian to Native American tribes. Despite the ruling, President Andrew Jackson and Martin Van Buren ordered the aggressive removal of Cherokee people. The *Trail of Tears* was a forced march of people from Cherokee, Choctaw, Muskogee, and Seminole tribes from the southeastern states to west of the Mississippi River. An estimated 2,000 to 6,000 Native American people died of communicable diseases, exposure to the elements, starvation, or violence suffered during the forced march.

In 1849, responsibility for Indian health was transferred from the War Department to the Department of the Interior. In 1867, the U.S. government purchased the Alaskan territory, expanding U.S. territory to include land inhabited by people of Inuit and Alaskan Native culture. In 1911, the federal government established a separate funding line for Native American health services. Despite the government's legal obligation to Native Americans and Alaskan Natives, indigenous people were not officially recognized as citizens. This means that they were not eligible for the same rights and privileges as other citizens. Exclusionary attitudes started to change with World War I when Cherokee and Choctaw code talkers were instrumental in transmitting classified military information. The Snyder Act of 1921 granted official U.S. citizenship to Native Americans who served in World War I. The act also highlighted the dire health needs of the Indian population by defining federal obligations for the "relief of distress and conservation of health of Indians" (IHS, 2005).

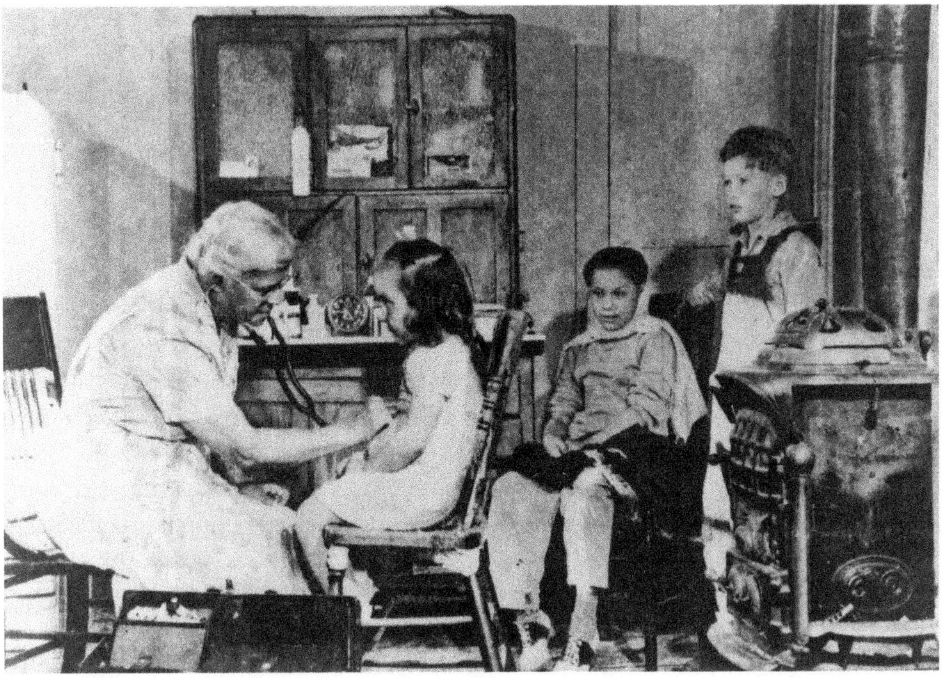

Dr. Lillie Rosa Minoka-Hill examines June Marie House in her kitchen clinic while Loretta House and Roger Dunks watch, 1947. Dr. Hill tended to members of the Oneida Nation of Wisconsin for almost 50 years. Dr. Hill's adopted name was Yo-da-gent, meaning "she who serves." (MPI/Getty Images)

The Hoover Commission (1947) was developed to recommend ways for the federal government to increase efficiency and decrease expenditures. The commission recommended eliminating duplicate government services, including services to Native Americans, and introduced the concept of *forced termination*. Forced termination involved repealing laws that differentiated Native Americans from other citizens, relocating native people from reservations to cities, assimilating Native Americans and Alaskan Natives into the larger population, dismantling the Bureau of Indian Affairs, and transferring any remaining Indian health or social programs to state governments. The legislature failed to pass. However, supporters developed other ways to achieve forced termination. The Transfer Act of 1955 established the Indian Health Service (IHS) as part of the U.S. Public Health Service (USPHS) within the Department of Health and Human Services. The USPHS offered centralized health services with care by white European American health care professionals. The combination of a paternalistic health care system and majority-culture professionals meant that caregivers could not or did not understand or respect differences between Native American medicine and Western medicine or between the medical practices of various tribes. Forced termination did not work. The concept deepened distrust among Native Americans and increased dependence on the federal government.

The civil rights movement of the 1960s empowered Native American/Alaskan Native (NA/AN) people. President Richard M. Nixon opposed the concept of forced termination. He believed that Indian health and social services were a "solemn obligation" forged by historic legal agreements (Kunitz, 1996). The Nixon administration passed the Indian Self-Determination and Education Assistance Act (1975) and the Indian Health Care Improvement Act of 1976. These laws empowered tribes to take control of their own health and social service programs and led to the creation of community health boards, hiring of Native American/Alaskan Native (NA/AN) professionals and paraprofessionals and culturally competent, decentralized services. Today, the Indian Health Service is a self-governed program which respects that tribal leaders and tribal members are in the best position to determine, direct, and administer health care needs. The system works through collaborative partnerships that assess health issues, the types of care needed, service delivery, and evidence-based care (IHS, 2005). The system is not perfect. It is extremely underfunded. Congress currently allocates $3,000 per person to IHS, significantly less than the budgeted $5,000 per person to prison inmates and $12,000 per person to Medicare beneficiaries (Davidson, 2017). This disparity raises questions of covert racism or care rationing.

The living history of North America's indigenous people presents unique health and social needs. Native Americans and Alaskan Natives started as nomadic hunter-gatherers who developed thriving settlements and cultures. European invasion brought infectious diseases, war, slavery, and oppression that almost decimated Native Americans. The people who survived represent ancient cultures dating back thousands of years and are one of the nation's most precious resources. The federal government, state governments, and descendants of European immigrants have a moral obligation to reconcile the actions of forefathers and preserve the unique culture of each tribe. IHS works to support and promote the biological, psychological, social, environmental, and spiritual health and well-being of indigenous people. Yet, their services are severely restricted by underfunding. Centuries of adversity and disease created populations with dire health needs that will require intensive, specialized resources to survive.

Sally Kuykendall

See also: Addictions; Cornely, Paul Bertau; Epidemic; Health Care Disparities; Health Disparities; Health Resources and Services Administration; Maternal Health; Smallpox; Spiritual Health; U.S. Department of Agriculture

Further Reading

Davidson, J. (2017). Staffing, budget shortages put Indian Health Service at "high risk." *Washington Post.* Retrieved from https://www.washingtonpost.com/news/powerpost/wp/2017/02/20/staffing-budget-shortages-put-indian-health-service-at-high-risk/?utm_term=.eaf628947972.

Indian Health Services (IHS). (2005). *The first 50 years of the Indian Health Service: Caring and curing.* IHS Gold Book Part 1, Department of Health and Human Services. Retrieved from https://www.ihs.gov/newsroom/factsheets/.

Kunitz, S. J. (1996). The history and politics of US health care policy for American Indians and Alaskan Natives. *American Journal of Public Health, 86*(10), 1464–1473.

INFANT MORTALITY

Infant mortality is the death of a baby within the first 12 months of birth. In the United States, an estimated 23,000 infants die each year (Centers for Disease Control and Prevention [CDC], 2016b). Data from vital statistics, birth, and death records are used to calculate infant mortality rate (IMR), the number of infant deaths per 1,000 live births. IMR is a standardized number serving as an important health indicator of human and social development. Public health professionals use the data to compare groups, communities, and nations in order to identify health needs. Monaco and Japan have the lowest IMRs at 1.8 and 2.0, respectively (Central Intelligence Agency [CIA], n.d.). IMR in the United States is 5.8 deaths per 1,000 live births. Most developing countries of Africa and Asia have higher IMRs. Infants in Afghanistan fare the poorest with an IMR of 112.8. The leading causes of infant death are birth defects, preterm birth, injuries, malnutrition, diarrhea, birth complications, infectious diseases, measles, and malaria (O'Brien, Usher, & Maughan 1966). Threats to infant health vary by geographic region, race, age, environmental conditions, and mother's level of education, socioeconomic status, and lifestyle. Quality prenatal services, medical care, good nutrition, immunizations, and home safety can prevent many of these untimely deaths.

Infant mortality is categorized as neonatal mortality and postneonatal mortality. *Neonatal mortality* is the death of a live-born baby within the first 28 days after delivery. *Early neonatal mortality* is death of a live-born baby within the first 7 days after delivery. *Neonatal mortality rate* (NMR) is the number of deaths of live-born babies within 28 days after delivery per 1,000 live births. NMR is used to assess prenatal, intrapartum, and neonatal care. *Postneonatal mortality* is the death of a baby from 29 days after birth to 12 months (364 days). Postneonatal mortality rate (PNMR or PMR) is the death of a live-born baby aged 28 days to less than 12 months (364 days) per 1,000 live births.

The major factors associated with neonatal mortality are congenital malformations, asphyxia and birth trauma, low birth weight, short gestation, and poor prenatal care. Factors associated with postneonatal mortality include maternal complications during pregnancy and delivery, sudden infant death syndrome (SIDS), infectious disease, premature births, unintentional birth injuries, congenital malformations, and malnutrition.

Every four and a half minutes in the United States, an infant is born with birth defects (CDC, 2016a). A defect may be mild or severe, structural or physiological, visible or invisible. Also referred to as congenital disorders, congenital abnormalities, congenital deformations, or congenital malformations, many defects develop during the first three months of pregnancy. This is a time when major organs form, and yet the woman may not realize she is pregnant. The causes of birth defects are often multifactorial, a combination of genetics, environment, paternal, and maternal health. Known risk factors include tobacco, alcohol, illicit drugs, acne medication, exposure to radioactive environment, sexually transmitted diseases (STDs), prenatal nutrition, and preexisting health conditions of the mother, such as obesity or diabetes. Alcohol and drug abuse significantly increases the risk of fetal deformation and birth complications. Environmental hazards include exposure to radioactive environment such as mines, chemicals, waste sites, and pesticides. Common nutritional causes are folate or iodine deficiency. In low and middle income countries, gonorrhea, rubella, hepatitis B virus (HBV), human immunodeficiency virus (HIV), and syphilis cause many congenital anomalies and infant death.

In some countries, low birth weight and short gestation birth account for up to 80 percent of infant mortalities (Andrews, Brouillette, & Brouillette, 2008; Stanley, Huber, Laditka, & Racine, 2016). In the United States, 8 percent of live births are low birth weight (CDC, 2016b). Low birth weight is defined as weighing less than 2,500 grams (5 pounds 8 ounces) at birth. Below 2,500 grams, the infant has difficulty with breathing, drinking, and fighting infections. At 1,000 grams (2.2 lb) or less, the infant struggles to survive the neonatal period. Low birth weight is typically associated with short gestation, less than 37 weeks. Causal factors include alcohol or drug use, poor nutrition, teenage pregnancy, poor prenatal care, maternal sickness, and multiple pregnancies.

Sudden unexpected infant death (SUID) or sudden infant death syndrome (SIDS) is the third leading cause of infant mortality in the United States (CDC, 2016c). SIDS is the unexpected, sudden death of a healthy infant aged less than 12 months. Over 1,500 such deaths occur each year in the United States. Ninety percent occur within the first six months of birth. SIDS is unexplainable. There are no known natural or physical causes or medical explanations. Medical examiners, forensic pathologists, autopsy and death scene investigators attribute SIDS to environmental stressors, accidental suffocation or strangulation in bedding materials, poor housing ventilation, poor sleeping position, or exposure to secondhand smoke. Genetic disorder, respiratory infections, premature birth, hypothermia, hyperthermia, neglect, low birth weight, and birth defects are also attributed as possible causes of SIDS.

Maternal complications are health problems experienced by the mother during pregnancy or after delivery. Maternal complications are associated with high infant mortality. Maternal complications may be due to previous illness, chronic disease, or disability, inadequate prenatal care, gestational diabetes, or placental abruption. Complications during delivery include mother to infant transmission of blood-borne infections or virus, asphyxia, birth trauma, or injury.

Infant mortality and IMR reflect the social, economic, and environmental development of a country. In 2015, the World Health Assembly (WHA) updated strategic plans to reduce infant and maternal mortality. "The Global Strategy sets out to ensure every woman, child and adolescent, in any setting, anywhere in the world, is able to survive and thrive by 2020" (World Health Organization [WHO] & UNICEF, 2017, p. 4). The global milestones include:

1. Establishing systems to gather accurate IMR data.
2. National policies and plans for quality health services.
3. Research and development in maternal and infant care.
4. Experts to champion the cause of maternal and infant health and welfare.

Many stillbirths of poor families are not recorded by birth or death certificate. Accurate data on births, deaths, and causes help identify areas for public health interventions. The WHA recommends that every country establish national policies and plans to provide quality health services to mothers and newborns. The WHO Quality of Care Framework defines quality services as following evidence-based practices in maternal and infant care, ensuring functional referral to other systems, offering clear and competent patient-provider communication, adhering to professional ethics of practice, offering emotional support, recruiting and retaining competent health care staff, and ensuring access to essential physical resources. Future research should focus on effective, innovative practices with special attention to stillbirth prevention. Pediatric champions are doctors, nurses, public health, or other medical professionals who commit to sharing best practices with colleagues and advocating for women and children who are not in a position to advocate for themselves.

Prevention and reduction of infant mortality are important health indices used to guide and formulate public health policies of maternal and infant care. Opportunities to improving maternal and infant care aim at increasing accessibility to prenatal, neonatal, and postneonatal care; addressing social determinants of health care coverage; educating expecting mothers on nutrition and lifestyle; promoting healthy postpartum behaviors; smoking and alcohol cessation; and breast feeding to provide nutrients and protection from infection during the critical first year of life.

Godyson Orji

See also: Baker, Sara Josephine; Birth Defects; Children's Health; Dunham, Ethel Collins; Ellertson, Charlotte Ehrengard; Family Planning; Health Care Disparities; Maternal Health; Measles; Polio; Sanger, Margaret Louise Higgins; Wegman, Myron Ezra; World Health Organization

Further Reading

Andrews, K. M., Brouillette, D. B., & Brouillette, R. T. (2008). *Mortality, infant.* Ipswich, MA: Elsevier, Inc. Gale Virtual Reference Library.

Centers for Disease Control and Prevention. (2016a). *Birth defects.* Retrieved from https://www.cdc.gov/ncbddd/birthdefects/facts.html.

Centers for Disease Control and Prevention. (2016b, January 12). *Infant mortality.* Retrieved from http://www.cdc.gov/reproductivehealth/maternalinfanthealth/infantmortality.htm.
Centers for Disease Control and Prevention. (2016c, June 8). *Sudden unexpected infant death and sudden infant death syndrome.* Retrieved from https://www.cdc.gov/sids/.
Centers for Disease Control and Prevention. (2017). *Infant mortality.* Retrieved from https://www.cdc.gov/reproductivehealth/maternalinfanthealth/infantmortality.htm.
Central Intelligence Agency. (n.d.). *Country comparison: Infant mortality rate. World FactBook.* Retrieved from https://www.cia.gov/library/publications/the-world-factbook/rankorder/2091rank.html.
Healthy Newborn Network. Retrieved from http://www.healthynewbornnetwork.org/.
O'Brien, J. R., Usher, R. H., & Maughan, G. B. (1966). Causes of birth asphyxia and trauma. *Canadian Medical Association Journal, 94*(21), 1077. Retrieved from http://www.ncbi.nlm.nih.gov/pmc/articles/PMC1935461/.
Stanley, W. A., Huber, L. R. B., Laditka, S. B., & Racine, E. F. (2016). Association of type of birth attendant and place of delivery on infant mortality in sub-Saharan Africa. *African Health Sciences, 16*(1), 1–9. doi:10.4314/ahs.v16i1.1
WHO & UNICEF. (2017). *Reaching the every newborn national 2020 milestones: Country progress, plans and moving forward.* Geneva: World Health Organization. Retrieved from http://apps.who.int/iris/bitstream/10665/255719/1/9789241512619-eng.pdf?ua=1.

INFECTIOUS DISEASES

Infectious diseases are illnesses caused by viruses, bacteria, or other pathogens, transmitted to a human host through water, food, rodents, insects, air, direct physical contact, or body fluids. The infectious diseases—cholera, smallpox, meningitis, influenza, and sexually transmitted diseases—were the scourge of ancient civilizations. Until the early 1900s, the average life span was 47 years, 33 years for African Americans (National Center for Health Statistics, 2011). The top three leading causes of death were pneumonia/influenza, tuberculosis, and diarrhea. Advancements in sanitation, microbiology, antibiotics, and vaccinations significantly affected health, increasing life span to 78 years (74 years for African Americans). Pneumonia/influenza dropped to eighth place as a leading cause of death. Despite progress against communicable diseases, ongoing vigilance is necessary. Infectious diseases are still the leading cause of death in many areas throughout the world, and pathogens are living organisms, capable of creative mutations involving drug resistance, mode of transmission, and lethality. Public health professionals are constantly surveilling for emerging and reemerging infectious diseases and working to control outbreaks throughout the world.

Infectious diseases have been the bane of humanity since early civilization. In 1346–1353, the bacterium *Yersinia pestis* killed an estimated 100 million people in the plague known as the Black Death. The caduceus, the medical symbol of two snakes wrapped around a pole, is an altered image of early treatment for guinea worm disease (GWD). The disease is contracted by ingesting water contaminated with the GWD nematode. The infected host remains asymptomatic for about a year after which time the mature female guinea worm blisters through the skin to discharge her larvae in water sources. Emergence is slow and painful, and efforts to pull the worm out more quickly can damage nerves or blood vessels. Forced removal could also break the nematode into pieces, leaving parts within the body to decay (putrefy) or harden (petrify). Ancient healers treated GWD by wrapping the emerging worm around a small stick, about the size of a matchstick. As the worm emerged, the stick was turned, successfully removing the intact organism. The symbol of a single serpent wrapped around a staff is the Rod of Asclepius, which was the original symbol of medicine and health care. The caduceus features two snakes around a pole with wings at the top of the pole. Both symbols indicate the significance of infectious diseases throughout history and ingenious methods devised by ancient healers to prevent or reduce the spread of such diseases.

Prior to the discovery of bacteria, people believed that infectious diseases were due to miasma, poisonous odors in the air. Soon after Dutch trader Anton van Leeuwenhoek refined glass lenses so that he could examine the delicate weave of linen, he turned his attention to nature. Through the microscope, van Leeuwenhoek and other scientists were able to view previously unknown organisms, and the fields of microbiology, epidemiology, and infection control were created. Today, many systems are in place to protect us from infectious diseases. Sanitation workers ensure that food in restaurants is properly stored and prepared, public health laboratories test for harmful microorganisms, and health practitioners administer vaccinations to guard against deadly childhood diseases. Yet, emerging and reemerging infectious diseases remain a threat to human existence. Infectious diseases commonly occur with deforestation, population movement, globalization, and overcrowding. Deforestation displaces animals and insects from their natural habitat. As the animals move to new areas, they bring organisms capable of causing disease. Population movement creates the same dynamic. Diseases that are endemic to a particular population move into new, unprotected populations. Globalization and overcrowding create interactions where formerly isolation may have prevented the spread of disease. World health officials are vigilant for catastrophic events, mass immigration, or global changes that could create new epidemics or pandemics.

The chain of infection, also known as the chain of transmission, is a schematic diagram showing how infections are passed to humans. The chain of infection is visualized as six links: pathogen, reservoir, portal of exit, mode of transmission, portal of entry, and susceptible host. The first link is the pathogen. Although many microorganisms are benign and fulfill important functions in nature, bacteria, fungi, viruses, helminths, protozoa, rickettsia, and prions can also cause disease. Pathogens are found in habitats that support their survival. Such habitats are known as reservoirs. In the case of GWD, the pathogen is *dracunculiasis medinensis*, and the reservoir is the human body that carries the nematode for over 12 months, providing nourishment for the larvae to mature (Office of Public Health Scientific Services, Center for Surveillance, Epidemiology, and Laboratory Services, and Division of Scientific Education and Professional Development, 2012). Other reservoirs are soil (*Clostridium botulinum*), animals (rabies), insects (*Yersinia pestis*), and water (*Legionella pneumophilia*). The portal of exit is how the pathogen leaves the host. Typical portals of exit from the human body are respiratory secretions, urine, feces, blood, or other body fluids. With GWD, the portal of exit is the outbreak through the skin. Means of transmission refers to how the pathogen moves to the new host. Direct contact is undeviating transmission between individuals through kissing, skin-to-skin contact, sexual intercourse, sneezing, coughing, or airborne droplets. Indirect contact refers to transfer by air currents, food, water, clothing, insects, or rodents. When the female guinea worm deposits her larva into water, they are ingested by copepods (small crustaceans). The copepods act as vectors, carrying the infective larvae. The portal of entry is how the pathogen enters the susceptible host. In most cases, the portal of exit is similar to the portal of entry. In the case of GWD, people drink water containing copepods contaminated with *dracunculiasis medinensis*. The final link in the chain is the susceptible host. In the normal healthy individual, skin, respiratory secretions, white blood cells, enzymes in tears, antigens, and acidic gastric juices will stop or contain many potential invaders. People who are struggling with compromised immune systems due to AIDS, leukemia, or other preexisting conditions are not able to combat pathogens as effectively. Additionally, certain behaviors, such as smoking marijuana or cigarettes, can impair the respiratory system increasing risk of infection. Susceptibility is also influenced by virulence and dosage of the pathogen. A minor exposure to the cold virus may be fended off with adequate rest and good nutrition. A major exposure where someone repeatedly coughs and sneezes in closed spaces may be harder to avoid. The beauty of the chain of infection is that it not only describes transmission from the original source to new hosts, but the diagram suggests multiple places to disrupt transmission.

Infection control measures seek to interrupt transmission at specific points. Antibiotics, antivirals, and other drugs interfere with pathogenic life cycle and replication. Reducing the number of pathogens in the environment reduces the potential for communicable disease transmission. Emptying standing water from old tires, pots, or stagnant pools (reservoirs) reduces West Nile virus. Good handwashing, personal hygiene, and cough etiquette intercepts pathogens at the portal of exit. Mode of transmission may be blocked by not sharing contaminated vehicles such as straws, needles, or cigarettes or through vector control, eliminating rats, roaches, fleas, and ticks. The human body has multiple natural defenses against pathogens. Immunity can be further enhanced through vaccinations, good nutrition, and adequate rest. Studying the chain of infection for each pathogen suggests numerous opportunities to control specific infectious diseases.

For many Americans, the days of overcrowded, unsanitary living conditions are long gone. The threat of losing loved ones to cholera, smallpox, polio, pneumonia, influenza, or typhoid is unfamiliar. One of the greatest advancements of public health in the past century is conquering communicable diseases through sanitation, food and water safety, infection control, and immunizations. Yet, as living organisms, pathogens are capable of interesting mutations, and public health professionals must remain vigilant for emerging and reemerging pathogens. The public can play an important role in securing health by following immunization guidelines, and employing good respiratory and personal hygiene including good handwashing.

Sally Kuykendall

See also: Ancient World, Public Health in the; Antibiotic Resistance; Cholera; Epidemic; Greco-Roman Era, Public Health in the; Human Immunodeficiency Virus and Acquired Immune Deficiency Syndrome; Immigrant Health; Meningitis; Pandemic; Public Health in the United States, History of; Renaissance, Public Health in the; Roosevelt, Franklin Delano; Smallpox; Snow, John; Vaccines; *Controversies in Public Health:* Controversy 3; Controversy 5

Further Reading

Centers for Disease Control and Prevention (CDC). (2012). *Respiratory hygiene/cough etiquette in healthcare settings.* Atlanta. Retrieved from http://www.cdc.gov/flu/professionals/infectioncontrol/resphygiene.htm.

National Center for Health Statistics. (2011). *Health, United States, 2010: With special feature on death and dying.* Hyattsville, MD. Retrieved from http://www.cdc.gov/nchs/data/hus/hus10.pdf.

Office of Public Health Scientific Services, Center for Surveillance, Epidemiology, and Laboratory Services, and Division of Scientific Education and Professional Development. (2012). *Principles of epidemiology in public health practice: An introduction to applied epidemiology and biostatistics* (3rd ed.). Atlanta: Centers for Disease Control and Prevention. Retrieved from http://www.cdc.gov/OPHSS/CSELS/DSEPD/SS1978/Lesson1/Section10.html#ALT120.

INFLUENZA

Influenza is a communicable disease caused by strains of the influenza virus. The pathogen is transmitted from the infected host to the potential host as respiratory droplets expelled during coughing, sneezing, or talking. Viral particles enter potential victims through the mouth or nose. Susceptible targets experience symptoms within one to four days after initial infection. Common symptoms include sore throat, cough, nasal congestion, fever, chills, body aches, headaches, and/or fatigue. Influenza, commonly known as the flu, is a serious public health problem. The disease causes widespread incapacitation and can progress to serious complications of pneumonia, sepsis (blood infection), myocarditis (inflammation of the heart muscle), encephalitis (inflammation of the brain), rhabdomyolysis (serious muscle injury), or multisystem organ failure. People with compromised immunity, children, the elderly, and those with preexisting health conditions are at high risk for infection and complications. The flu can be fatal, especially within these vulnerable populations. Fortunately, the disease is highly preventable through vaccination, basic infection control (public health) practices, and early treatment to limit continued transmission. Influenza is a classic example of how tiny, microscopic particles can pose an enormous threat to public health and how simple efforts can effectively prevent or control such threats.

The flu pandemic of 1918 was one of the worst public health disasters in modern history. An estimated one-fifth of the world's population, 50 to 100 million people, died. Experts are unsure where the virus originated. The first report is in an article in the British medical journal, *The Lancet*. The article describes an outbreak of severe respiratory infection at the Etaples military base in 1916 (Oxford et al., 2002). Located on the coast of northern France, Etaples was a strategic military base during World War I (1914–1918). Historians estimate that over one million allied troops moved through the Etaples base during World War I. With 22 hospitals, Etaples treated soldiers from around the world. The massive population movement combined with the stressful conditions of the battlefields (malnourishment, overcrowding, poor hygiene, and limited access to health and medical care) were ideal for infectious diseases. The first recorded flu case in the United States presented in January 1918 at Camp Devens (Auerbach, 2014). Devens was a military hospital and training base near Boston, Massachusetts. This case was followed by a minor epidemic that went largely unnoticed. The war was coming to an end, and people looked forward to celebrating the return of surviving sons, brothers, fathers, and boyfriends. A second wave of infection struck Devens on September 7, 1918. A soldier in D Company, 42nd Infantry presented with symptoms of meningitis. The following day, 12 other patients appeared. Within a week, the number of cases rose to 599. The virus strain, later identified as H1N1 avian influenza A, was unusual and lethal. Although most flu strains attack children and the elderly, this strain attacked young, healthy adults. Within a few hours of the initial symptoms, the victim's lungs filled with respiratory secretions and the patient would slowly drown. The infection spread quickly within the body and between victims. Healthy men and women died within hours of the initial complaints. Bodies were stacked in makeshift morgues. The Devens epidemic peaked on September 20, 1918, with 1,543 cases admitted on this one day, alone. Yet, Devens was not unique. Military bases, hospitals, and communities across the world were hit as 70 million military personnel returned from Europe, Asia, Africa, the Middle East, the Pacific Islands, and the Indian Ocean. In remote Brevig Mission, Alaska, 72 residents died within five days (Carroll, 2013). The only survivors were eight children and teenagers. Nurses and physicians were already in short supply because just about anyone with medical training had been deployed to field hospitals overseas. Desperate government officials implemented whatever measures they deemed appropriate. Curfews, bans on public gatherings, bans on commercial sales that might entice shoppers, and bans on spitting, sneezing, or coughing in public were implemented. By the end of 1919, the virus mutated to a less lethal form, and the pandemic subsided almost as quickly as it started. Within this one year alone, the flu pandemic reduced overall life expectancy by 12 years in the United States.

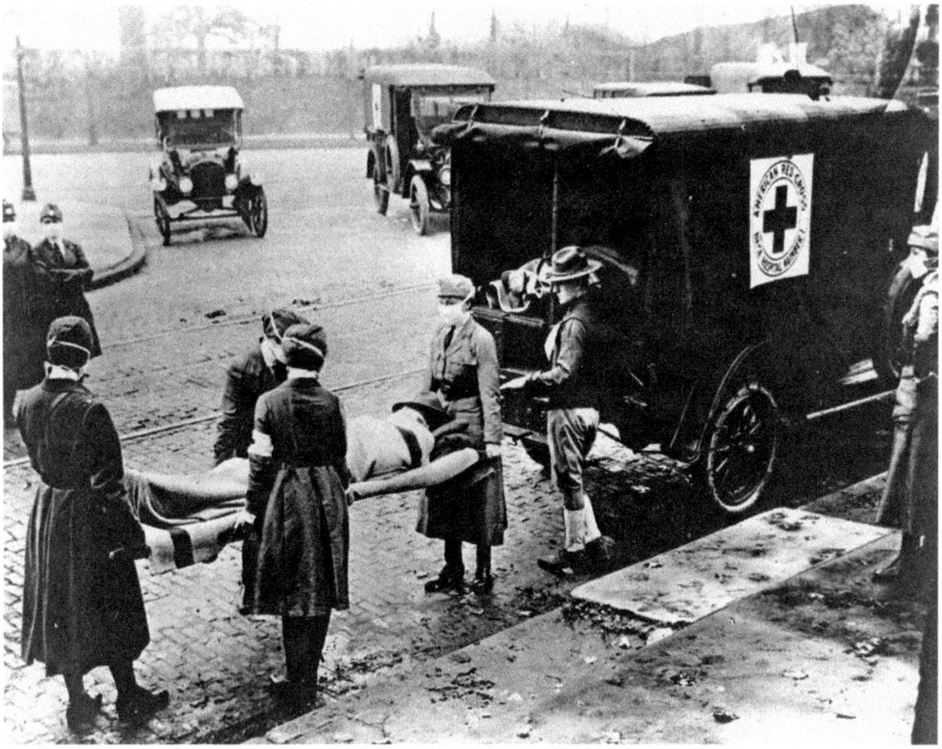

Nurses load St. Louis residents into a Red Cross ambulance during the flu pandemic of 1918. Closing all schools, churches, businesses, and public gathering places, health commissioner Dr. Max C. Starkloff secured a death rate of half that of other major cities. (American Red Cross)

In 1918, there was no treatment for flu. People resorted to a variety of mixtures, tonics, or herbs. Other "treatments" included rolling in the snow, hot baths, or inebriation with alcohol. In Great Britain, authorities asked factories to "fumigate" the air with industrial smoke (Semiatin, 2012). Today, public health officials recommend three (more effective, less harmful) steps to flu prevention and treatment: (1) vaccinate, (2) stop germs, and (3) treat with antiviral medicine. The Centers for Disease Control and Prevention (CDC) recommends that everyone should get the flu vaccine every year and especially high-risk populations of young children (older than six months), pregnant women, people with chronic illnesses, adults over the age of 65, and health care staff (CDC, 2016). The vaccine should not be used in infants under six months. People with severe allergies to eggs or other vaccine ingredients should only get the vaccine under strict medical supervision. Flu vaccinations are manufactured to protect against specific strains of the virus. The seasonal flu vaccine protects against viruses that are predicted to strike in the upcoming year. Trivalent flu vaccines protect against influenza A (H1N1) virus, influenza A (H3N2) virus, and influenza B virus. Vaccinations work on two levels. They protect the individual from illness, and they prevent the microorganism from spreading within a community. When the flu vaccine matches the strain of virus presenting in the community, vaccination reduces flu-related doctors' visits by 50–60 percent (CDC, 2016). When 80–90 percent of people in a community are vaccinated, it is much harder for a pathogen to find susceptible hosts. In this way, vaccines also protect children and adults who are unable to get the vaccine. To prevent the spread of influenza, *Healthy People 2020* recommends that 70 percent of children and adults and 90 percent of health care professionals obtain the seasonal flu vaccine. During the early part of the 2016 flu season, 40 percent of children and adults and 69 percent of health care professionals obtained the flu vaccine (CDC, 2016). Thus, there is a need to increase flu vaccination rates among all people.

Basic infection control practices can reduce susceptibility to infectious diseases and prevent transmission to friends, family members, or coworkers. To prevent flu outbreaks, the CDC (2016) recommends:

1. *Optimize immunity:* Create a strong immune system through regular physical activity, nutritious diet, and stress reduction activities.
2. *Limit exposure:* Prevent infection by avoiding contact with people who are coughing, sneezing, or have a fever. Disinfect your work spaces at school or the office. Use good handwashing techniques and avoid touching your eyes, nose, or mouth.
3. *Protect others:* When you are sick, stay home from work, school, and other public spaces. Get plenty of rest, stay hydrated, and eat healthy foods. Cover your mouth and nose with a tissue when coughing or sneezing, use good handwashing techniques, and disinfect your living or working spaces to avoid contaminating others.

These simple methods can effectively break the transmission of a pathogen from one person to another and stop flu epidemics.

Antiviral drugs are prescription drugs used to treat people with the flu. The medicine works by binding to the neuraminidase protein of the flu virus and preventing replication. For best results, treatment should start within the first two days (36–48 hours) of infection. When used as prescribed, antivirals can lessen the symptoms of the flu, shorten illness by one to two days, and/or reduce complications. As with any prescription drug, antiviral medications can have adverse side effects and should only be used under medical supervision.

The influenza virus has the potential to disable schools, workplaces, communities, and nations. And yet, it can be stopped with simple techniques of vaccination, good hygiene, and early, effective treatment. Public health efforts to prevent this annual scourge focus on increasing vaccination rates, protecting at-risk populations, and early detection.

Sally Kuykendall

See also: Epidemic; Epidemiology; Handwashing; Infectious Diseases; Koch, Heinrich Hermann Robert

Further Reading

Auerbach, M. P. (2014). An army physician on the 1918 flu pandemic. *Defining Documents: World War I*, 267–269.
Carroll, A. (2013). An Alaskan village holds the key to understanding the 1918 Spanish flu. *American History*, *48*(4), 29–30.
Centers for Disease Control and Prevention (CDC). (2016). *Seasonal influenza: Flu basics.* Retrieved from https://www.cdc.gov/flu/about/disease/index.htm.
Morens, D. M., & Taubenberger, J. K. (2015). Historical review. A forgotten epidemic that changed medicine: Measles in the US Army, 1917–18. *The Lancet Infectious Diseases*, *15*, 852–861. doi:10.1016/S1473-3099(15)00109-7
Oxford, J. S., Sefton, A., Jackson, R., Innes, W., Daniels, R. S., & Johnson, N. S. (2002). World War I may have allowed the emergence of "Spanish" influenza. *The Lancet Infectious Diseases*, *2*(2), 111–114.
Semiatin, S. (2012). The great flu pandemic of 1918. *History Magazine*, *14*(2), 31–33.
Soper, G. A. (1918). The influenza pneumonia pandemic in the American army camps during September and October. *Science*, *48*(1245), 451–456.

INJURIES

Injuries are a category of health issues characterized by damage to the body caused by an external force or forces. Injuries are the leading cause of death among young people and create huge economic, social, and emotional burdens. More than 199,000 people die annually due to injuries, the equivalent of one person every three minutes (National Center for Injury Prevention and Control [NCIPC], 2016). In 2013, injuries cost an estimated $671 billion (NCIPC, 2016). The most common injuries are prescription drug overdoses, falls, motor vehicle crashes, traumatic brain injury, child abuse and neglect, and violence. In the past, injuries were referred to as accidents. The term "accident" is misleading because it infers that health-related incidents occur by random and are unavoidable. When someone gets drunk and gets behind the wheel of an automobile, the resulting crash is not an accident. When a child finds a loaded, unlocked gun, the subsequent shooting is not an accident. And when a worker fails to follow instructions on Material Safety Data sheets, chemical burns are not an accident. Injuries are not random and are easily prevented. In public health, injuries are classified as intentional or unintentional. Intentional injuries are violence-related. Physical and emotional harm caused by child abuse and neglect, youth violence, intimate partner violence, sexual violence, and self-directed violence are intentional injuries. Unintentional injuries include prescription drug overdose, falls, motor vehicle crashes, and traumatic brain injuries. Grouping injuries into categories enhances prevention efforts and may impact several health issues simultaneously. For example, alcohol and substance abuse increases risk of both intentional and unintentional injuries. Policies and education on substance abuse decreases homicides, suicides, intimate partner violence, child abuse, motor vehicle crashes, workplace injuries, and falls.

The causes of injuries and potential prevention mechanisms may be understood through physics. When kinetic, thermal, chemical, electrical, or radiation energy exceeds the threshold of body defenses, injury is likely to result. Kinetic energy is the energy created by motion. A car moving at 15 mph has less kinetic energy than a car moving at 100 mph. The faster a car moves, the harder it is to stop and the greater the risk of injury to pedestrians, the driver, and passengers. Speed limits control kinetic energy, thereby reducing injuries. Thermal energy is energy from heat. Burns from hot food or drinks or frostbite are examples of thermal injuries. To protect customers from scalds and still ensure a satisfactory product, scientists recommend that restaurants serve coffee, tea, or other hot drinks at 136°F or 57.8°C (Brown & Diller, 2008). Chemical injuries occur when chemicals are ingested, injected, inhaled, or come in contact with the body at the level where toxicity or impaired body function occurs. Examples include carbon monoxide poisoning, heroin overdose, or corrosive burns due to high acid or alkali content. Poison control centers provide free emergency information and prevention materials to avoid household poisonings. Electrical injuries are caused by electrical shock from a high-voltage or low-voltage source and can result in tingling, burn, respiratory paralysis, or cardiac shock. Electrical safety standards of the Occupational Safety and Health Administration (OSHA) are designed to protect electricians, engineers, and other workers from electrical shock, electrocution, fires, and explosions. Although the majority of exposures are acute and may be cared for at home, repeated exposure can lead to chronic health problems. For example, jolts to the head after a concussion may lead to more severe brain injury; ongoing exposure to asbestos can lead to lung cancer, mesothelioma, or asbestosis; and repeated exposure to sunlight may lead to skin cancer.

Public health addresses injuries through systematic approaches using surveillance, identifying risk and protective factors, developing and evaluating strategies, and encouraging widespread adoption of evidence-based programs. Applying the example of falls, surveillance indicates that 2.8 million people are treated in the emergency room every year due to falls (CDC, NCIPC, Division of Unintentional Injury Prevention, 2016). Elderly people are at highest risk. One out of four elderly people will experience a fall each year. The program STEADI (Stopping Elderly Accidents, Deaths, and Injuries) was developed to prevent falls in the elderly. STEADI provides resources for patients and their health care providers to evaluate individual risk of falling and potential for injury. Interventions include the following: reviewing medications to see whether prescribed medications cause dizziness or sleepiness; regular eye exams, keeping eyeglass prescriptions up to date; regular exercises to increase strength and balance; calcium and vitamin D supplements to strengthen bones and reduce the risk of fracture if a fall does occur; and removing home hazards, such as loose rugs or uneven pavement, and installing handrails or extra lighting. The cost of an evidence-based prevention program such as STEADI is minimal in comparison to the $31 billion currently spent on annual medical costs due to falls.

Injuries are one of the most pressing public health concerns of the nation. Current prevention efforts employ policies, laws, education, engineering, and science at the federal, state, and local levels. Efforts have been highly successful in improving community and occupational health. Between 1925 and 1997, advances in road and vehicle safety decreased motor vehicle fatalities from 18 per 100 million vehicle miles traveled (VMT) to 1.7 per 100 million VMT (Centers for Disease Control and Prevention [CDC], 1999a). Occupational safety and health policy and programs decreased unintentional work-related fatalities from 37 per 100,000 workers in 1933 to 4 fatalities per 100,000 workers in 1997 (CDC, 1999b). Through collaborative efforts, the Centers for Disease Control National Center for Injury Prevention and Control, public health professionals, National Highway Traffic Safety Administration (NHTSA), National Institute of Occupational Safety and Health (NIOSH), businesses, workplaces, schools, communities, hospitals, and many other organizations are working to further reduce the physical, emotional, social, and financial burden of injuries through research, education, and practice.

Sally Kuykendall

See also: Aging; Agricultural Safety; Centers for Disease Control and Prevention; Child Maltreatment; Elder Maltreatment; Epidemiology; Healthy Places; Home Safety; Infant Mortality; Intimate Partner Violence; Kelley, Florence; Men's Health; Middle Ages, Public Health in the; Motor Vehicle Safety; National Center for Injury Prevention and Control; Prevention; Sports-Related Concussions; Violence

Further Reading

Brown, F., & Diller, K. R. (2008). Calculating the optimum temperature for serving hot beverages. *Burns, 34*, 648–654. doi:10.1016/j.burns.2007.09.012

Centers for Disease Control and Prevention. (1999a). Achievements in public health, 1990–1999 motor vehicle safety: A 20th century public health achievement. *Morbidity and Mortality Weekly Reports, 48*(18), 369–374. Retrieved from https://www.cdc.gov/mmwr/preview/mmwrhtml/mm4818a1.htm.

Centers for Disease Control and Prevention. (1999b). Achievements in public health, 1990–1999: Improvements in workplace safety—United States, 1990–1999. *Morbidity and Mortality Weekly Reports, 48*(22), 461–469. Retrieved from https://www.cdc.gov/mmwr/preview/mmwrhtml/mm4822a1.htm.

Centers for Disease Control and Prevention, National Center for Injury Prevention and Control, Division of Unintentional Injury Prevention. (2016). *Important facts about falls.* Retrieved from http://www.cdc.gov/HomeandRecreationalSafety/Falls/adultfalls.html.

National Center for Injury Prevention and Control. (2015). *CDC Injury Center research priorities.* Atlanta: U.S. Department of Health and Human Services, Centers for Disease

Control and Prevention. Retrieved from http://www.cdc.gov/injury/pdfs/researchpriorities/cdc-injury-research-priorities.pdf.

National Center for Injury Prevention and Control. (2016). *Cost of injuries and violence in the United States*. Atlanta: U.S. Department of Health and Human Services, Centers for Disease Control and Prevention. Retrieved from http://www.cdc.gov/injury/wisqars/overview/cost_of_injury.html.

INTERVENTION

An intervention, typically a health program, is a systematically planned effort or set of activities intended to bring about a health improvement to a specific community or population. Interventions are developed to address a need that was formally identified by a needs assessment. The vast majority of interventions aim at changing three major factors that affect health: knowledge, attitudes, and behavior (Gilbert, Sawyer, & McNeil, 2011). The population targeted by an intervention differs based on the need being addressed, and may include, among others, neighborhood residents, organization directors or staff members, community leaders, or policy makers. By influencing the people and factors that impact health, the intervention can improve the long-term wellness of a population. There is a plethora of intervention strategies, such as media campaigns or public service announcements, conveying health information, modifying public policy, restructuring how organizations operate, and creating partnerships between organizations. Interventions can vary widely; they can use any of these strategies independently or several strategies in combination. For example, an intervention to prevent skin cancer might consist of a poster explaining the negative consequences of direct sun exposure or a program that offers free skin cancer screenings in local community centers.

There are many examples of interventions throughout the history of public health. One landmark example is that of Dr. John Snow in London, England. During the mid-1800s, Snow observed that many individuals were suffering from cholera, an intestinal disease that can result in death. Those who were most affected lived in Soho, an area of the West End of London. On investigation, Snow believed that contaminated drinking water may have caused many of the cholera-related deaths. At that time, sewage was disposed of in the Thames River. Water from the river mixed with water in nearby communal wells, which was the source of water for most local townspeople. Snow recommended that the pumps of contaminated wells be removed to prevent individuals from drawing up the water. Once implemented, the number of cholera-related deaths decreased dramatically. The action by Snow to eliminate hand pumps was considered an intervention. He changed the way individuals could obtain clean drinking water and successfully reduced deaths and improved the health of Londoners. Other examples of public health interventions throughout history include the widespread addition of fluoride into public drinking water to prevent tooth decay and anti-smoking laws that prohibit indoor smoking to prevent the negative consequences of secondhand and side stream smoking.

There are four main phases in public health interventions: assessment, planning, implementation, and evaluation (Bartholomew, Parcel, Kok, Gottlieb, & Fernandez, 2011). In the assessment phase, project collaborators perform needs and assets assessments. The needs assessment identifies the specific health problem that needs to be addressed, the number of people impacted by the issue, and the short- and long-term impact of the problem on individuals and the community. During the planning phase, key stakeholders decide which program or actions may be most effective for the people or community experiencing the health issue. The program planners may obtain existing program materials or design a new intervention. Planning requires a great deal of time and consideration. Multiple factors must be taken into consideration, such as competing priorities, engaging key stakeholders and participants, and securing resources. Implementation is the time period when the program activities are delivered. The program evaluation involves assessing the activities that were delivered and the outcomes, or changes, the intervention sought to achieve. Although the components seem to appear in chronological order, all of the components occur as ongoing and iterative processes. For example, if participant attendance is low during implementation, program planners may need to adjust the original implementation plans.

Thoughtful planning is critical to the success of an intervention. Planning begins with selecting a program-planning model, theory, or evidence-based practice that will guide the intervention. There are a wide variety of systematic program planning models and frameworks available to develop health interventions. In many of these models, a systems thinking approach, such as the social ecological model, is utilized to provide a big picture view of the issue. That is, the health of individuals is impacted by various factors, such as their knowledge and beliefs, their family and friends, their community, and state and federal laws. Interventions are most successful when they target the modifiable factors that influence health. For example, an intervention that changes people's attitudes, knowledge, and behavior toward using sunscreen is more feasible, and will be more successful, than an intervention that creates a law requiring individuals to wear sunscreen when outdoors. Other important tasks in the planning phase are identifying key stakeholders, creating a working group, developing goals and objectives, and identifying safe, convenient, and appropriate locations for program implementation.

Public health interventions are most effective when they are based on a recognized model or theory. Theories help explain why people do or do not become involved in particular health-related behaviors and the most effective ways to modify health behaviors. Evidence-based practices are those techniques that have proven to be effective through empirical research and evaluation. For example, if previous research suggests that training lifeguards is effective at reaching and educating members of a community about skin cancer, then it would be considered an evidence-based practice. Thus, training and employing lifeguards could be used in the development of other beach and pool based interventions, as it has been proven to work. Evidence-based practices and programs tend to be more effective than programs not based on scientific theory.

Interventions that are developed using a framework and informed by theories and evidence-based practices are more successful at achieving their stated outcomes. The logic model is one of the most common ways to organize information and plan an intervention. The logic model is a visual representation of the intervention that outlines the connections between the underlying public health theory and specific components of the intervention. For example, one widely used theory in intervention planning is the health belief model, which describes why people may or may not engage in certain health-related behaviors. Such an understanding would help a public health practitioner to understand the problem better and devise solutions accordingly as part of the intervention. One construct of the health belief model is *perceived susceptibility*. Perceived susceptibility describes how much individuals believe they are at risk of a condition. If individuals do not believe they are at risk for skin cancer, then they may not use sunscreen when at the beach or pool. Thus, they have low perceived susceptibility of skin cancer. Using the health belief model, the interventionist might aim to increase perceived susceptibility by designing messages and materials to increase awareness of risk factors for skin cancer. The logic model draws the link between perceived susceptibility and health education to increase awareness of the risk factors of skin cancer.

The third phase of conducting an intervention is the implementation phase. In the implementation phase, those who will be delivering the intervention are trained and instructed on the curriculum or protocols. Participants are recruited from the target community, and the intervention is delivered to the participants. Leading or administering an intervention requires a fine balance between staying true to the original program design and customizing the intervention to meet the needs of the participants. The program coordinator must make sure that the intervention meets the needs of the participants and must also work to achieve buy-in of the participants and key stakeholders. Multiple demands on people's time can interfere with attendance and participation. To ensure that interventions are implemented in the way that they were meant to be implemented, fidelity of implementation may be measured. Fidelity of implementation measures how faithful the intervention is to the original program design.

The final phase of performing an intervention is to conduct an evaluation. There are two types of evaluations, process evaluation, which assesses how well the intervention was delivered, and outcome evaluation, which measures how well the intervention achieved its intended objectives. The process evaluation is an ongoing assessment that occurs *during* the implementation of the intervention and measures how many people are interacting with the intervention and whether people find the materials helpful. The final outcome evaluation is conducted *after* the intervention has been delivered and measures if and how participants' knowledge, attitudes, or behaviors changed after the intervention. The evaluations' results inform decisions about modifying the current health program or developing future health interventions.

The gold standard for evaluation is a randomized controlled trial design. That is, there is one group of individuals who receives the intervention, known as the intervention group, and one group who does not, known as the control group. By using such a design, the public health practitioner can compare the two groups and effectively understand if observed outcomes were a result of the intervention or simply by chance. For example, an intervention that aims to decrease skin cancer within a community distributes brochures about safe sun practices and free bottles of sunscreen to individuals at one community pool (intervention group), but not to others at another pool within the same community (control group). If a comparison between the two groups shows that those in the intervention group engaged in more safe sun practices than those in the control group, then it could suggest the intervention was successful. However, if the comparison between the two groups does not reveal such findings, then it could suggest the intervention was not successful. Though the randomized controlled trial is usually the gold standard, in many other instances it may be unethical to deny a group of individuals access to a program that could help them; thus, other implementation designs can be used.

Public health interventions are programs and practices designed to improve the knowledge, attitudes, or behaviors of individuals or groups of individuals in order to improve health and well-being. Interventions are planned and designed by public health professionals, and they are based on scientific theory and practices. Implementation requires sensitivity to the needs of the target population and understanding of the core program components. The most effective interventions are evidence-based programs and practices, which have been studied and proven to work in various communities.

Noora F. Majid and Nadav Antebi-Gruszka

See also: Cholera; Community Organizing; Evaluation; Emergency Preparedness and Response; Evidence-Based Programs and Practices; Fluoridation; Health Education; Logic Model; Needs Assessment; Prevention; RE-AIM (Reach, Effectiveness, Adoption, Implementation, and Maintenance); Risk-Benefit Analysis; Snow, John; Social Ecological Model; Syringe Service Programs; Transtheoretical Model

Further Reading

Bartholomew, L. K., Parcel, G. S., Kok, G., Gottlieb, N. H., & Fernandez, M. E. (2011). *Planning health promotion programs: An intervention mapping approach.* San Francisco: Jossey-Bass.

Centers for Disease Control and Prevention. (2014, February 4). *Assessment and planning models, frameworks and tools.* Retrieved from http://www.cdc.gov/stltpublichealth/cha/assessment.html.

Community Preventive Services Task Force. (2015, March 5). *The community guide, what works to promote health: Plan an intervention.* Retrieved from http://www.thecommunityguide.org/toolbox/plan-an-intervention.html.

Gilbert, G. G., Sawyer, R. G., & McNeil, E. B. (2011). *Health education: Creating strategies for school and community health.* Sudbury, MA: Jones & Bartlett.

INTIMATE PARTNER VIOLENCE (IPV)

Intimate partner violence (IPV) is a serious, preventable health problem, defined as "any behavior within an intimate relationship or former relationship that causes physical, psychological, or sexual harm" (Feder, 2016). Such harm includes:

- Physical aggression, such as hitting, kicking, and beating.
- Psychological violence, such as intimidation and humiliation.
- Controlling behaviors, such as isolation from family and friends, monitoring of movements, and controlling finances.
- Sexual violence, such as forced intercourse.

The term is often used synonymously with domestic violence (DV). Differences are that DV refers to acts of violence committed by any family member, including intimate partners (Garcia-Moreno et al., 2012) whereas IPV occurs among heterosexual or same-sex couples with or without sexual intimacy (Feder, 2016). More than 32 million men and women experience IPV in the United States. Females who report IPV at least once in their lifetime have three to four times more emotional distress, suicidal thoughts, and suicide attempts than nonabused women (Ellsberg et al., 2008).

American attitudes toward violence against women (VAW) originated from England where women were traditionally viewed as personal property of the husband. Most legal and social structures established prior to the 19th century supported IPV against wives as a right of the husband. During the mid-1800s, social views began to change. By 1871, Alabama and Massachusetts prohibited IPV. In 1878, England passed the Matrimonial Causes Act giving both women and men the right to legal separation, custody of their children, and earnings from the separation in cases of cruelty, desertion, or adultery. As female empowerment grew through feminism, so did recognition of IPV as a health issue. Today, cases of IPV have captured widespread media attention, increasing awareness of the issue as a public health problem.

IPV affects people of all ages, socioeconomic classes, ethnicities, gender identities, and sexual preferences. The World Health Organization (WHO) surveyed 24,097 women in 10 countries about experiences with physical and sexual IPV. Lifetime prevalence ranged from 15 to 75 percent and in 6 of 15 study sites, prevalence was 50 percent or greater (WHO, 2013). Physical violence was the most common form, and 30 to 56 percent of women experienced both physical and sexual violence. In reviewing homicide data from 66 countries, researchers found that 39 percent of female homicides and 6 percent of male homicides were committed by an intimate partner (Feder, 2016; Stöckl et al., 2013). IPV is the second leading cause of homicide for women in the workplace (Tiesman, Konda, & Amandus, 2012). Victims can change their telephone number, address, and appearances. It is harder to change one's workplace. Data show that IPV is a pandemic problem. Furthermore, only about one out of five female sexual assault victims, one out of four physical assault victims, and one of two stalking victims report the aggression; male victims are even less likely to report (Tjaden & Thoennes, 2000). Reasons for nonreporting originate from outdated attitudes and legal systems that viewed female partners as property to be mistreated at will. Public service announcements and media campaigns are working to change attitudes toward IPV and increase victim willingness to report. The next steps are to incorporate strategies to prevent and respond to IPV within workplace safety programs.

A combination of individual, relationship, community, and societal factors are associated with victimization and perpetration; however, they are not in themselves causes of IPV (Heise & Garcia-Moreno, 2002). Individual factors for victimization include young age (less than 24 years), heavy drinking, depression, low academic achievement, low income, and exposure to violence in childhood. Relationship factors are poor family functioning, marital instability, male dominance, and economic stress. Community factors are weak sanctions against violence, poverty, and economic inequality. Societal factors include rigid gender norms and positive attitudes toward violence (Abramsky et al., 2011; Feder, 2016). Risk factors for perpetration include exposure to childhood violence, unresolved post-traumatic stress disorder, recent job loss, and substance abuse (Renner & Whitney, 2012). Childhood history of maltreatment is a risk factor for both victimization and perpetration. Although it is important to be aware of risk factors in order to identify those at risk, a growing number of public health and medical professionals routinely screen for IPV during the history and physical exam.

Patients typically do not present with the chief complaint of IPV. Instead, practitioners might notice a history of multiple injuries, injuries that are not consistent with the patient's explanation, or delays in seeking medical care (Feder, 2016). The most common injuries related to IPV are trauma to the head, face, neck, teeth, or genital area. Victims also present with musculoskeletal injuries, sprains, fractures, or dislocations. Injuries often reflect the mode of attack, with marks suggesting strangulation, or hitting by a hand or household object. Use of a knife or gun is comparatively less common (Feder, 2016). Many victims have no signs of obvious trauma and instead present with chronic somatic complaints of headache or backache, or nonspecific complaints of difficulty with daily activities, memory loss, or dizziness (Ellsberg et al., 2008). Irritable bowel syndrome, fibromyalgia, and various chronic pain syndromes are commonly associated with victimization (Heise & Garcia-Moreno, 2002). Victims of sexual violence suffer from a range of sexual and reproductive health effects, including unintended pregnancy, abortion, sexually transmitted infections, and sexual dysfunction. Psychosocial problems, such as difficulty in negotiating contraceptive or condom use with a partner, can be harder to identify but are important health consequences that demand consideration (Garcia-Moreno et al., 2012). Violence will often escalate with the stress of pregnancy or childbirth, and violence against pregnant women is of particular significance due to the risk of harm to both mother and fetus. Patterns of injury during pregnancy tend to be more central, such as blunt trauma to the head, torso, abdomen, breasts, and genitalia (Feder, 2016). Miscarriage, late entry into prenatal care, perinatal death, and preterm labor and birth are associated with IPV (Garcia-Moreno et al., 2012). The effects of abuse do not end when the abuse ends. Abused women are twice as likely as nonabused women to self-report poor health and physical and mental health problems, even if the violence occurred years before (Garcia-Moreno et al., 2012). Children in families with IPV also exhibit symptoms, regardless of whether they are also victims of violence. Children of abused mothers exhibit significantly more internalizing, externalizing, and total behavioral problems than children of nonabused mothers. When a patient presents with unexplained injuries or nonspecific complaints, health care practitioners will first rule out medical causes.

Without realizing it, the victim is caught up in a controlling cycle of abuse, consisting of romance, tension building, and abuse and returning to romance. In the romance or honeymoon phase, the partner is attentive and charming. As life's struggles and difficulties overwhelm, the abuser views the victim as either the cause of the problem or an acceptable scapegoat. The batterer responds to tensions with physical, verbal, sexual, or emotional violence directed at the victim. After an abusive incident, the batterer will blame the victim, apologize, try to console the victim with promises or gifts, or pretend that the abuse never happened. The romance phase confuses the victim into thinking that the abuse never happened, was somehow his or her fault, or was simply a one-off occurrence. The romance phase also confuses friends and family members who question the victim's judgment of the situation. The cycle is difficult to break for reasons mentioned previously. Through childhood experiences, the victim may have a distorted view of relationships, not knowing or understanding respect between partners. Rigid gender norms, lack of economic opportunity, and disparities in earning potential motivate female partners to stay with male abusers, especially when children are involved. Internally, the victim believes that the partner regrets the abuse and intends to change. The health care practitioner must respond to suspected IPV in ways that protect and support the victim. Recognizing that the victim may not be prepared to make major life changes by leaving the relationship, public health professionals can refer the victim to a hotline or onsite domestic violence counselor who can provide practical safety tips to de-escalate the violence and protect the victim. Numerous programs exist for both batterers and victims.

Given the long-lasting and detrimental effects of intimate partner violence, increased efforts toward prevention are under way. Active screening in clinical settings contributes to greater identification of victims. The national hotline is available for victims in the United States (http://www.thehotline.org/). Multiple organizations and coalitions, such as the Battered Women's Justice Project, Child Welfare League of America, National Coalition Against Domestic Violence, Institute of Domestic Violence in African American Communities, and women's shelters are focused on combating IPV through awareness, prevention, and victim support. An effective approach toward alleviating the public health burden of intimate partner violence requires continued collaboration of individuals, communities, and institutions as well as changes in social norms.

Nooshin Asadpour and Maria DiGiorgio McColgan

See also: Adverse Childhood Experiences; Child Maltreatment; Children's Health; Family Planning; Injuries; Lesbian, Gay, Bisexual, and Transgender Health; Maternal Health; Violence; Women's Health

Further Reading

Abramsky, T., Watts, C. H., Garcia-Moreno, C., Devries, K., Kiss, L., Ellsberg, M., & . . . Heise, L. (2011). What factors are associated with recent intimate partner violence? Findings from the WHO multi-country study on women's health and domestic violence. *BMC Public Health, 11*(1), 109–125.

Battered Women's Justice Project. (2017). Retrieved from http://www.bwjp.org.

Dobash, R., & Dobash, R. (1992). *Women, violence & social change.* New York: Routledge.

Ellsberg, M., Jansen, H. M., Heise, L., Watts, C. H., & García-Moreno, C. (2008). Intimate partner violence and women's physical and mental health in the WHO multi-country study on women's health and domestic violence: An observational study. *The Lancet, 371*(9619), 1165–1172.

Feder, G. (2016). Beyond identification of patients experiencing intimate partner violence. *American Family Physician, 94*(8), 600.

Feder, G., & Macmillan, H. (2012). 249: Intimate partner violence. *Goldman's Cecil Medicine*, 1571–1574.

Feder, G., Wathen, C. N., & MacMillan, H. L. (2013). An evidence-based response to intimate partner violence: WHO guidelines. *Journal of the American Medical Association, 310*(5), 479–480.

Garcia-Moreno, C., Guedes, A., & Knerr, W. (2012). *Understanding and addressing violence against women: Intimate partner violence.* World Health Organization.

Heise, L., & Garcia-Moreno, C. (2002). Violence by intimate partners. In E. G. Krug, L. L. Dahlberg, J. A. Mercy, A. B. Zwi, & R. Lozano (Eds.), *World report on violence and health* (pp. 87–121). Geneva: World Health Organization.

National Domestic Violence Hotline. (2017). Retrieved from http://www.thehotline.org and 1.800.799.SAFE (7233).

Renner, L. M., & Whitney, S. D. (2012). Risk factors for unidirectional and bidirectional intimate partner violence among young adults. *Child Abuse & Neglect*, *36*, 40–52.

Stöckl, H., Devries, K., Rotstein, A., Abrahams, N., Campbell, J., Watts, C., & Moreno, C. G. (2013). The global prevalence of intimate partner homicide: A systematic review. *The Lancet*, *38*(2), 859–865.

Tiesman, H. M., Konda, S., & Amandus, H. E. (2012). Workplace homicides among U.S. women: The role of intimate partner violence. *Annals of Epidemiology*, *22*(4), 277–284.

Tjaden, P. G., & Thoennes, N. (2000). *Extent, nature, and consequences of intimate partner violence*. Washington, DC: U.S. Department of Justice, Office of Justice Programs, National Institute of Justice.

World Health Organization. (2013). *Responding to intimate partner violence and sexual violence against women: WHO clinical and policy guidelines*. Retrieved from http://apps.who.int/iris/bitstream/10665/85240/1/9789241548595_eng.pdf.

J

JENNER, EDWARD (1749–1823)

Edward Jenner was a British physician and ornithologist (a person who studies birds) who lived in the late 18th and early 19th centuries. Jenner contributed to the field of natural history and human medicine, and he was a noted philanthropist and promoter of public health initiatives. He is best remembered for his pioneering work in the discovery and propagation of the smallpox vaccination.

Jenner was born in 1749, the eighth son of the Reverend Steven Jenner, in the predominantly rural area of Berkeley, Gloucestershire, in England. Reverend Jenner's prominent position in the community allowed Edward to pursue a classical education. At the age of 14, Edward began an apprenticeship with a local surgeon that lasted seven years. In 1770, he continued his studies under the Scottish surgeon John Hunter (1728–1793), who during his tenure at London's St. George's Hospital advocated the use of observation and scientific method in medicine. In 1773, Jenner returned to his native Berkeley where he established a successful medical practice.

Jenner was a respected pillar of his local community. He helped establish scientific societies such as the Fleece Medical Society or Gloucestershire Medical Society. In 1788 he was elected to the prestigious Royal Society for his work on the nested cuckoo. Through diligent observation and dissection he challenged the long-held belief that the adult cuckoo pushed the eggs and hatchlings of its host from the nest, demonstrating that it was the newly hatched cuckoo instead.

Shortly after his election into the Royal Society, in 1792 Jenner completed his medical studies and received his doctorate from the distinguished medical faculty of the University of St. Andrews in Scotland. His work centered on *Angina pectoris,* or chest pain related to obstruction or spasm of the arteries around the heart.

Jenner was not the first to discover an immunological connection between the benign bovine disease of cowpox and the immunity of milkmaids to deadly smallpox. Observers throughout Europe suggested the idea as early as the 1760s but with few tangible results. On May 14, 1796, Jenner took scrapings from cowpox blisters on the hand of Sarah Nelmes, a milkmaid, and inoculated an eight-year-old boy named James Phipps. Later, when exposed to smallpox, the child did not catch the disease. After subsequent experimentation, Jenner reported to the Royal Society the immunological importance of vaccination.

By 1803 the combined efforts of doctors and governments witnessed the increase of vaccination throughout Europe and the world. That year Jenner became president of the Jennerian Society, the purpose of which was to promote the eradication

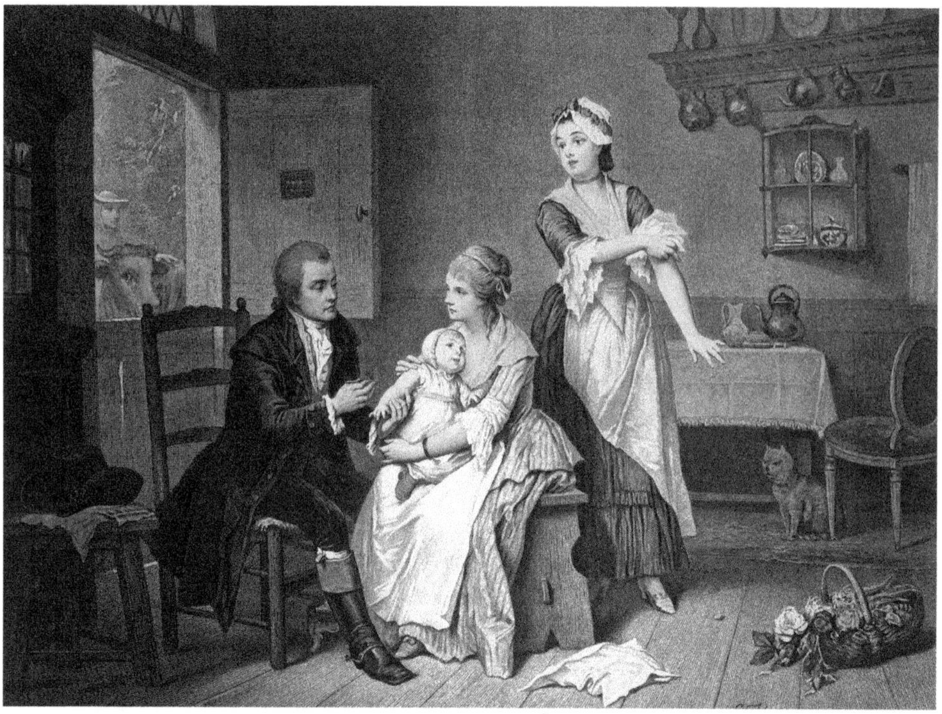

Dr. Edward Jenner transfers cowpox virus from dairymaid to young patient. Jenner carefully studied and tested his hypothesis that inoculation with weaker viral material protects against deadly infectious disease. (Wellcome Collection)

of smallpox through vaccination. The society was dissolved in 1809 and replaced by the National Vaccine Establishment, whose conflicts in leadership convinced Jenner to return to his practice in Berkeley.

Jenner was instrumental in the creation of the Medical and Chiurgical Society of London, which became the Royal Society of Medicine. King George IV granted him the honorary post of physician extraordinary in 1821. The remainder of Jenner's life was dedicated to further work in ornithology before his death from stroke complications at the age of 73 in 1823.

Sean P. Phillips

See also: Bioterrorism; Infectious Diseases; Prevention; Smallpox; Vaccines

Further Reading

Bazin, H. (2000). *The eradication of smallpox: Edward Jenner and the first and only eradication of a human infectious disease.* London: Academic Press.

Dawtrey Drewitt, F. (2013). *The life of Edward Jenner M.D., F.R.S.: Naturalist, and discoverer of vaccination.* Cambridge, UK: Cambridge University Press.

Riedel, S. (2005). Edward Jenner and the history of smallpox and vaccination. *Proceedings (Baylor University, Medical Center)*, *18*(1), 21–25.

K

KELLEY, FLORENCE (1859–1932)

Florence Kelley was a social reformer of the Progressive Era who studied and documented the living and working conditions of America's poor and immigrant men, women, and children. Her political strategy was to "investigate, educate, legislate, and enforce." Initially, Kelley worked with politicians to legislate protections for women and children in the workplace. When these efforts failed, she encouraged civic leaders and consumers to use their economic power to create and maintain protections against abuse. Kelley was instrumental in developing the 1921 Sheppard-Towner Maternity and Infancy Protection Act, the first law that allocated federal funds for health care. Some of the most important occupational health and safety laws today are the result of Kelley's tenacious efforts.

Florence Kelley was born on September 12, 1859, to Caroline Bartram-Bonsall and William Durrah Kelley. Mr. Kelley was a powerful member of the Philadelphia community. He served as a judge, 15-term congressman, founding member of the Republican Party, and friend of President Abraham Lincoln. Religiously and politically, he was a Quaker with a deep commitment to the abolition movement and the rights of African Americans. Florence's great-aunt, Sarah Pugh, was also a social reformer. Pugh founded the Philadelphia Female Anti-Slavery Society (PFASS) and promoted the boycott of sugar and cotton, goods made by slave labor. The PFASS lobbied for emancipation, supported the Underground Railroad, and started a school for African Americans. As a young girl, Florence's father taught her to read using a book that described the horrific working conditions of children. Within a few years, she read her father's entire library. Through her young eyes, she started to notice injustices and atrocities that even the adults failed to see. Florence recalled joining her father on late night tours of Pennsylvania's steel mills and glass factories. While her father was awestruck by the sight of huge, bright, burning cauldrons and loud, massive machines, Florence was horrified by young boys working in dangerous jobs in dark, dirty, and hot factories. Kelley recalled "the utter unimportance of children compared with products, in the minds of the people whom I am among" (Child labor reforms and the National Child Labor Committee, n.d., p. 24)

In 1882, Florence graduated from Cornell University where she studied Greek, Latin, algebra, and children and the law. She wrote and published her senior thesis on legal policies affecting children and founded the New Century Guild for Working Women in Philadelphia. She hoped to continue her studies at the University of Pennsylvania but was denied admission because University of Pennsylvania refused to accept females. Instead, she moved to Switzerland to study law at the University of Zurich. Zurich was a refuge for Europe's anarchists, socialists, and political radicals. Here, Florence was introduced to Frederick Engels. Socialism validated Florence's early impressions of the exploitive conditions suffered by the working class. It also opened her eyes to how capitalism pits worker against worker in order to control discourse, the economy, and politics (Clark & Foster, 2006). Florence's translation of Engels's *Condition of the Working Class in England in 1844* provided the English-speaking world with new perspectives on the Industrial Revolution. The book documented the hardships, diseases, and mortality rates of workers in Manchester and Liverpool, England before and during the Industrial Revolution. Problems were not specific to England. Worker oppression by wealthy businessmen was a universal problem in the industrial age. Engels wrote the preface to Kelley's translation, recommending shorter working days, legal limits on overtime for females and children, and breaking up the monopolies that enabled worker abuse.

In 1884, Florence met and married Lazare Wischnewetzky, a Russian-Polish medical student. Within three years, Mrs. Wischnewetzky gave birth to three children. The family moved to New York in 1886. However, Lazare was physically abusive and after five years Florence fled with her children to Hull House in Chicago. Hull House was an organized community founded by Jane Addams to provide social support, education, and cultural opportunities to new immigrants. The settlement attracted many famous social reformers, such as Alice Hamilton, Clarence Darrow, John Dewey, and Julia Lathrop. Florence worked evenings as a librarian and continued using the title "Mrs." so that her children would not be stigmatized as illegitimate. She reverted to her original name of "Kelley."

Chicago was a major gateway between the East and the West, home to thriving railroad, garment, and meatpacking industries. The city attracted new immigrants and free men and women from the southern states, disadvantaged populations who were highly vulnerable to financial abuse. Poorly paid workers and their families lived in slums and suffered high rates of disease. For many years, wealthy business owners hired private henchmen to prevent organized labor. In 1886, workers protested in Haymarket Square. What started as a peaceful rally with workers demonstrating for an eight-hour workday quickly turned into a massacre. Eleven people died after someone threw a bomb and the police opened fire. In 1894, Pullman railroad workers went on strike in response to company cutbacks. Pullman reduced wages and laid off employees without a commensurate reduction in the monthly rent of company housing.

Kelley was interested in the garment industry. Originally, all clothing was made by skilled tailors who sewed individual items from start to finish. The combination of machines and cheap, unskilled labor opened the possibility of manufacturing less expensive clothing using assembly lines. The problem was that machines moved at much higher rates than humans. Workers had to work faster plus endure 10- to 12-hour days without a break in order to keep up with the machines. The factories were hot from the steam driven machines, and the work was repetitive and constant. In order to meet consumer demand for cheap clothing, business owners cut corners. They ran businesses out of converted basements, attics, or homes to avoid paying rent. They crowded as many workers as they could into small quarters, and they demanded long hours from the cheapest labor possible, women and children. The heat from the machines, overcrowding, and cramped and exhausting working conditions created sweatshops where communicable diseases spread easily.

In 1892, Kelley convinced the Illinois Bureau of Labor Statistics to hire her to investigate the garment industry. She discovered three-year-old children working in sweatshops along with exhausted adults, high rates of occupational injuries, workplaces with no bathroom facilities, and areas that doubled as living and working areas. Her reports described horrific working conditions in graphic detail. She escorted politicians and civic leaders on tours so that they could see conditions firsthand. In 1893, Illinois passed legislature that limited women's workday to eight hours, prohibited employment of children under 14 years old, and required a signed work affidavit by parent or guardian for youth aged 14–16. The state hired Kelley as the chief factory inspector. Her efforts were frequently met with obstructionism. At one point, someone tried to shoot her. Angry and frustrated by the political and

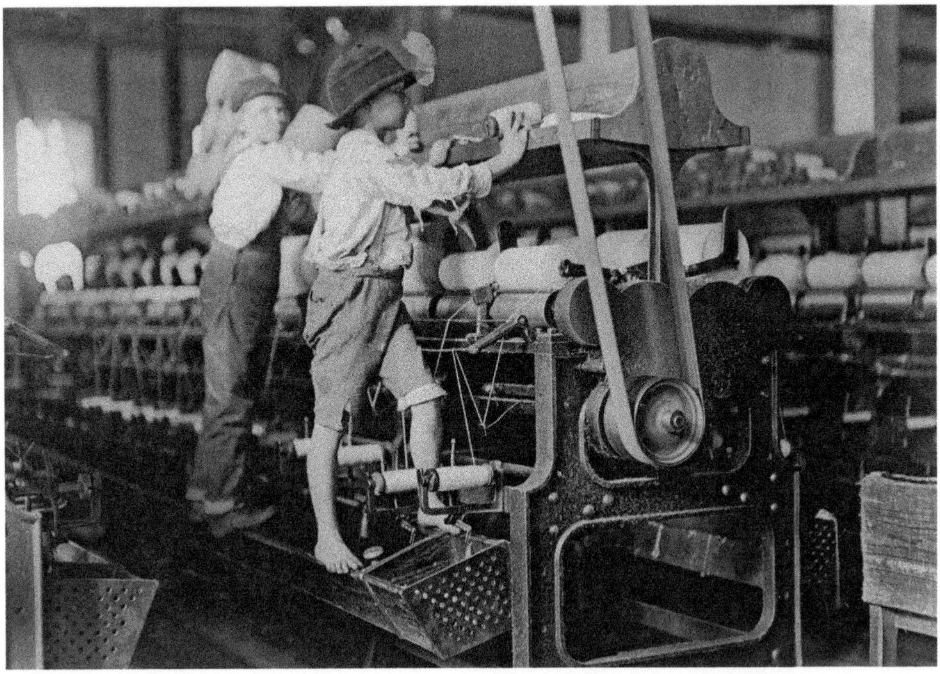

Young children fixing broken threads and empty bobbins on a spinning frame at a textile mill in Macon, Georgia, 1909. To meet consumer demand for inexpensive clothing the garment industry exploited poor and immigrant women and children. Minimum wage and child labor laws were developed to protect Americans from hazardous working conditions. (Library of Congress)

legal system, Kelley took night classes to earn her law degree, and in 1894 she graduated from Northwestern University School of Law. In 1895, the Illinois Supreme Court struck down the eight-hour day ruling as unconstitutional and with a subsequent change in political administration, Kelley was fired as chief inspector.

In 1898, Kelley collaborated with Ellen Henrotin to form the Illinois Consumers' League. The group encouraged women to use their purchasing power to pressure factories into improving working conditions. A year later, she moved to the Henry Street Settlement in New York to develop and manage the National Consumers' League (NCL). The NCL compiled lists of factories that paid living wages, limited workdays to no more than 10 hours per day, did not hire children, and provided safe working conditions. These factories used *white labels,* labels that noted the garment was made in a factory that obeyed state labor laws. Leveraging the economic power of consumers turned out to be a successful ploy. Over the next few years, Kelley helped to establish 64 local consumer leagues and collaborated with labor unions to develop stricter regulations. When a businessman in Oregon challenged the 10-hour workday rule, Kelley worked with Josephine Clara Goldmark to develop the *Brandeis Brief*. The *Brandeis Brief* was a lengthy report that presented health data to highlight the adverse health effects of repetitive tasks and long workdays. The report focused on women's health and used the (outdated) argument that women were weaker than men and therefore needed special protections. Supreme Court Justice Louis Brandeis used the *Brandeis Brief* to support the rights of states to enact laws limiting women's workday. The *Brandeis Brief* is noteworthy because it relied on medical and health data to determine law rather than legal arguments. Based on the information in the report, the Supreme Court determined that Oregon's laws did not violate the constitution.

Throughout the remainder of her life, Kelley continued her efforts advocating for minimum wage laws for women, campaigning against child labor, helping to create the Federal Children's Bureau and the 1921 Sheppard-Towner Maternity and Infancy Protection Act. Her efforts served as the foundation for the 1938 Fair Labor Standards Act and the allocation of federal funds for health care. She also helped organize the National Association for the Advancement of Colored People (NAACP). In her later years, she was criticized for opposing the Equal Rights Amendment (ERA). Kelley believed the ERA would undermine many of women's rights that she had fought so hard to earn.

Florence Kelley grew up in a time when the United States was moving toward a mechanized, consumer-driven society. People who immigrated to the United States came for opportunity and were greeted with poverty, overcrowding, and physically and emotionally abusive working conditions. Women and children were forced to work long hours at low pay to meet consumer demand for cheap clothing. Following her Quaker formation, Kelley was determined to improve the lives of vulnerable populations. Many of the laws on minimum wage and child labor trace back to Kelley.

Sally Kuykendall

See also: Bowditch, Henry Ingersoll; Children's Health; Immigrant Health; *Controversies in Public Health:* Controversy 5

Further Reading

Child labor reforms and the National Child Labor Committee. (n.d.). Retrieved from https://www.upress.pitt.edu/htmlSourceFiles/pdfs/9780822943778exr.pdf.

Clark, B., & Foster, J. B. (2006). Florence Kelley and the struggle against the degradation of life: An introduction to a selection from modern industry. *Organization and Environment, 19*(2), 251–263.

Dreier, P. (2012). Florence Kelley: Pioneer of labor reform. *New Labor Forum, 21*(1), 71–76. doi:10.4179/NLF.211.0000011

Fee, E., & Brown, T. (n.d). Florence Kelley: A factory inspector campaigns against sweatshop labor. *American Journal of Public Health, 95*(1), 50.

Flannery, J. (2009). *The glass house boys of Pittsburgh.* Pittsburgh: University of Pittsburgh Press.

Kelley, F., & Sklar, K. K. (1986). *Notes of sixty years: The autobiography of Florence Kelley; with an early essay by the author on the need of theoretical preparation for philanthropic work.* Chicago: Published for the Illinois Labor History Society by C. H. Kerr.

Spargo, J. (1916). *The bitter cry of the children.* New York: MacMillan. Retrieved from https://archive.org/details/bittercryofthech029787mbp.

The Sweating System. (2005). *American Journal of Public Health, 95*(1), 49–52.

KOCH, HEINRICH HERMANN ROBERT (1843–1910)

The identification and control of infectious diseases is one of the greatest public health accomplishments of the 19th and 20th centuries. Prior to vaccinations, antibiotics, and the sanitation movement, outbreaks of cholera, dysentery, tuberculosis (TB), typhoid fever, influenza, yellow fever, and malaria regularly appeared and claimed many lives. Advancements in the treatment and prevention of infectious diseases were possible because of the early microbiologists who identified bacteria and demonstrated the association between pathogens and disease. German physician and bacteriologist Robert Koch isolated and identified the causal agents of tuberculosis and cholera and made numerous scientific advances in the study of anthrax, plague, malaria, and sleeping sickness. Koch's staining and culture methods enabled others to study microorganisms and eventually find ways to control infectious diseases. Koch's postulates outline conditions that must be met in order to prove that a particular pathogen causes a specific disease. The postulates are still used in medical research today. In 1905, Koch was awarded the Nobel Prize in medicine.

Early Life and Research

Heinrich Hermann Robert Koch was born on December 11, 1843, in Clausthal, Germany. Robert was 1 of 13 children born to Mathilde Julie Henriette (Biewend) and Hermann Koch. Robert's father was a mining official who earned a respectable salary and worked diligently managing mines. Robert spent a lot of time with his uncle, Eduard Biewend. Biewend was a well-educated man who took Robert on field trips to collect plants, insects, and minerals. The specimens were examined by magnifying glass, classified, and photographed. Robert planned to study linguistics in college. However, the school headmaster encouraged him to study natural sciences. He attended the University of Göttingen where he initially majored in botany, physics, and mathematics before changing to medicine. The University of Göttingen is a world-renowned university, claiming 40 Nobel Prize winners. Koch studied under Professor Friedrich Gustgav Jakob Henle, an early proponent of the germ theory of disease. In 1866, Koch completed his medical degree, married Emmy Fratz, and worked at the General Hospital in Hamburg. From 1870 to 1871, Koch served as military surgeon in the Franco-Prussian War, gaining expertise in wounds and septicemia. After leaving the military, he was appointed district physician in the small, rural town of Wollstein. Isolated from libraries, equipment, and the scientific community, Koch set up his own laboratory and launched vigorously into studying bacteria. With Emmy working as an unpaid laboratory assistant, Koch developed innovations such as the hanging-drop method for microscopic investigations and, later, the use of photography and staining techniques to study bacteria.

By the middle of the 19th century, no diseases had been conclusively traced to bacteria. However, there was growing evidence that anthrax was bacterial in origin. Anthrax was an ideal microorganism for Koch to study. Wollstein was surrounded by fields and potentially infected farm animals. The anthrax bacillus is gigantic in comparison to other bacteria, making it relatively easy to observe. Preventing the disease would have enormous economic ramifications for Koch and the European livestock industry. Koch isolated Bacillus anthracis and traced the life cycle from large rodlike bacterium to tiny spore and back to bacterium. He presented his research to Ferdinand Cohn, professor of botany at the University of Breslau. Cohn immediately recognized the significance and published Koch's work in his botanical journal.

Koch continued his research in Wollstein until 1880 when he accepted an appointment at the Imperial Gesundheitsamt (Imperial Health Bureau) in Berlin. The bureau provided Koch with equipment and qualified research assistants. Agar, the jelly-like substance used as a growth medium for bacteria and fungi, was the idea of Fannie Hess. Hess worked as an unpaid assistant alongside her husband, Walther Hesse. The flat dish that holds agar, a petri dish, was invented by Koch's laboratory assistant Julius Richard Petri. The solid-culture media allowed Koch to cultivate pure cultures and to develop *Koch's postulates*. Koch's postulates expanded on work by Henle, defining necessary conditions to prove that a particular pathogen causes a specific disease. The postulates are: (1) the microorganism must be found in abundance within or on the infected organism (animal or human body) and is not present in healthy organisms; (2) the microorganism can be collected from the organism, isolated, and grown in pure culture; (3) inoculation of the cultured microorganism into a healthy organism causes disease; and (4) microorganisms collected from the inoculated, diseased organism are identical to the original microorganism. Once Koch adopted the postulates, he repeatedly insisted that only by following those steps could causation be conclusively established.

Conflict with Pasteur

Koch's anthrax research brought him into direct competition with French microbiologist Louis Pasteur who, in contrast to the young and aspiring Koch, was at the crest of a long and distinguished career. At first, Pasteur praised Koch's innovations, but later, largely because of Koch's harsh and often personal attacks, their relations became hostile. Ultimately, each claimed to have provided the final proof that the anthrax bacillus caused anthrax. Pasteur's argument rested on isolating the suspected causal organism and on inoculating pure strains into otherwise healthy animals—a procedure matching Koch's postulates. Ironically, at no point in his work on anthrax did Koch ever actually follow the postulates. In fact, his failure to isolate and inoculate the organism was one basis for Pasteur's criticism of Koch's purported proof.

Work on Tuberculosis

In the late 19th century, tuberculosis was the single most prominent disease in the Western world. There had been repeated, but unsuccessful, attempts to show that it was bacterial in origin. Koch began studying the disease in August 1881. His work was kept absolutely secret and was conducted at a frantic pace. Relying, as usual, on technological innovations, Koch identified the causal organism and proved causation by meticulously following the postulates.

His first paper on tuberculosis, which was presented on March 24, 1882, in a meeting of the Berlin Physiological Society, was a stunning success. The younger biologist Paul Ehrlich described the meeting as his greatest experience in science. Within two

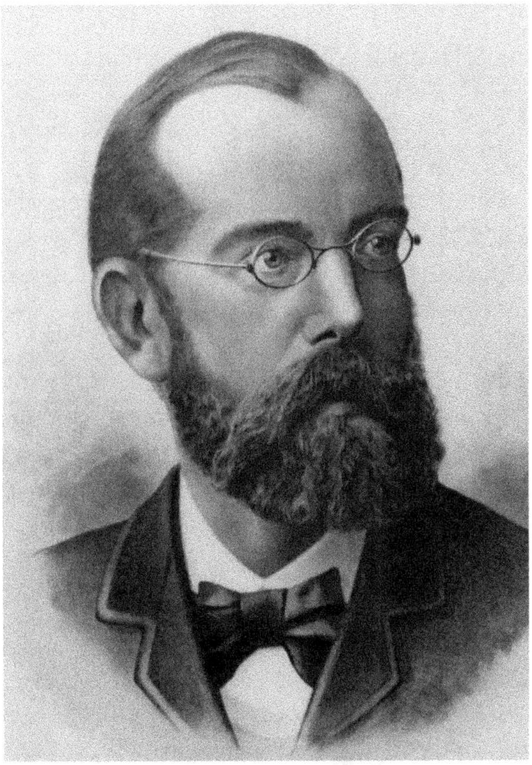

Dr. Robert Koch contradicted popular miasma theory by isolating pathogens that cause cholera and tuberculosis. Koch's postulates name four criteria necessary to match causal pathogen with disease. (Library of Congress)

years, Koch had also identified the causal organism for cholera. These achievements, together with Pasteur's successful anthrax and rabies inoculations, which came at about the same time, probably did more than anything else to persuade the world of the germ theory of disease in particular and of what has been called the etiological research program in general.

Recognition and Setbacks

In 1891, the German government opened the Institute for Infectious Diseases and appointed Koch as the first director. Among Koch's students and colleagues at the institute were Emil Adolf von Behring, who discovered diphtheria antitoxin; William Henry Welch, who was central to the rise of American bacteriology; Shibasaburo Kitasato, who helped develop tetanus antitoxin and identified the plague bacillus; Gerhard Hansen, who discovered the leprosy bacillus; Christiaan Eijkman, whose work led to the discovery of vitamins; and August von Wasserman and Paul Ehrlich, who made important contributions to immunology.

All of this work brought world recognition to Koch, but there were clouds on the horizon. Probably hoping to emulate Pasteur's heralded and lucrative anthrax inoculations, in 1890 Koch had prematurely announced discovery of a substance, called tuberculin, which was expected to have prophylactic (preventive) or therapeutic significance for tuberculosis. As evidence accumulated that tuberculin was ineffective, Koch's professional credibility was tarnished. His reputation was also compromised by developments in his personal life. Around 1890, Koch fell in love with a 17-year-old actress named Hedwig Freiberg; he hastily divorced Emmy and married Freiberg. Society ostracized the couple.

Embarrassed by professional setbacks, rejected by Berlin society, and dogged by endless squabbles with competitors and former students, Koch spent more and more time away from Berlin. In 1896 he was invited to investigate rinderpest, a disease that was ravaging cattle in the British colony of South Africa. He next traveled to Asia to study the bubonic plague. In 1898 and 1899, he visited Italy, Indonesia, and New Guinea. Between 1902 and 1907, he made several trips to Africa to investigate a range of human and animal diseases. In 1908, Koch visited America and Japan. After suffering a severe heart attack, Koch died on May 27, 1910, in Baden-Baden, Germany. His ashes were deposited in a mausoleum in the Institute for Infectious Diseases in Berlin.

K. Codell Carter and Sally Kuykendall

See also: Bioterrorism; Cholera; Emergency Preparedness and Response; Infectious Diseases; Pasteur, Louis; *Controversies in Public Health:* Controversy 3

Further Reading

Brock, T. D. (1988). *Koch: A life in medicine and bacteriology.* Madison, WI: Science Tech.

Byrne, J. P. (Ed.). (2008). *Encyclopedia of pestilence, pandemics, and plagues.* Westport, CT: Greenwood Press.

Carter, K. Codell. (Trans.). (1987). *Essays of Robert Koch.* Westport, CT: Greenwood Press.

Carter, K. Codell. (2003). *The rise of causal concepts of disease.* Burlington, VT: Ashgate.

Centers for Disease Prevention and Control. (1999). Achievements in public health, 1900–1999: Control of infectious diseases. *Morbidity and Mortality Weekly Report, 48*(29), 621. Retrieved from https://www.cdc.gov/mmwr/preview/mmwrhtml/mm4829a1.htm.

Gradmann, C. (2000). Money and microbes: Robert Koch, tuberculin and the Foundation of the Institute for Infectious Diseases in Berlin in 1891. *History and Philosophy of the Life Sciences, 22*(1), 59–79. Retrieved from http://www.jstor.org.ezproxy.sju.edu/stable/23332275.

Kaufmann, S. E. (2001). Koch's dilemma revisited. *Scandinavian Journal of Infectious Diseases, Supplement, 33*(12), 14–17. doi:10.1080/003655401753382468

Koch, R. (1891). Professor Koch's remedy for tuberculosis. *The British Medical Journal, 1*(1568), 125–127.

Koch, R. (1900). The combating of tuberculosis in the light of the experience that has been gained in the successful combating of other infectious diseases. *Public Health, 13,* 764–777. doi:10.1016/S0033-3506(00)80175-4

Koch, R. (1901). An address on the fight against tuberculosis in the light of the experience that has been gained in the successful combat of other infectious diseases. *The British Medical Journal, 2*(2117), 189–193. Retrieved from http://www.jstor.org.ezproxy.sju.edu/stable/20269087.

Koch, R., Brock, T. D., & Fred, E. B. (1982). The etiology of tuberculosis. *Reviews of Infectious Diseases, 46*(6), 1270–1274.

Lienhardt, C., Glaziou, P., Uplekar, M., Lönnroth, K., Getahun, H., & Raviglione, M. (2012). Global tuberculosis control: Lessons learnt and future prospects. *Nature Reviews Microbiology, 10*(6), 407. doi:10.1038/nrmicro2797

Ligon, B. L. (2002). Biography. Robert Koch: Nobel laureate and controversial figure in tuberculin research. *Seminars in Pediatric Infectious Diseases, 13,* 289–299. doi:10.1053/spid.2002.127205

Morens, D. M. (2003). Characterizing a "new" disease: Epizootic and epidemic anthrax, 1769–1780. *American Journal of Public Health, 93*(6), 886–893.

Tuberculosis: A menace and a mystery and $4,500,000 in Christmas Seals. (1937). *Life, 3*(22), 30–37.

L

LEADING HEALTH INDICATORS

Health indicators are behaviors and characteristics that can be used to gauge quality of life, health, or wellness of a community. For example, high levels of tobacco use suggest the presence of cancer, heart disease, stroke, chronic obstructive pulmonary disease (COPD), birth defects, and sudden infant death syndrome (SIDS). Public heath efforts to reduce and prevent smoking would significantly improve health within the community. *Healthy People 2020* outlines 1,200 health objectives for the nation. Health and medical experts from the U.S. Department of Health and Human Services (DHHS) Office of Disease Prevention and Health Promotion (ODPHP) analyzed the most important health issues of the nation and reduced the problems into related categories. The 12 Leading Health Indicators (LHIs) are access to health services; clinical preventive services; environmental quality; injury and violence; maternal, infant, and child health; mental health; nutrition, physical activity, and obesity; oral health; reproductive and sexual health; social determinants; substance abuse; and tobacco use. Public health professionals use the LHIs to identify program priorities, policies, partnerships, and progress toward goals. Reducing and improving the LHIs is an important step toward reducing disease and improving health across the nation.

The 12 LHIs are described in detail by *Healthy People 2020* resources. This entry will highlight the LHI of tobacco. Tobacco use is the leading cause of death in the United States. Tobacco causes more deaths than HIV, alcohol, illicit drug use, violence, and motor vehicle crashes, combined. Preventing the initiation of tobacco use, promoting cessation, eliminating exposure to secondhand and sidestream smoke, and eliminating tobacco-related disparities will go a long way toward preventing disease, disability, death, and health disparities (Office on Smoking and Health, 2017). *Healthy People 2020* lists 21 tobacco use (TU) objectives that range from reducing smoking (individual level) to increasing and expanding medical screening for tobacco use (health systems level) or increasing cigarette taxes (policy level). More recent surveys indicate positive progress toward reducing cigarette smoking. Tobacco Use Objective 1.1 (TU-1.1), "Reduce cigarette smoking by adults," started at a baseline with 20.6 percent of adults reporting smoking and has decreased to 18.2 percent of adults (ODPHP, 2017). The target is to reduce cigarette smoking to 12 percent of adults by 2020. Meanwhile, adolescent smoking (TU-2.2) has shown no significant change. The goal is to reduce adolescent smoking to 16 percent. Most recently, 18.1 percent of adolescents smoke.

One area to focus public health efforts is cigarette smoking by race. Among adults, mixed race and white, non-Hispanic populations have the highest rates of smoking (24.5 percent and 20.6 percent, respectively), twice the rate of Asian American populations (10.2 percent). Focusing efforts within high-risk communities ensures good stewardship of limited public health resources and maximizes impact.

The Office of Smoking and Health's Tips from Former Smokers program presents the life stories of real people whose lives were altered due to tobacco. The cases are presented by ethnic group, social group, person's name, or disease. For example, Ellie was a bartender who worked in a bar catering to LGBT patrons. Tobacco companies actively targeted certain communities, including the LGBT community with cigarette advertising. Although Ellie never smoked, her parents and patrons did. Exposure to secondhand smoke resulted in asthma and severe, disabling attacks. In order to stay alive, she had to quit her job. The Tips campaign offers free resources to quit smoking (1-800-QUIT-NOW). The campaign is very successful. An estimated 500,000 people have quit smoking at a cost of $480 per person. Considering that asthma cost approximately $3,300 per person per year between 2002 and 2007, the cost benefit of the Tips campaigns is enormous (American Academy of Allergy Asthma and Immunology, 2017). The Tips campaign demonstrates how targeting one LHI has the potential to decrease many diseases, to help people live more productive, healthier lives, and yield significant cost savings to individuals and communities.

LHIs are useful tools to guide planning and implementing public health policy, intervention, and prevention. LHIs allow public health professionals to ascertain the leading health problems within communities, determine who is impacted the most, and evaluate efforts.

Sally Kuykendall

See also: Birth Defects; Cancer; Care, Access to; Children's Health; Goals and Objectives; *Healthy People 2020*; Heart Disease; Nutrition; Social Determinants of Health; *Controversies in Public Health:* Controversy 2

Further Reading

Academy of Allergy Asthma and Immunology. (2017). *Asthma statistics.* Retrieved from http://www.aaaai.org/about-aaaai/newsroom/asthma-statistics.

National Center for Health Statistics. (2016). *Health, United States, 2015: With special feature on racial and ethnic health disparities.* Hyattsville, MD: Author. Retrieved from https://www.cdc.gov/nchs/data/hus/hus15.pdf#053.

Office of Disease Prevention and Health Promotion. (2017). *Healthy People 2020.* Retrieved from https://www.healthypeople.gov/.

Office on Smoking and Health, Centers for Disease Control and Prevention. (2017). Retrieved from https://www.cdc.gov/tobacco/.

LESBIAN, GAY, BISEXUAL, AND TRANSGENDER (LGBT) HEALTH

Nonheterosexual and transgender populations are at greater risk for many health problems, such as bullying victimization, substance abuse, depression, sexually transmitted diseases, intimate partner violence, and suicide. Lesbian, gay, bisexual, and transgender (LGBT) health refers to the mental and physical health of people of minority sexual orientation as well as transgender individuals. Many of the health problems experienced by LGBT populations—of which there are 5 million in the United States (Ward, Dahlhamer, Galinsky, & Joestl, 2014)—are directly related to lack of social acceptance and support. Due to persistent social rejection, LGBT youth and adults are more likely to self-medicate with risky behaviors and are less likely to access and use health care systems. Improving the health of this vulnerable population is an important goal of *Healthy People 2020.*

The first step toward alleviating the health disparities of LGBT individuals is to accurately identify the prevalence rates of sexual orientations (National LGBT Cancer Network, n.d.). Since questions about LGBT identity were not included in national, population-based surveys, it is difficult to estimate what percentage of the population is LGBT. Given the multidimensional nature of sexual orientation, surveys use different ways to capture this information (Institute of Medicine, 2011). The four main methods are (1) self-identification as LGBT, (2) past or current sexual activity, (3) sexual attraction, and (4) sexual fantasies (thoughts). Each form of measurement yields different rates. Current estimates suggest that approximately 2 to 4 percent of U.S. adults self-identify as LGBT (Gates, 2011; Ward, Dahlhamer, Galinsky, & Joestl, 2014). When assessing sexual orientation by sexual activity, approximately 25 percent of U.S. adults report same-sex or bisexual behavior (Gates, 2011). It appears that some individuals may engage in homosexual or bisexual behaviors, yet still self-identify as heterosexual. Obtaining accurate prevalence rates is an important first step toward improving public health. This means that individuals must feel comfortable disclosing sexual behaviors and trust that disclosures will not result in judgment, rejection, or stigma. Public health communities strive to recognize the difficulties and complications posed by coming out to multiple health providers and overcome obstacles using LGBT liaisons within advisory and planning committees.

Historically, there has been confusion regarding the health status of LGBT people. In the early 1960s, LGBT identity was framed as a health problem by the American Psychiatric Association (APA) when homosexuality was classified as a mental disorder in the *Diagnostic and Statistical Manual of Mental Disorders* (*DSM*), which is one of the most commonly used and recognized resources by medical professionals around the world.

In the 1960s, it was believed that gay and lesbian individuals were internally disordered and that homosexuality may be caused by traumatic events or psychological issues in early childhood or young adulthood. The listing of homosexuality as a pathological problem was based on popular thought rather than rigorous science. The *DSM* listing was eventually challenged by gay-affirmative research, which showed that gay men are not psychologically different from their heterosexual counterparts. In 1973, homosexuality was removed from the *DSM* as a mental disorder. Although mental health professionals now recognize homosexuality as a healthy expression of human sexuality, the stigma of homosexuality as a mental disease continues. In 1980, the third edition of the *DSM* listed transsexualism as a mental disorder. Transsexualism was defined as a continuous desire to transform one's physical body to match self-ascribed gender identity. The fifth edition of the *DSM* (2013) was updated to focus on the mental health aspects of transgendered individuals. The updated term "gender dysphoria" describes the discontent and distress that transgender individuals experience as a result of the mismatch between sexual anatomy at birth and cognitive identity. Past rejection, misdiagnosis, and maltreatment by such notable and prestigious medical organizations as the APA left a scar on the LGBT community, which makes the stigmatized individuals reluctant to seek treatment. Securing the health of the LGBT population requires health professionals to acknowledge and compensate for past traumas.

Following the removal of homosexuality from the *DSM*, LGBT health research shifted from studying homosexuality as a disorder to studying the health problems experienced by LGBT people (Meyer & Northridge, 2007). LGBT health disparities refer to the differential health status between LGBT populations and non-LGBT populations, specifically heterosexual and cisgender (nontransgender) populations. Compared to heterosexual/cisgender individuals, LGBT individuals have higher rates of many different mental and physical health problems. Health problems vary by subgroup (Institute of Medicine, 2011). Men who have sex with men (MSM) as well as transgender women are among the most vulnerable populations for human immunodeficiency virus (HIV). Seventy-eight percent of new HIV infections in 2010 were among MSM (Centers for Disease Control and Prevention, 2012). The risk of obesity and obesity-related diseases are two times higher among lesbian women compared to heterosexual and bisexual women (Boehmer, Bowen, & Bauer, 2007). All LGBT individuals are at greater risk for substance abuse and other mental health problems. Cigarette smoking rates are twice as high among LGBT individuals (American Lung Association, 2010). Alcohol abuse, depression, and suicide attempts also run approximately two times higher among LGBT adolescents (Russell & Joyner, 2001). Public health addresses the unique needs of LGBT individuals by ensuring the use of culturally competent health education materials and health promotion activities. For example, smoking cessation materials should contain images and language that include people from across the sexual orientation spectrum. Inclusive materials demonstrate respect and concern for sexual minorities.

One of the most widely used theories to explain health disparities among LGBT individuals is the *minority stress model*. According to this theory, people who self-identify as LGBT are members of a stigmatized group. Although everyone experiences some degree of stress, stigma and discrimination increase stress over and above other normal life stressors. This additional burden increases the likelihood of high-risk or escapism behaviors such as smoking, drinking alcohol, illicit drug use, or high-risk sexuality. Over time, these behaviors increase the risk of other health problems, such as sexually transmitted diseases, intentional and unintentional injuries, and heart and lung diseases. To apply the minority stress model, many LGBT individuals report harassment, teasing, and bullying in school. These stressful incidents are on top of the normal stressful life events such as concerns about dating partners, finances, or future. Experiencing verbal or physical attacks and other social injustices can lead to running away, truancy, or substance abuse. Avoiding or dropping out of school robs LGBT youth of educational opportunities that may limit future earning potential. A significant percentage of the homeless youth are LGBT. Homelessness leads to other health problems, such as substance use and limited access to health care services.

Other factors may compound the health disparities. Racial or ethnic identity, nationality, education level, income, social class, religion, disability status, obesity, and gender nonconformity can inflame social stigmas. These factors complicate and further increase the likelihood of health problems. For example, gay and bisexual men and transgender women of color are more likely to become HIV-positive compared to white gay and bisexual men and transgender women. LGBT people of color are at a higher risk of experiencing health problems due to the negative consequences of both homophobia and racism.

When considering the health status of LGBT individuals, it is crucial to consider protective factors and personal resilience. Protective factors guard against the adverse health effects that accumulate from negative life experiences. For the LGBT individual, protective factors may counteract the consequences of stigma and discrimination. Some known protective factors are connectedness to community, social support, family support, and self-accepting the LGBT identity. Research shows that LGBT individuals who are accepted and supported by their friends and family are better able to cope with and manage stigma and discrimination. In fact, the strength of parental acceptance is alarming. LGB adolescents rejected by their families are eight times more likely to report attempted suicide, six times more likely to report depression, three times more likely to report illegal drug use, and three times more likely to report unprotected sex in comparison to LGB adolescents with low or no family rejection (Ryan, Huebner, Diaz, & Sanchez, 2009). An emerging field of study is in the area of resilience. It is believed that because of their exposure to stigma and discrimination, LGBT individuals may develop positive psychological attributes that benefit society as a whole. Experiences with stigma and discrimination create a heightened sense of empathy and compassion toward the suffering of other people. This knowledge and attitude promote connection with others in the community and may, in turn, diminish the negative consequences of stigma and discrimination for other disadvantaged groups. Future research may focus on how to foster resilience without subjecting people to damaging experiences.

LGBT individuals are at risk for a plethora of mental health disparities compared to heterosexual and cisgender counterparts. Many of the health problems are directly related to the stigma, discrimination, and prejudice associated with LGBT identity. The goal of public health is to ensure the safety and social acceptance of all individuals in order to promote health and well-being. The next steps are to educate the general public on diverse sexual orientations and gender identity in order to reduce and eliminate discrimination and ensure that all members of society have an opportunity to reach their maximum potential.

Nadav Antebi-Gruszka

See also: Addictions; Health Disparities; *Healthy People 2020*; Human Immunodeficiency Virus and Acquired Immune Deficiency Syndrome; Prevention; Substance Abuse and Mental Health Services Administration

Further Reading

American Lung Association. (2010). *Smoking out a deadly threat: Tobacco use in the LGBT community.* Retrieved from http://www.lung.org/assets/documents/research/lgbt-report.pdf.

Boehmer, U., Bowen, D. J., & Bauer, G. R. (2007). Overweight and obesity in sexual-minority women: Evidence from population-based data. *American Journal of Public Health, 97*(6), 1134–1140. doi:10.2105/AJPH.2006.088419

Centers for Disease Control and Prevention. (2012). Estimated HIV incidence in the United States, 2007–2010. *HIV Surveillance Supplemental Report 2012, 17*(4). Retrieved from http://www.cdc.gov/hiv/topics/surveillance/resources/reports/#supplemental.

Gates, G. J. (2011). *How many people are lesbian, gay, bisexual and transgender?* UCLA: The Williams Institute. Retrieved from http://escholarship.org/uc/item/09h684x2.

Institute of Medicine. (2011). *The health of lesbian, gay, bisexual, and transgender people: Building a foundation for better understanding.* Washington, DC: The National Academies Press.

Meyer, I. H. (2003). Prejudice, social stress, and mental health in lesbian, gay, and bisexual populations: Conceptual issues and research evidence. *Psychological Bulletin, 129*(5), 674–697.

Meyer, I. H., & Northridge, M. E. (2007). *The health of sexual minorities: Public health perspectives on lesbian, gay, bisexual, and transgender populations.* New York: Springer.

National LGBT Cancer Network. (n.d.). *Best practices in creating and delivering LGBTQ cultural competency trainings for health and social service agencies.* Retrieved from http://www.cancer-network.org/downloads/best_practices.pdf.

Russell, S. T., & Joyner, K. (2001). Adolescent sexual orientation and suicide risk: Evidence from a national study. *American Journal of Public Health, 91*(8), 1276–1281. doi:10.2105/AJPH.91.8.1276

Ryan, C., Huebner, D., Diaz, R., & Sanchez, J. (2009). Family rejection as a predictor of negative health outcomes in white and Latino lesbian, gay, and bisexual young adults. *Pediatrics, 123*(1), 346–352.

Savin-Williams, R. C. (2009). *The new gay teenager* (Vol. 3). Cambridge, MA: Harvard University Press.

Ward, B. W., Dahlhamer, J. M., Galinsky, A. M., & Joestl, S. S. (2014, July 15). Sexual orientation and health among U.S. adults: National health interview survey, 2013. *National Health Statistics Reports, 77*. Hyattsville, MD: National Center for Health Statistics. Retrieved from http://www.cdc.gov/nchs/data/nhsr/nhsr077.pdf.

LOCUS OF CONTROL

Locus of control is a principle that describes a person's perception of the factors that influence his or her life. *Locus* is Latin, meaning "place.". *Locus of control* means the "place of control." The concept of locus of control traces back to ancient religions when people believed that disease was generated by supreme beings as punishment for sin or misdeed. In the treatise *On the Sacred Disease* (400 BCE) Hippocrates proposed that the brain, not supernatural powers, effected disease and infirmity. Scientific discoveries in bacteriology, virology, and pathophysiology proved that many diseases are preventable and unrelated to what society dictates as moral or immoral. Dr. Julian B. Rotter developed the modern concept of locus of control. As a clinical psychologist, Rotter was interested in personality types and motivation for achievement. Rotter defined internal versus external control as "the degree to which persons expect that a reinforcement or an outcome of their behavior is contingent on their own behavior or personal characteristics versus the degree to which persons expect that the reinforcement or outcome is a function of chance, luck, or fate, is under the control of powerful others, or is simply unpredictable" (Rotter, 1990, p. 489). For example, an individual with cardiovascular disease (CVD) may perceive that the disease is the result of genetics (fate) and there is little that can be done to prevent or control disease progression. This person demonstrates an external locus of control. Another individual with CVD may perceive that the disease is related to personal lifestyle, and increasing physical activity and healthy diet can prevent adverse consequences. This person demonstrates an internal locus of control. Locus of control is a fundamental principle of behavioral health because the person with internal locus of control starts from a place of personal empowerment. It can be more difficult to motivate behavioral change among people with external locus of control. Although locus of control is often presented as a dichotomous scale, Rotter believed that perspectives exist on a continuum and may vary, depending on the circumstances. This concept was confirmed by researchers in Scotland who found that patients undergoing coronary bypass surgery scored higher on external locus of control during the perioperative period and higher on internal locus of control during rehabilitation (Rideout, Tolmie, & Lindsay, 2017). The concepts of locus of control apply to many health topics, such as dietary supplements, brain exercises, dental visits, violent offenders, and occupational health. The principle is often used as a construct of health behavior theories and models, most notably social cognitive theory. Imbedding the idea of locus of control within a broader theory allows program planners and health educators to consider other factors that influence locus of control. Overall, locus of control is a good starting point to understanding why some people are able to change behavior while others appear resistant to change.

Sally Kuykendall

See also: Greco-Roman Era, Public Health in the; Hippocrates; Self-Efficacy; Social Cognitive Theory

Further Reading

Lefcourt, H. M. (1982). *Locus of control: Current trends in theory and research.* Hillsdale, NJ: Erlbaum.

Rideout, A., Tolmie, E., & Lindsay, G. (2017). Health locus of control in patients undergoing coronary artery surgery—changes and associated outcomes: A seven-year cohort study. *European Journal of Cardiovascular Nursing, 16*(1), 46–56. doi:10.1177/1474515116636501

Rotter, J. B. (1954). *Social learning theory and clinical psychology.* Englewood Cliffs, NJ: Prentice Hall.

Rotter, J. B. (1966). Generalized expectancies for internal versus external control of reinforcement. *Psychological Monographs: General and Applied, 80*(1), 1–28. doi:10.1037/h0092976

Rotter, J. B. (1990). Internal versus external control of reinforcement: A case history of a variable. *American Psychologist, 45*(4), 489–493. doi:10.1037/0003-066X.45.4.489

LOGIC MODEL

A logic model is a tool used to define, develop, and evaluate public health programs. The program planner draws the various program components as a flowchart, and the chart becomes an organizational tool, providing an overview of the program. Similar to a road map, a logic model helps users to see where they are and the path they need to take to achieve a desired goal. By presenting the program as a sequential arrangement, the logic model allows the viewer to map connections between the efforts required to implement the program and the intended outcomes. Public health professionals use logic models to represent the activities, functions, and goals of a program. This valuable tool may be used to map one-time health promotion events, programs, interventions, working groups, organizations, or health communication brochures or other materials. It is a useful tool to outline the connections between program parts in order to show how the program activities work.

There are different kinds of logic models. Most models are presented as tables or flowcharts and consist of four sections. The sections may be presented vertically (from top to bottom) or horizontally (from left to right). The main sections are inputs, activities, outputs, and outcome/impact. Inputs refer to the main resources that are necessary for the program to occur, and they might include the staff, funding, an advisory board, infrastructure, or equipment. Activities are the tasks that must be conducted in order to plan and deliver the intervention. Development activities might include involving stakeholders, creating training manuals or other program materials, or training those who will implement the program. Delivery activities are related to the intervention itself, such as inviting individuals to participate in the program, hosting workshops, or distributing brochures. Outputs are the products of the activities and include the number of people trained or number of people participating. Outcomes and impacts describe the desired changes as a result of the project. Outcomes are the benefits and goals that the intervention aims to achieve, and they are subdivided into three types: short-term, medium-term, and long-term. Short-term outcomes describe changes in health opinions, attitudes, knowledge, and skills. Medium-term outcomes refer to action-related changes such as behavioral changes, changes in public health policy, or social changes. Long-term outcomes, referred to as impacts, describe the sustained influence that the program has on the individual or community. By stating the activities of the project, the program planner, the funder, and the evaluator can track the program to ensure that it is progressing as expected. If the project is not progressing, adaptations may be made early, ensuring that any problems are corrected and conserving precious resources. Program outcomes state the desired benefits and goals of the program, defining how and what the program evaluator will study to ensure that the program achieved what it promised to achieve.

The main benefit of using the logic model tool is that the public health practitioner can visualize the intervention in its entirety, from the beginning to end. For example, as an intervention against skin cancer, public health professionals decide to design a poster to educate individuals about the harmful effects of direct sun exposure and to encourage individuals to wear sunscreen. Health educators, funding, and a graphic designer (inputs) come together to plan and produce a poster (output). The poster is displayed at local community pools (activities). Through the outreach, sunbathers learn about skin cancer and the benefits of sunscreen (short-term outcome), use sunscreen (medium-term outcome), and ultimately reduce the number of people in the community diagnosed with skin cancer (long-term outcome/impact). The logic model is a useful tool that defines a public health project, identifies the resources and activities needed, and determines the desired outcomes of the project.

Noora F. Majid

See also: Administration, Health; Centers for Disease Control and Prevention; Collaborations; Community Organizing; Evaluation; Intervention

Further Reading

Logic models in public health program management. (2012). *Centers for Disease Control's National Public Health Improvement Initiative.* Retrieved from http://www.doh.wa.gov/Portals/1/Documents/1000/PMC-Logic%20Models%20May_16_12forWeb.pdf.

Pell Institute. (2015). *Using a logic model.* The Pell Institute and Pathways to College Network. Retrieved from http://toolkit.pellinstitute.org/evaluation-guide/plan-budget/using-a-logic-model/.

W. K. Kellogg Foundation. (2006, February 2). *Using logic models to bring together planning, evaluation, and action: Logic model development guide.* East Battle Creek, MI: Author. Retrieved from https://www.wkkf.org/resource-directory/resource/2006/02/wk-kellogg-foundation-logic-model-development-guide.